FED & FIT

a **28-day** food & fitness plan to jump-start your life
with over **175** squeaky-clean paleo recipes

Cassy Joy Garcia, NC

with
New York Times bestselling author
Juli Bauer

VICTORY BELT PUBLISHING
Las Vegas

First Published in 2016 by Victory Belt Publishing Inc.

ISBN-13: 978-1-628601-03-9

Interior and cover design by Yordan Terziev and Boryana
Yordanova

Printed in Canada
TC 0320

For my mom,
the strongest woman I know.

I'm forever a work-in-progress, but here are a few of the things she's taught me:

- Cook with love and a sense of adventure.
- Never show up empty-handed.
- Leave a place cleaner than you found it.
- Silliness is the fountain of youth.
- Stand up for what's right.
- Trust.

table of contents

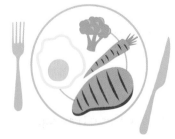

foreword

It's impossible not to love Cassy Joy Garcia.

Moreover, it's impossible not to love the incredible program she's created. Because *it works.*

She—along with the thousands of people she's mentored through her online community—is the gorgeous, happy, fit, living proof.

When you learn from Cassy, you're learning from someone who's been in the trenches and found her way out. Cassy will tell you point-blank— she went from being in pain, unhappy, and at an unhealthy weight to losing *ten dress sizes* and becoming the glowing, happy, well-fed person she is today—and she achieved all that *without dieting.*

Are you kidding me? Sign me up!

No, seriously. Sign me up. Immediately. Because whatever she's doing, I want to do it, too.

Actually, I felt this way from the moment I met Cassy at a book signing in Houston, Texas—I wanted to know what her secret was. I was instantly blown away by her warmth and her knowledge, and most of all by the way she radiates joy. (FYI, Joy actually is her middle name. Fitting, right?)

See, when you're dieting, starving, and punishing your body with stressful workouts and self-hatred and not enjoying the process of getting healthy and fit, it shows. In my work as a Nutritional Therapy Practitioner, I've met countless people who are clearly not enjoying their journey. In fact, many of them are flat-out miserable. Some of them haven't reached their aesthetic goals and are stuck in an endless diet-crash-diet loop; others look good on the outside but are still plagued by physical pain, self-doubt, extreme hunger, and unhappiness.

Shouldn't the goal be to get healthy *and* happy? What's a fit body worth if you feel miserable, tired, and afraid it won't last?

All of those people are missing the key components to changing their bodies and their lives and making it stick: having a smart, *individualized* plan, knowing what really works (hint: you need more than just food and exercise), and, above all, finding joy in the process.

That's why I knew immediately that Cassy was the real deal. She wasn't tired or run-down. She wasn't obsessive. She wasn't suffering through crash-diet torture or stressful workouts. She'd completely changed her life by using methods that were targeted to her needs, that worked long-term, and that actually *added* to her happiness. She was on top of her game, both personally and as a sought-after Nutrition Consultant—and I knew that if I could ever get involved with her mission, I'd jump at the chance.

In *Fed & Fit,* Cassy has put together everything you need to reach your goals. This is the blueprint for designing your *life*—your "Perfect You Plan"— complete with an *actionable* 28-day "squeaky-clean" food and fitness plan that will get you what you want without having to suffer through the same diet and lifestyle mistakes again and again.

And the recipes. Oh, the recipes! Whether you're an ace in the kitchen or totally clueless, Cassy has you covered. She's crafted more than 175 Project-compliant recipes to keep you 100% on track; and not only does it all taste amazing, but *it's all made from real food.* No trying to trick your taste buds or pull a fast one on your hunger hormones. It's all designed to work *with* your body.

Bonus: The amazing Juli Bauer of PaleOMG has added her insanely amazing workout wisdom to the fitness section. There's literally *nothing* you need that this book doesn't give!

Built around the four pillars of mindset, rest/ hydration, food, and fitness (aka what you *really* need to implement to get permanent results), Cassy's plan is customizable, it evolves with your goals and your needs, and most important, it works. And with bonus tools like the Fed & Fit app and the Project Online, you've got everything you need to go beyond the book and make your transformation last well beyond the final page. Cassy has truly created something fabulous, amazing, intuitive, and, most of all, incredibly effective.

The food and fitness industry has needed a book like this for a very, very long time. Now smile—because thanks to Cassy, you're about to be the healthiest *and* happiest you've ever been.

Liz Wolfe, NTP
Author of *Eat the Yolks*
Wall Street Journal Bestseller

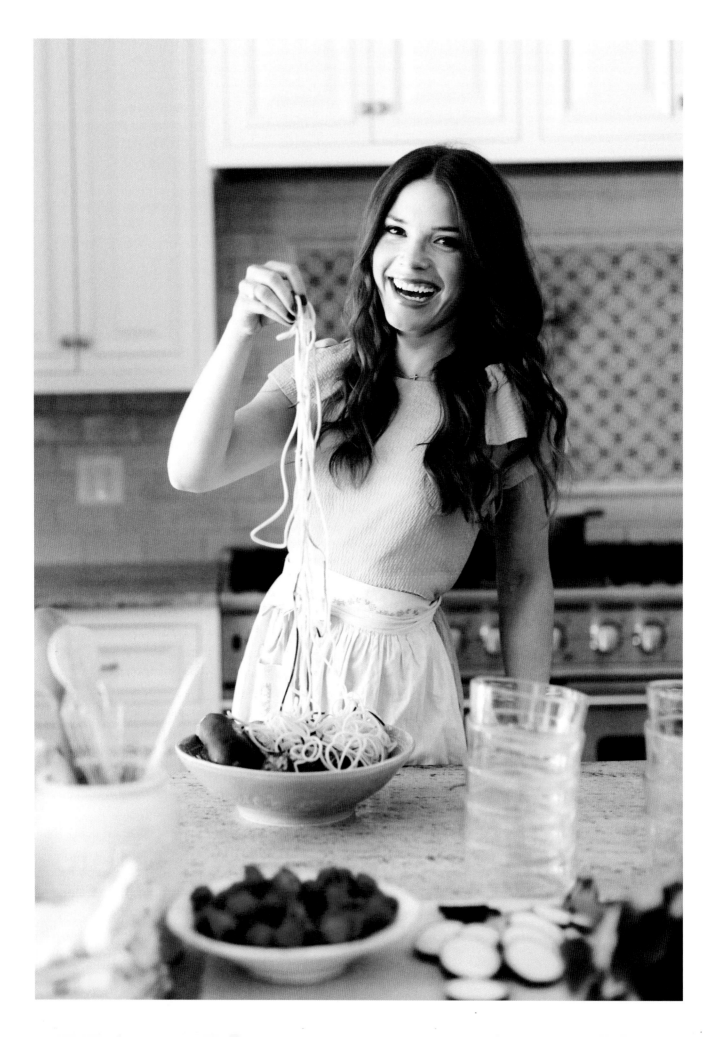

INTRODUCTION

Howdy and welcome!
My name is Cassy Joy.
I changed the things
I couldn't accept.

I want to tell you a story. Actually, I want to tell you all kinds of stories! Being a storyteller is woven into the fiber of my heart and soul. I want to tell you about the time all of the peaches on our two brand-new peach trees (almost 200 of them) mysteriously went missing, about how I married the best guy I know in the pouring rain, and about the epic friendship between my Great Pyrenees, Gus, and the neighborhood bunny rabbit. I've drafted children's books that follow the adventures of a wily little turtle named Pete (a just-for-fun hobby), published hundreds of short stories on my blog (in the form of an introduction to each recipe) , and shared the story of my life and business through photos and short narratives on social media.

I prefer stories over other dry presentations because they're much more fun and seem to have a more lasting effect. While the details may fade *(how many peaches did she say went missing?)*, the lessons and feelings linger. They strike a deeper chord, and if we're really paying attention, they can shift the lens through which we view the world. Adventure stories can strike fun in the heart of a reader, mystery strikes wonder, struggle strikes a relatable comfort, and triumph can strike inspiration. A fresh perspective on the world and how we fit within it is ours at the end of a good story. We can visualize new possibilities, and if we encourage the feeling, excitement can take over, telling us that new and wonderful things are possible.

The story I want to tell you here is about a girl (me) who decided that she'd had *enough*. It's a story that encompasses fun, mystery, struggle, adventure, and eventually triumph. It's a story that has it all, though I guess a story can't help but have it all when it spans ten years of a person's life.

The first part is the story is a bird's-eye view, picture book–style recounting of me before I was Fed & Fit. I want to share this part of my story because I want you to know where I'm coming from. My transformation didn't happen overnight. I was an average girl who just wanted to feel healthy, have fun, eat tasty foods, and love my body. I didn't think I was asking for much.

Once upon a time, between the years of 2007 and 2011 . . .

- I had the time of my life at Texas A&M University, then graduated with a bachelor of science degree and a strong appetite to make something happen. Gig' em, Aggies!

- I learned to love ice-cold India pale ale and discovered that I'm the opposite of a natural snowboarder.

- I ate more pizza (with ranch dressing) than you can shake a stick at.

- I balanced my (admittedly unhealthy) pizza intake with (what I thought was healthy) whole-wheat pasta and low-calorie yogurt.

- I couldn't jog a mile—or 400 meters, for that matter.

- I bought one size bigger in all my favorite Express pants, then went back for one size bigger, and then decided I'd just buy two sizes bigger so I wouldn't have to feel like I was squeezing myself into too-small pants ever again. That feeling is the worst.

- I threw out every piece of clothing in my closet that wasn't a size 12/14 so I could further embrace "the new me" without feeling misplaced longing for my younger, smaller self.

- I endured such debilitating joint pain that I couldn't walk without wincing.

- I couldn't stay awake during a drive, lecture, or movie. I thought this was normal.

- Despite honest efforts to embrace my new size, I still felt like I was walking around in someone else's body.

- I threw myself into every diet I could find in an effort to slim down and feel like myself again. While I did slim down some (because I was starving), nothing stuck. I was confused.

- I thought that a skinny vanilla latte was the healthier option.

- I thought I just needed more cardio. So I trained for and eventually ran six half-marathons. Didn't help.

- I went vegan for almost a full year. Didn't help.

- I decided that *enough was enough*.

After four years of emotional, bodily, and dietary turmoil, I put my foot down. I was done not feeling like myself. I was done accepting the pain and exhaustion. I was done throwing myself into possibly well-meaning but ultimately ineffective diets. I was done with my goals and my priorities. Something needed to change—something deeper than my vanity, deeper than my emotions, and deeper than my belief about what is or isn't possible.

The time had come to *change the things I couldn't accept*. I couldn't accept that the nutrition advice I'd received was the best available, that cardio was the best way to lose weight, or that healthy food was the most boring food. Accepting "the new me" felt like settling, like throwing in my chips after the first hand or like giving up after a tough nine holes. With a new sense of grit, I went back to the drawing board. I leaned heavily on my science background and embraced the belief that nutrition likely holds the answer. I dug deep into the research, learned a tremendous amount, swallowed my pride, and humbly took myself on as my first client.

Here's what finally worked:

• I put healing before weight loss and happiness before skinny jeans. In other words, I got to work on my attitude. Joint pain and chronic fatigue were signs of sickness, so I focused on those symptoms and let my body be.

• I learned that chronic inflammation could be the root cause of my ailments.

• I learned that I would heal faster with more (read: adequate) sleep and more (read: adequate) water. So I slept more and drank more water.

• I started to put foods into two categories: inflammatory and anti-inflammatory. I omitted the first group and built a diet around the latter.

• I swallowed my fear of free weights and group classes and joined CrossFit. My efforts to slowly build healthy muscle were made even healthier when I added yoga to the mix.

I now stand before you a healthy, happy woman who finally feels like she's in the right body. I've managed to maintain my results with relative ease. Slow, intentional, and healthy, my transformation spanned a full year. While I did lose a whopping ten dress sizes and (a surprisingly few) ten pounds, *I value my new attitude above all.* This new attitude is the reason I'm still Fed & Fit six years later and counting.

My life completely changed. Things I thought were out of reach suddenly became possible. I took life by the horns, chased goals that used to intimidated me, and realized that I'm worthy of all my wildest dreams. I stopped settling and started living the example of a person who works hard, takes responsibility, enjoys silly fun, and believes that anything is attainable. This attitude transformation is available to anyone, and you don't need to lose weight to achieve it. You just need prove to yourself that you're not stuck.

Okay, attitude aside, how exactly did I do it? How did I lose the weight and inches? How did I heal my body? Well, first I want to tell you what I *didn't* do. I didn't count calories or track macros, although I won't deny that these things do work for some people. I didn't starve myself or work out to the point of exhaustion. I didn't step on a scale (until a full year later), and I didn't take body measurements. I didn't learn very quickly, which was compounded by the fact that I went at it alone. It was a long process of trial, error, and small victories.

Well, then, what *did* I do? I followed a strict Paleo template (as outlined in this book) and educated myself about portion sizes. I learned to interpret when my body was actually hungry as opposed to stressed, sleepy, thirsty, or just in need of more of a certain nutrient. I learned to rest well, hydrate, and cook healthy foods that kept my plates entertaining (like the recipes in this book), and I learned how to design a fitness program that I really love. I learned that my now-healed body is more forgiving when I do indulge, that I can't "get fat" from one night out (that's probably just inflammation), and that choosing the right carbohydrates is *really* important. I learned that the healthiest foods are free from pesticides, antibiotics, hormones, preservatives, and other lab-crafted ingredients. I learned that saturated fats aren't bad, but trans fats are. I learned that the moment I shared my progress and my story with another person, it became even more real.

Looking back, I see that there are ways I could have fine-tuned my efforts to transform myself, making the process even more efficient and effective. I boiled down the lessons I learned over the years into a concise but powerful how-to that I could share with others. I realize now that every single experience, struggle, success, and failure was working to prepare me for my job—the job I didn't even know was coming: the job of sharing, leading, and motivating anyone who wants to live Fed & Fit.

the 28-day Fed & Fit project (aka the project)

How exactly do you become Fed & Fit? I think definitions can be wonderfully helpful. So let's set the stage by defining what becoming Fed & Fit means.

A person who is Fed & Fit:

1.
is living healthily and happily in his or her own skin.

2.
is well nourished and active, with abundant energy.

3.
has broken free from dogmatic dietary chains and instead lives a consistently healthy lifestyle centered around a positive outlook, adequate rest and hydration, regular nourishment, and fun physical fitness activities.

4.
after arriving at his or her own "Perfect You Plan," observes any indulgences as a part of life, not as a counter to healthy efforts.

Sounds like a pretty neat way to live, doesn't it? It's essentially the "have your cake and eat it too" plan. By "have your cake," I mean that you feel your best, and by "eat it too," I mean that you get to live like a normal person who enjoys the occasional slice of birthday cake or Friday night cocktail without fear (or suppressed fear) of sabotaging otherwise healthy efforts or intentions.

How do we get to this holy grail of a healthy lifestyle? It requires a little work, but I'm confident that in just 28 days, you'll have the answers you seek. I'm going to lead you through a program that will equip you with all of the tools you need to solve the mystery for yourself.

I want us to rethink diets and detoxes. Let's reconsider the purpose of nutrition challenges and protocols. What if we leave the meanings of those terms behind and instead think of a healthy lifestyle breakthrough as a new venture? There is no grade, no failing, no winning, no cheating, and no bandwagon to be on or off.

My 28-Day Fed & Fit Project is designed with your success in mind. It's the jump-start, the leg up, the training wheels that will help you get from your "enough is enough" moment to a lasting healthy lifestyle that *you really love living*.

project tools

The process of designing, transitioning to, and living a healthy lifestyle is both straightforward and complicated. There are a number of components to consider, but at the end of the day, all you really need is determination. To provide you with as much support as possible, I've crafted a wealth of resources for you to keep in your Project toolbox:

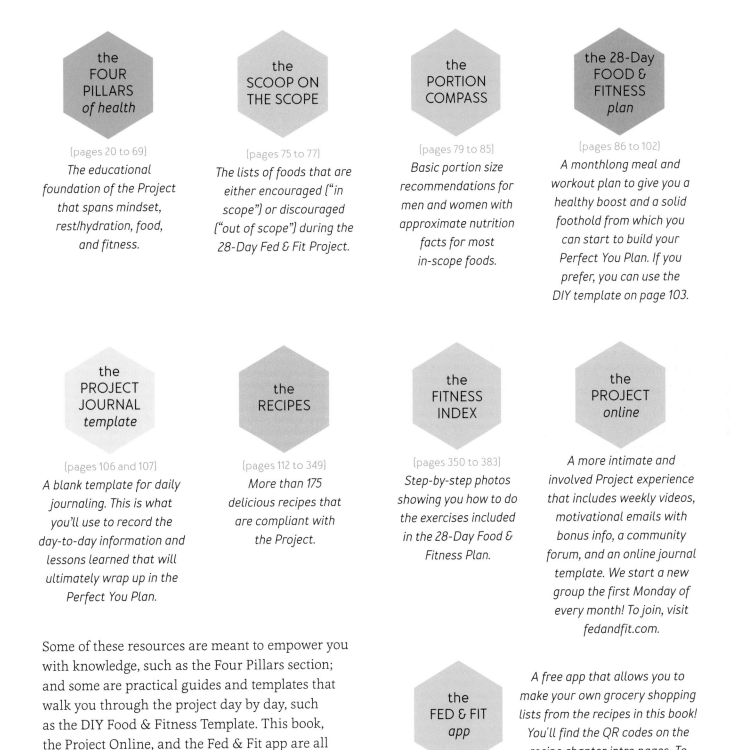

the FOUR PILLARS *of health*

[pages 20 to 69]

The educational foundation of the Project that spans mindset, rest/hydration, food, and fitness.

the SCOOP ON THE SCOPE

[pages 75 to 77]

The lists of foods that are either encouraged ("in scope") or discouraged ("out of scope") during the 28-Day Fed & Fit Project.

the PORTION COMPASS

[pages 79 to 85]

Basic portion size recommendations for men and women with approximate nutrition facts for most in-scope foods.

the 28-Day FOOD & FITNESS *plan*

[pages 86 to 102]

A monthlong meal and workout plan to give you a healthy boost and a solid foothold from which you can start to build your Perfect You Plan. If you prefer, you can use the DIY template on page 103.

the PROJECT JOURNAL *template*

[pages 106 and 107]

A blank template for daily journaling. This is what you'll use to record the day-to-day information and lessons learned that will ultimately wrap up in the Perfect You Plan.

the RECIPES

[pages 112 to 349]

More than 175 delicious recipes that are compliant with the Project.

the FITNESS INDEX

[pages 350 to 383]

Step-by-step photos showing you how to do the exercises included in the 28-Day Food & Fitness Plan.

the PROJECT *online*

A more intimate and involved Project experience that includes weekly videos, motivational emails with bonus info, a community forum, and an online journal template. We start a new group the first Monday of every month! To join, visit fedandfit.com.

the FED & FIT *app*

A free app that allows you to make your own grocery shopping lists from the recipes in this book! You'll find the QR codes on the recipe chapter intro pages. To download the app, visit fedandfit.com or your favorite app store.

Some of these resources are meant to empower you with knowledge, such as the Four Pillars section; and some are practical guides and templates that walk you through the project day by day, such as the DIY Food & Fitness Template. This book, the Project Online, and the Fed & Fit app are all great places to start, but making healthy lifestyle improvements happen is up to *you!*

you can't "fail" the project

Though the Project includes some pretty distinct lists of encouraged (and discouraged) activities and foods, they are not the main focus. The main focuses are that you make an effort (not follow the steps perfectly) and that you use each of your decisions, both "in scope" and "out of scope," as an opportunity to journal so that you can learn more about what's right for you.

Here's what the Fed & Fit Project is actually asking of you:

1.
Make an effort to restructure your lifestyle so that sleep and hydration become higher priorities.

2.
Make an effort to redirect your diet to focus on healing, anti-inflammatory foods.

3.
Make an effort to rethink your fitness routine so that it is full of regularly scheduled activities that both benefit you physically and bring you true enjoyment.

4.
Journal all your work both in scope and out of scope so that you have a personalized reference manual to help explain how you're feeling and why.

5.
Do not criticize yourself or feel as if you've fallen off the wagon if your personal journey doesn't perfectly match the plan provided. You're still working in the Project!

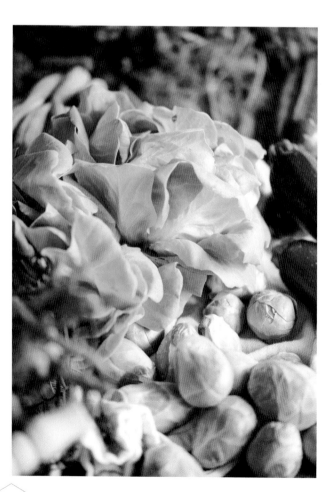

The Fed & Fit Project is essentially a set of practical instructions for writing a healthy lifestyle manual that is specific to your individual needs. I'm giving you a process, a set of recommended tools, and a list of the materials that typically work best. How you personally interpret my instructions and put the plan into action will determine your own unique experience and result in your own unique manual. Your manual will be a collection of your journal entries—your goals, adventures, self-discoveries, successes, food favorites, and fitness favorites. Your finished manual won't look like anybody else's, and it'll be filled with a unique set of knowledge that you can truly rely on in the future.

what if you still feel like you're doing it wrong?

1. What if I've missed a lot (or all) of the to-date journal entries?

You're still *in* the Project! If you are finding it daunting to make journal entries as I've outlined, simply jot down notes when you can and when you feel they're significant. For example, if you notice that you have an unusual amount of energy and clarity one day, reflect on your activities over the two days prior and highlight what was unique and what you believe contributed most. Or if you wake up with a headache, find that you are digesting food more slowly, and have mental fog, think back on the previous two days to identify the contributing factors.

2. What if I haven't actually implemented any changes to lifestyle, food, or fitness?

You (too) are still *in* the Project! I want to meet you where you are. Come find us at the Project Online and share the troubles or questions that are holding you back. All questions related to the Four Pillars (pages 20 to 69), the Scope (pages 75 to 77), and the process of establishing your Ideal Fitness Fit (IFF) are welcome. Share your biggest roadblock or fear so that we can help clear it up and get you on a path that feels comfortable.

the Perfect You Plan

The Perfect You Plan (PYP) is the state of living that strikes *your* perfect balance between healthy choices and indulgent choices. Your PYP also accounts for the foods that work for you and the foods that don't. For example, some people do well when they omit nuts altogether, and others find that they feel especially great when they enjoy a cup of cooked kale each day. Your Daily Sleep Number (DSN) and Daily Water Need (DWN) are priceless data points, as is the discovery of the workout routine that gets you excited to break a sweat. These customized dos and don'ts are the lessons learned that ultimately boil down to the Perfect You Plan.

I'm thrilled that you're here, and I want to encourage you to proceed empowered. Know that the Fed & Fit Project is a commitment. Extensive journaling, self-reflection, delicious foods, and fun new fitness activities lie ahead. When these 28 days are over, you will walk away with a (literal) book on yourself and a refreshed perspective of what is right for *you*. I suggest that you begin when you're really ready to strap on that thinking cap and commit. You are in the driver's seat, and I am your esteemed copilot.

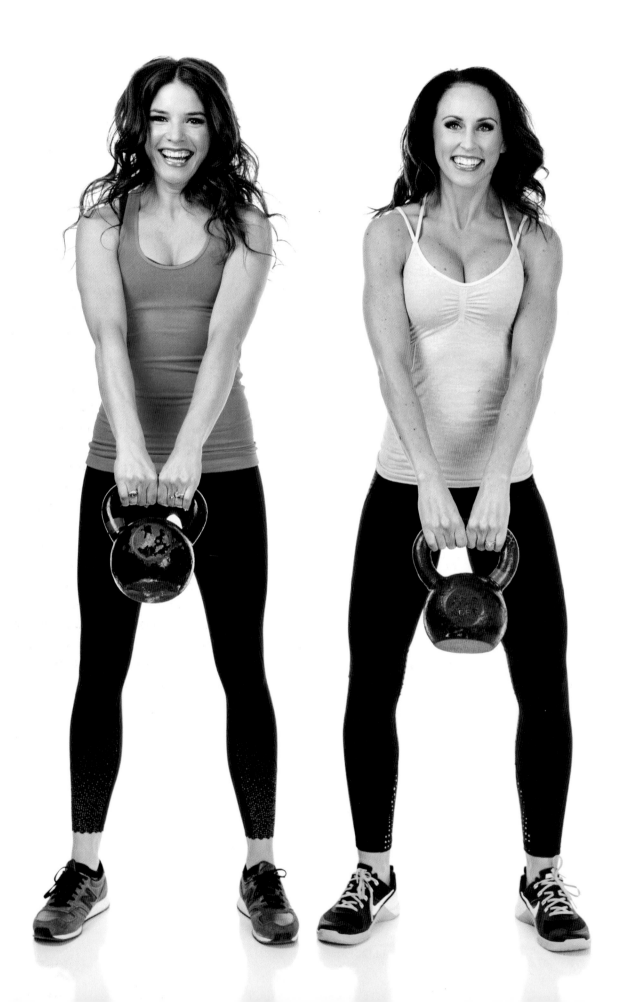

meet Juli!

I want to equip you with the most significant information that I've collected over the years. I want to design the most inclusive program and make you feel as welcome as possible. I want to present you with my best recipes. There is one area, however, where I still defer (almost completely) to outside experts: fitness.

Though I've managed to work up to a decent golf game, it took me almost 15 years of coaching to get there; though I can hang in a CrossFit class, I'm by no means competitive and still ask a lot of questions; and though I can semi-confidently bend and snap my way through a yoga class, I've not yet been asked to guest-lead. What I'm getting at is that while I'm highly coachable, I still put the fate of my exercise routines in the hands of other experts. I place a high value on mixed fitness, I choose my coaches carefully, and I trust their programming. I wanted to incorporate that outside coaching element in the Project. I wanted to bring someone in not just to bolster, but to *revolutionize* the 28-day fitness plan.

So I put my thinking cap on. I asked myself who, in the great big world of fitness, would I entrust with a Fed & Fit Project member's exercise routine? Who embodies the positivity, commitment, self-confidence, Paleo-friendly qualities that signify a Project graduate? Who would create a fun, challenging, thoughtful, exciting workout series that produces real results?

Her name is Juli Bauer.

I'm a lucky gal because I get to call her a friend, and now I'm even luckier because I get to call her a business partner as well.

I've asked Juli to step in as your other copilot for the Project because I want you to have the best of the best. She is one of the most motivating people I've ever had the pleasure of knowing, and she's a darn good coach. A certified CrossFit coach for the past six years, Juli is a confident, knowledgeable, balanced trainer who knows her way around a month of fitness programming designed to change lives.

Juli is the blogger behind the wildly popular blog PaleOMG, and she's also a *New York Times* bestselling author. She's the person you call when you want an honest opinion and someone to inspire your rear into shape.

In addition to her 28-day fitness program, Juli has offered up insight in several other arenas. You can catch her thoughts in Pillar #4: Fitness (beginning on page 17), in her detailed workouts (pages 90 to 97, with a breakdown of how to do each exercise on pages 350 to 383), and in the morning newscaster–style video clips that we created to walk you through all four weeks of the Project's Four Pillars. In those videos you will find weekly expectations, bonus nutritional insights, extra fitness tips, and motivational thoughts. To view them, visit fedandfit.com.

what's in it for me? (WIIFM)

Ah, the million-dollar question: *"WHY should I do the 28-Day Fed & Fit Project?"* I knew it was coming! So by now you've got a pretty good understanding of why I created the Project, and you know what the major components are. You've heard me throw around the terms *healthy lifestyle* and *Perfect You Plan.* You understand that committing to this detailed four-week program, working through the journaling exercises, and carrying those lessons learned past the 28 days will help you feel healthier and happier. But is there more? What else are you going to get out of it?

I'm so glad you asked! Let's review the obvious and (sometimes) not-so-obvious benefits:

- Clearer, more supple skin
- A greater ability to manage stress
- A more positive attitude
- Stronger nails and faster hair growth
- Flexibility, strength, and endurance
- More energy throughout the day
- Clearer thinking
- An easier time falling asleep at night
- Healthier, more regular bowel movements
- Confidence and prowess in the kitchen

- Prevention or reversal of chronic pain
- Prevention or reversal of chronic disease
- Lower cholesterol
- Lower blood pressure
- A reduction in body fat
- Naturally balanced, healthy hormone levels
- Increased muscle mass
- A stoppage of bone deterioration
- "Cleaned-up" taste buds (meaning that food will taste better than ever before)

Remember that the real goal of the Project is to provide you with a tool set that enables you to solve the mystery of your Perfect You Plan for yourself. You will walk away knowing your ideal sleep pattern and ideal daily water intake, and with a list of foods that make you feel great and a list of foods that make you feel crummy. Add to that a personal knowledge of how much food to eat and when to eat what and an understanding of which fitness activities fit you, your goals, and your fun-meter best. Even better than all of the above, you will walk away with the knowledge that you have the power and the tools to *realize your own dreams.*

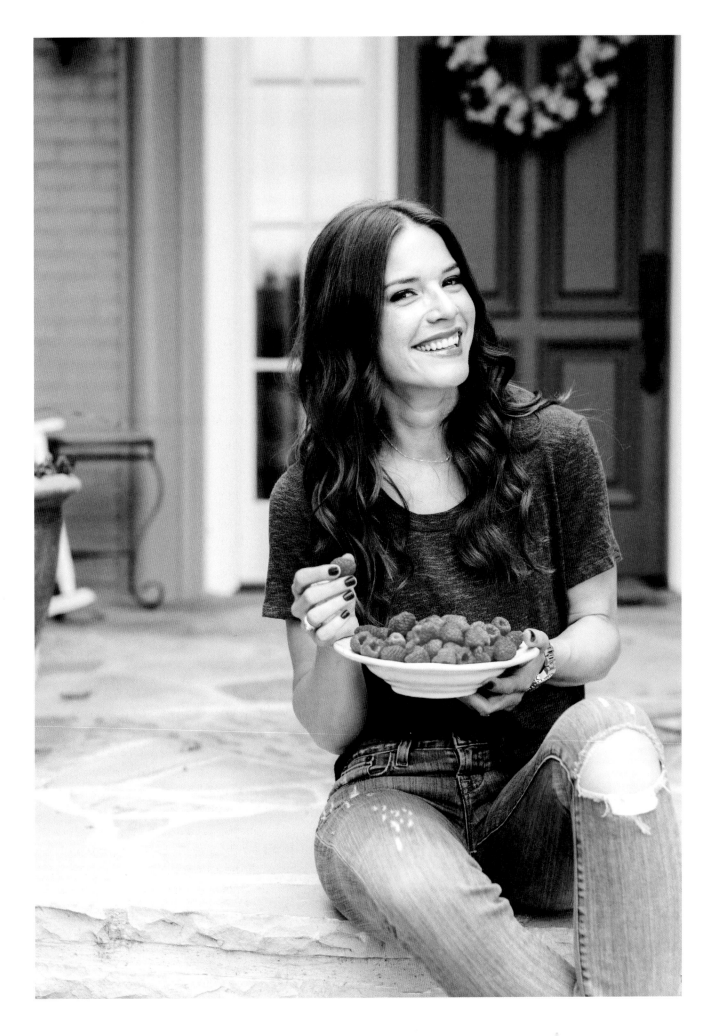

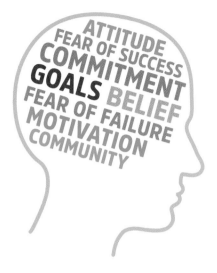

MINDSET:

LEARN HOW TO CRAFT A VISION
AND SET GOALS.

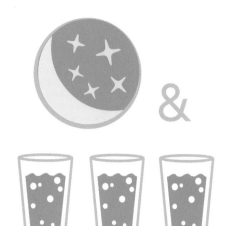

SLEEP & HYDRATION:

LEARN YOUR DAILY SLEEP NUMBER (DSN)
AND DAILY WATER NEED (DWN).

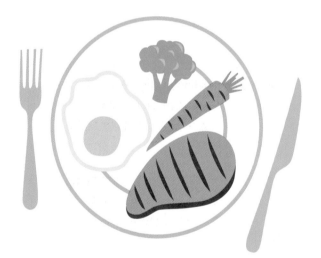

FOOD:

LEARN WHY WE'RE SICK AND
HOW WE CAN HEAL.

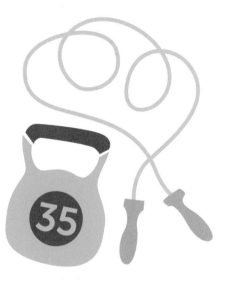

FITNESS:

LEARN HOW TO FIND YOUR
IDEAL FITNESS FIT (IFF).

THE FOUR PILLARS

After years of thinking over the reasons for my own success and observing the success stories of my nutrition clients, I decided to organize the most pertinent stepping-stones into four priorities. I like to call them the Four Pillars.

1. Mindset: Learn how to craft a vision and set goals.

2. Sleep & Hydration: Learn your Daily Sleep Number (DSN) and Daily Water Need (DWN).

3. Food: Learn why we're sick and how we can heal.

4. Fitness: Learn how to find your Ideal Fitness Fit (IFF).

The pillars work to circumvent pitfalls and offer up a wide safety net so that you're fully equipped to take on this transformation with confidence and the knowledge that you're in great hands. Whose hands exactly? *Hint:* They're holding this book you're reading. Within each pillar, you'll find answers to most of your what, why, and how questions. The pillars are meant to:

- *Assertively organize simple priorities to help ensure that you make efficient strides toward your personal healthy lifestyle— also known as the Perfect You Plan.*

- *Offer just enough background and other scientific information so that you have a solid grasp on why the Project is structured as it is.*

- *Provide you with simple exercises that help turn lofty concepts into live action.*

Let's jump in!

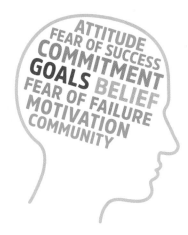

PILLAR #1:

MINDSET

I've (almost accidentally) made a career out of mindset coaching. Sure, nutrition and fitness are the more obvious mainstays of my job, but mindset has evolved to become the topic that I spend the most time on. Why has mindset found its way into my business and up to the top of my Four Pillars list? Because a healthy, balanced outlook is, without a doubt, the most important secret to success. Mindset also happens to be the most difficult component to address. With so many varieties of personal experiences and starting points (you're all so wonderfully, perfectly unique), it can be a challenge to articulate a single strategy.

So I've kept notes—for years. I've written down the tips that have resonated the most with my clients and readers. Like a quality reduction, I kept this pot of ideas simmering on the stove until I was left with the most concentrated list of effective tricks. I hope that you find it helpful, and I hope that you take a deep breath after it's all over, because after all, you've got this. You have totally and completely got this.

Before I jump into the meat of this topic, I'd like to set the stage.

What if we liken a healthy lifestyle transformation to learning a new sport—say, soccer. I just love soccer! Though I was far from the best player on my middle school team, soccer still lovingly occupies a piece of my heart.

Let's say you decide that you want to learn how to play soccer. You're probably going to start by equipping yourself with the tools needed: a ball, a goal, some shin guards, a pair of shoes with cleats. You also need to find a place to run around and a coach to instruct you. It seems like a complete picture! You eventually find a community, known here (of course) as your teammates, who share your interest for learning and playing the game. In addition to making the sport more fun, your teammates become a part of an accountability system. They take note when you're absent, encourage your progress, and remind you that mistakes are normal.

After several lessons, your skills advance. Dribbling becomes second nature, you can skillfully throw a ball back into play with confidence, and the flow of the game becomes intuitive. You eventually note that your curiosity for the sport has matured into a true passion. Soccer becomes a part of your life; it's both a part of your identity *and* something you represent. No longer a beginner, a novice, or a person who just

wants to learn a new skill, you've become a full-fledged soccer player.

Who (or what) is to credit for this newfound identity?

Though the ball, goal, cleats, field, and coach seemed like the complete picture at the beginning of your journey, you've come to understand that your identification with the sport isn't derived solely from the tangible components of the game. Your newfound identity doesn't live on the field; it lives in you. The credit belongs to *you*.

As with soccer, there are plenty of tools that you can employ to help you on this journey of learning to eat and exercise for optimal health. Meal plans, recipes, nutrition knowledge, cooking skills, a purposefully stocked refrigerator and pantry, a fitness routine, and a coach are all critical components—but they're not the whole picture.

Learning a sport, just like any other new skill or habit, takes time and practice. You've got to experience successes and failures before you can achieve mastery. In other words, regardless of the venture, new pursuits are always uncomfortable, and then one day the uncomfortable becomes slightly more comfortable. The clouds part, and this foreign new skill, habit, or mindset feels like an old friend. It seems to require less effort and less planning, and your mind shows less resistance. This is the sweet spot—the holy grail of new habits. This is what we're working toward in the Project.

the key components of a healthy mindset

Why is Mindset our first pillar? Because although you can power through a monthlong food and fitness challenge, experience success, and learn a few things, upselling those short-term lessons and experiences into a long-lasting healthy lifestyle is possible only when you nurture the mind and its components: goals, attitude, community, motivation, fear of failure, fear of success, belief, and commitment.

Let's break it down!

GOALS · ATTITUDE · COMMUNITY · MOTIVATION · FEAR OF FAILURE · FEAR OF SUCCESS · BELIEF · COMMITMENT

attitude

At the risk of oversimplifying, I want to address just two kinds of attitudes: can-do and can't-do. I'm talking about MacGyver versus Chicken Little; positivity versus negativity; silver lining–seeker versus fault-seeker; go-getter versus woe-is-me; and my personal favorite, Dory of *Finding Nemo* versus Eeyore of *Winnie-the-Pooh*.

I believe that a negative attitude can stem from a collision of confused priorities and unclear plans. Positive, can-do people tend to have a relatively firm grasp on their priorities and take steps to align their time and actions accordingly. When priorities are unclear and efforts to improve are disorganized, it can be difficult to track progress in a constructive, positive manner.

The solution I propose is incredibly simple; follow the exercise below and repeat it as often as necessary:

1.

Make a list, in no particular order, of all the things in your life that consume your time. *Think: family, friends, career, blog, spirituality, pets, bird-watching, gardening, fitness, health, TV, golf, shopping, travel, cooking, etc. Next, write down the number of hours that you spend on each item. Some activities may overlap, like quality time with your significant other and cooking, so don't worry about being too precise. As an example, these include the hours dedicated to family time or catching up with friends and the hours spent at work, blogging, working out, watching your favorite show on TV, taking pets for a walk, maintaining a spiritual practice, etc.*

2.

On a separate sheet of paper, rewrite your list but in order of priority, starting with the most important. *Reapply the hours spent on each task next to the now-organized priorities.*

3.

Review your priorities and the time you spend on them. *Does the time you spend on each item reflect its significance? Take note of where you spend the most and least time and where those priorities fall in importance.*

4.

Set an intention to exchange time spent on low-priority items for more time on items at the top of your priority list. *If you see that high-priority fitness is receiving only two hours of your time each week but low-priority TV watching receives eight hours, consider exchanging three hours of TV time for a few more hours at your favorite fitness studio. Wherever you find a discrepancy between priority and time spent dedicated to that task, consider making an effort to reorganize how you spend your time.*

Deep-seeded positivity doesn't necessarily stem from a feeling of being in control of life. It stems from a feeling we get when our actions align with our priorities. It speaks to a life in sync with purpose. Spending (or making) more time for the things at the top of your list leads to a feeling of purposeful living. Sunny-side attitudes follow closely behind clear intentions and thoughtful actions.

goals

Getting clear on *why* you want to pursue a healthier way of living is mission critical. Goals help set the tone, calibrate our motivational compass, and give us something to focus on when developing a new habit feels especially difficult. When we imagine ourselves as the embodiment of our goals, inspiration seeps in, and we're even more ready to make. it. happen.

It's important to note that *not all goals are created equal.* Some goals are skin-deep, and some speak directly to our identities as people. If your goal is to impress your classmates at your ten-year reunion, that's completely okay! Just manage your expectations of that goal's staying power. The motivational power it holds will likely fizzle after the event, or even beforehand if you encounter an obstacle that seems larger than the reunion. For example, what if it becomes increasingly more challenging to spend time preparing food? You may find yourself asking, "Is the reunion really worth all this time?" The answer is likely no, the reunion isn't worth it—but *you* are. Hence the need for setting at least one deep-seated goal.

Here's how to set a balance of meaningful goals that will last:

1.

If you have a goal that relates to the look, size, or feel of your body, write it down. *There's nothing wrong with goals related to weight, clothing size, or energy. Just make sure that you don't stop there. Challenge yourself to set a goal from the second category (Step 2) so that you have a deeper investment to turn short-term gains into long-term living.*

2.

Brainstorm goals that relate to your top priorities. *Dig deep and hold nothing back! Do you want to have more energy to chase grandkids? Do you want to be a healthier, happier version of yourself for your significant other, your kids, or yourself? Do you want to prevent or reverse chronic disease? Do you want to become the person your heart tells you you're meant to be? Write these goals down. Pin them on the wall or fold them into your day planner. They are worth holding on to.*

community

A truly magical thing happens when you put an ambitious, motivated, determined person in a room with like-minded people: that person becomes even more unstoppable. She becomes more comfortable, more at home, more excited, and more invested. A community offers accountability, support, and excitement. Find your community as soon as possible!

Here are some avenues:

Start this journey with a friend, family member, group from the gym, etc. *Working through the Project with a companion can remind you that you're not the only one struggling to adjust to a new lifestyle. The two of you can share tips, favorite recipes, and daily successes.*

Join the online Fed & Fit Project! *We have a solid community of people working through this exact material.*

Join a gym! *Though the other members of the gym may not be working through this exact material, they offer a regular dose of community geared toward health and well-being.*

Start a blog! *Share your story, put yourself out there, and see who comes to the table. It's incredibly motivating to be held accountable to people who have come to rely on you for inspiration.*

motivation

Motivation can come in any number of forms, but I've found that we tend to experience a deeper buy-in when the motivation is tailored to us—to *our specific* journey. Who can we find who knows us so incredibly well, so deeply, that they can handle the responsibility of providing us with constant, tailored, perfect motivation that speaks directly to our goals and experiences?

You're hired.

It's you! You're the best person. You know yourself better than anyone else. You already know your favorite excuses and deepest desires. You've got your own number, which makes you the absolute best person for the job.

Now that you're hired, let's talk about the job.

Your job as a self-motivator is to provide fresh, supportive, tailored motivation as often as you need it. Note that this may require a larger investment of time at the beginning of a new healthy lifestyle journey, but the workload eventually tapers off as you start to build your own library of personal success stories.

Here are some ways to find inspiration and keep yourself motivated:

Research healthy lifestyle transformation stories! *In today's world, there is no shortage of incredible people sharing their incredible stories online. Keep digging until you find three or four that you relate to, print or save them somewhere you can access easily, and reread them whenever you're in need of a little motivation. Note that the Fed & Fit Project community forum is a great place to find some of these stories!*

*WARNING:
Know thyself. If you know that photos and measurements will open a door for you to body-shame yourself, then skip this step altogether. Before/during photos and measurements are highly effective motivational tools when placed in the right hands. In the wrong hands, they can have the opposite effect. This distinction is up to you to make; choose wisely.

Document your progress. This is done in one of two ways, though you can absolutely employ both*:

1. Take a before picture and a during picture!

a. **Before:** *Put on a pair of athletic pants or shorts and your favorite sports bra (gentlemen, modify accordingly). Stand in bright natural light (by a window works) and either snap a photo looking in a mirror or ask someone to take it for you. Be sure to smile; you're beautiful.*

b. **During (not "after"):** *Whether it's every two weeks, at the end of a 28-day Project, or six months later, I encourage you to snap a "during" photo. Try to wear the same or similar clothing and stand in the same place under the same light. Look at the photos side by side and see for yourself the progress you've made.*

2. Take measurements!

a. **Before:** *Break out that measuring tape and write down the circumference of your waist, hips, thigh, upper arm, and bust. Record those numbers and then give them no more thought. They hold no power right now.*

b. **During:** *After you feel that you've made some progress, feel free to measure the same body parts. If the Delta is negative, congratulations! You likely had some inflammation and possibly excess body fat. You're doing a great job; keep it up! If the Delta is positive, congratulations! You likely had very little inflammation and very little excess body fat. In fact, you may be gaining muscle and becoming a stronger, healthier you. Keep it up!*

My point here is that the lasting motivation that embeds itself in your heart doesn't necessarily come from a quote that you quickly read online or how you think you look in the mirror. It comes from stories and experience—the more personal, the better.

So, back to your job description. Part of your job of motivator is to *keep* motivated over the long haul, even if you find yourself going off-track or falling into a funk caused by something like:

- An indulgent weekend
- The feeling that you're not making any or fast-enough progress
- A general lack of motivation

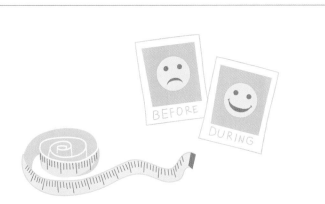

Document lessons learned / start your own story narrative. *Either via the Project daily journal or in your own notebook, document the lessons you've learned at day's end. These lessons can offer a goldmine of motivation. I encourage you to be both specific and general. For example, I would document both of the following:*

- *I learned that three eggs, a side of cooked greens, and a half a small sweet potato for breakfast gave me plenty of energy during my morning, and I wasn't hungry until lunch! I wasn't even tempted by the break room candy bowl. That hasn't happened in months!*

- *I had high energy and a sunny outlook today. I don't even care if I go down a dress size in time for my high school reunion. I love feeling this way. Today was a win.*

The best way to shake off a feeling of funk is to take an objective look at your progress. Whether your progress has been incremental or monumental, let it fuel your fire. Let it show you (despite that "you're doing this wrong" voice in your head) that you are, in fact, on the right track. Keep up the good work!

fear of failure

I need you to know that you're going to fail. It's just going to happen! As soon as you acknowledge that hiccups, mistakes, and feelings of falling behind are inevitable, they lose their crippling power over you. Don't let a fear of an imperfect journey keep you from taking tremendous strides toward a healthier, happier you. The healthy distinction of working toward progress, not perfection, can be your saving grace.

fear of success

Stay with me; this one digs deep. I'm going to briefly talk about a forbidden feeling that haunts so many of us—the unmentionable questions "Am I even worthy? Am I worth the effort, the trials, the errors, the grace, the patience, and the success?" Ask yourself these questions out loud or on paper and give yourself the answer you deserve: yes. Yes, you *are* worth every single minute and every single effort. You're worth it all, and you need to remember that. Don't let a fear of success keep you from living a life you deserve to live.

Write it on your bathroom mirror in lipstick, plant handwritten notes in your jacket pockets, and set a "you are *so* worth it" daily alarm on your phone for when you need reminding.

belief

This one is pretty simple. Do you believe in your goals? Your dreams? The science, the success of the people who've come before you, and the Project? Articulate it and then put this arrow into your mindset quiver. There's no knowing when or where you may need to employ your belief, but it's a smart concept to think through in the early stages. Determining belief helps align our subconscious—making our daily conscious decisions easier to make and even more in line with our true goals.

Note that if you'd like a review of the science, the successes, and the Project, this book has you covered. As for your goals and dreams, those are up to you! Make sure to write them down. Handwritten words have power over the spoken and unspoken.

commitment

Commitment is the final piece of the healthy mindset puzzle. This last piece is what helps you hit the proverbial ball out of the great big park. Commitment encompasses your determination, plan, follow-through, and consistency. The determination is something you have to find for yourself, the plan I've carefully constructed for you, the follow-through requires grit and a decision you make for yourself, and the consistency is the true key that unlocks your success.

Note that failed perfection and unmet expectations are commitment's kryptonite. Therefore, let's start with manageable expectations and the understanding that we're working toward *progress*, not perfection.

Consistency is key, determination your fuel, and the Project your map. Stay the course and keep working at it every day. It will feel like work at first, but just like building muscle or learning a new sport, it gets easier and more intuitive with time.

You've got this.

When the Project lessons learned are combined with a solid healthy mindset, you become unstoppable. You emerge as one of those "naturally healthy" people. I know this because I went through the journey myself. Having gone from an unhealthy serial dieter in chronic pain to a person who is regularly accused of being "just naturally healthy," I remember that none of it was by accident.

If you take nothing else away from this pillar, I want to stress the point that success is hardly ever an accident. A professional athlete makes her sport look easy, but even the pros have to start somewhere. The secret to becoming a master of healthy living is to become a master of healthy perspective. A transformation of our bodies requires a transformation of our minds.

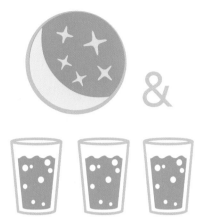

PILLAR #2:

SLEEP & HYDRATION

Could it be so simple? Are we really going to devote a whole pillar to Sleep & Hydration? "Surely there's a catch," you might be thinking. "Surely I need to buy a special mattress, diffuse essential oils in my bedroom, and drink special water at certain times of the day in order to be the healthiest version of myself."

My answer: NOPE! You'll find no snake oil sales pitch here. I'm a strong believer in hard science and proven practices. It just so happens that the strongest science lines up with the simplest practices. Our bodies need good old-fashioned sleep (and plenty of it) plus good old-fashioned hydration (and plenty of it).

Let's break it down and strategically discuss these wonderful, fundamental principles.

sleep

the circadian rhythm

It's impossible to address the science of sleep without mentioning the circadian rhythm. The circadian rhythm is essentially the internal clock, set on a 24-hour cycle, that regulates biological processes in all animals, plants, fungi, and even some bacteria. It refers to the timing and balancing of the body's regulatory hormones (like sleep and wake hormones). It tells us when it's daytime, when it's nighttime, when we should have energy, when we should feel sleepy, when it's time for food, and when it's time for activity. A finely tuned circadian rhythm is like a finely tuned clock. You can almost set your watch to the exact time you wake each morning and the exact time you fall asleep at night. Your body knows when to expect a meal and when to expect activities.

If this sounds completely foreign, think about a pet. Our sweet dog Gus, a four-year-old Great Pyrenees, wakes up at exactly 6:30 a.m., stands by his bowl for breakfast at exactly 7:00 a.m., and then demands a walk at 7:30 a.m. He then naps, barks, and loafs around until exactly 3:45 p.m., when he demands another walk. He stands by his bowl for dinner at exactly 5:30 p.m. and then passes out in his bed at exactly 8:00 p.m. This is a sign of a healthy pup. Gus can't tell time, but his routine is never off by more than five minutes. His circadian rhythm, nurtured by a healthy routine, navigates his day.

This healthy, predictable, dependable routine is possible for you, too. In fact, I highly recommend it.

I want to highlight a few of the main circadian rhythm players:

- Melatonin—sleep hormone
- Cortisol—wake hormone
- Sunlight/Blue light—cortisol stimulator
- Darkness/Orange light—melatonin stimulator

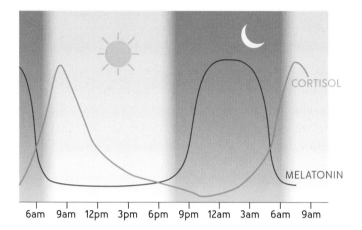

In one circadian rhythm example, melatonin would peak in the middle of the night and cortisol just after waking. When melatonin starts to rise in the early evening, the body starts to feel tired and ready for sleep. As melatonin continues to climb and cortisol continues to drop, we get closer and closer to falling asleep. In the morning, melatonin starts to drop off and cortisol starts to rise, causing us to feel more and more awake.

Which came first, the chicken or the egg? Do our hormones dictate our day, or does the day dictate our hormones?

YES.

Cortisol and melatonin are mostly courteous gentlemen who will wait their turn to take a pretty lady out on the floor for a few spins. They don't like to compete. They prefer to step in when the other steps out. Melatonin likes to dance all night, and cortisol likes to dance all day. There are times, however, when they can get a little mixed up. Cortisol *can* occupy the dance floor during the night and melatonin during the day, throwing their predictable turn-taking cycle out of balance.

While sunlight helps stimulate the rise of our wake hormone, we can keep cortisol levels unnaturally high through uncontrolled stress, exposure to sun-mimicking light (like that from a computer or phone screen), and caffeine (which I address below). Elevated cortisol levels into the night prevent melatonin levels from rising, which prevents us from naturally becoming ready for rest. The side effects of the imbalance continue into the next morning, when we find it more difficult to wake up, as melatonin is still present in our system. Maybe we require an extra cup of coffee before we jump back into another day filled with stress.

Why does this matter so much? The lack of sleep, chronically elevated cortisol levels, and exhaustion put our bodies in a prime position for additional stress, weight gain, and illness. The good news is that there is a way to correct your personal rhythm! And it's more accessible than you may think.

well-rested body versus tired body

A WELL-RESTED BODY:	A TIRED BODY:
Experiences consistently high amounts of energy throughout the day.	Has low energy or inconsistent bursts of energy throughout the day.
Doesn't necessarily need caffeine in the morning.	Must have caffeine in the morning, and sometimes even throughout the day.
Finds it easier to fall and stay asleep at night.	Finds it incredibly difficult to fall and stay asleep at night.
Finds it easier to keep off excess body fat.	Finds it difficult to lose excess body fat.
Experiences fewer non-hunger-based food cravings.	Endures numerous non-hunger-based food cravings throughout the day as a way to cope with exhaustion.
Experiences even, positive moods throughout the day.	Experiences moodiness, both highs and lows, throughout the day.
Finds it easier to handle stress.	Finds it difficult to handle stress, which often leads to more stress.
Has healthy skin, nails, and hair.	Has under-eye bags, dull skin, thinning hair, and weak nails.
Tends to experience less chronic pain.	Is more susceptible to chronic pain.
Tends to get sick less.	Tends to get sick more often.
Has plenty of energy for workouts.	Often feels tired and sluggish during workouts.
Recovers from intense workouts more quickly.	Takes a long time to recover from intense workouts.

your daily sleep number (DSN)

Getting your body set up on a healthy sleep schedule tailored to your needs is possible and, better yet, relatively straightforward. First, you need figure out your personal Daily Sleep Number (DSN)! Your DSN is the number of hours you need to sleep at night in order to feel fully rested and function at your best. Because so many of our sleep habits are constantly interrupted by dinging cell phones, significant others who like to watch TV in bed, pets who want to be let out, and children who wake throughout the night, it can be difficult to know how much sleep we really need. So I've come up with a homework-style analysis. Asking others to let you sleep in may seem like an indulgent practice, but remember—sleep is a crucial foundation of your health.

To determine your DSN, you'll need to get at least one full night's sleep data point. Here's how it works:

1. Choose a night plus the following morning out of the week that allows for the most flexible schedule. Weekends are the most popular choice, so for the sake of this example, let's say that we're looking at a Friday evening and a Saturday morning.

2. Ask your spouse, children, roommate, etc. to let you sleep undisturbed so that you can wake up naturally. Leave your pets at a friend's house for the night, suggest that your spouse take the kids out for an early breakfast, and ask your roommate to hold off on her early-morning kickboxing fitness video until you surface.

3. Follow all of the everyday sleep best practices below and as many of the bonus practices as you like.

4. Get tucked in for sleep at a logical time. Typically, I would recommend no later than 10:00 p.m. for most folks who like to start the day between 6:00 and 7:00 a.m. If you follow a different schedule, adjust accordingly. Whatever bedtime you set, write it down.

5. If you have a hard time falling asleep or you wake up during the night, do your best not to look at a clock. Just quiet your mind until you fall back asleep.

6. Sleep until you wake up naturally and feel fully rested, but be sure that you actually get out of bed when you wake up naturally. Forcing yourself back to sleep after a full night's rest will skew the results of this test.

7. Record the time at which you woke up fully rested, then determine the number of hours you slept. This becomes your Daily Sleep Number! Your DSN may be 7, or 8, or even 9. Don't worry about what your number means—just know that your body requires that much sleep for optimal function.

A COUPLE OF NOTES:

• If you already know that you're sleep deprived, I recommend performing the above test three or four evenings in a row. This way, your body can recover from a possible sleep deficit in the first couple of days. I then recommend that you take an average of the last two nights to determine your DSN.

• Do your best to comply with these steps, but if you truly can't escape all responsibilities, try to get as close as possible. Remember: progress, not perfection, is the name of the game.

Just like your personal Daily Water Need, which you'll read about in a bit, your Daily Sleep Number becomes a daily goal. If you must start your day by 6:00 a.m., subtract your DSN and write down your bedtime. This may be earlier than you're used to, but do your best to end your day and be in bed on time.

After a few weeks of honoring your new bedtime and following healthy sleep practices, you will likely find yourself waking up more rested, on time, without the help of an alarm clock.

restful sleep best practices

EVERYDAY PRACTICES:

 ⊗8 HOURS BEFORE BED

Avoid caffeine for at least eight hours before you plan to go to bed.

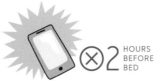 ⊗2 HOURS BEFORE BED

Avoid looking at blue light (from a television, cell phone, or computer) for at least two hours before bed.

If you don't already keep the temperature in your bedroom a little cooler than the rest of your house or apartment, turn the temperature in your bedroom down a couple degrees.

Choose a logical bedtime and make sure that you're tucked in on cue.

If you have a hard time falling asleep, try reading a print book (not an eBook) by lamplight until you start to grow tired.

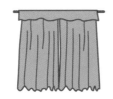

Turn off your cell phone, point your bedside clock away from your line of sight when lying in bed, and cover any other ambient light in your room with a blackout curtain, blanket, or towel.

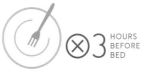 ⊗3 HOURS BEFORE BED

Avoid eating for at least three hours before bed.

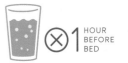 ⊗1 HOUR BEFORE BED

Avoid drinking liquids for at least one hour before bed (so that you don't have to get up in the middle of the night to relieve yourself).

Make sure that your bed sheets are clean and tidy before you climb in.

Do your best to avoid working or watching TV in bed.

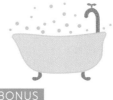

BONUS
Before bed, relax in a warm bath for at least 15 minutes. Add Epsom salts or calming oils if you like.

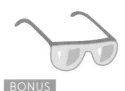

BONUS
Wear amber-tinted goggles after the sun goes down. This will help prepare your body for rest by blocking the cortisol-stimulating blue light emitted by computers, televisions, and cell phone screens.

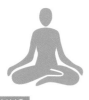

BONUS
Develop a winding-down pre-bed practice to calm your mind. This can include a short meditation, journaling, or light yoga or stretching.

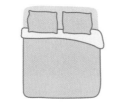

BONUS
Invest in high-quality sheets.

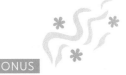

BONUS
Invest in an ambient noise machine to help drown out other sounds.

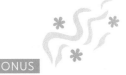

BONUS
Invest in a humidifier or an essential oil diffuser for the bedroom.

caffeine 101

I'm tucking this information on caffeine here in the Sleep section because uncontrolled use/abuse can sabotage healthy sleep efforts. While moderate use is perfectly healthy, uncontrolled or mindless consumption throughout the day can prevent your body from finding quality rest. Before I jump into some details about caffeine, let's briefly review some super fun science!

What happens to caffeine in the body?

This is fascinating but slightly anti-intuitive stuff. Stay with me!

Most of us think of the morning cup of coffee as giving us a needed jolt of speed to get the day going. But in reality, caffeine doesn't cause the body to speed up; instead, it tells the body not to slow down. To understand how this works, you need to get to know a little compound called adenosine. Naturally produced by the body, adenosine's main function is to act as an inhibitory neurotransmitter. This means that it attaches itself, via its very own personalized receptor, onto a nerve ending in the brain. Once it attaches, it tells (by inhibiting) the neurons to *slow down*. This is a totally natural process. The body will present a higher concentration of adenosine while it prepares for rest (coinciding with a rise in melatonin and a drop in cortisol) and a lower concentration while active.

To the body, caffeine happens to look a lot like adenosine! In fact, you could almost call it an adenosine impostor. It attaches to the special adenosine receptor on the nerve ending but does not trigger the same slowdown effect. Therefore, the neurons (which have a natural inclination to go fast) keep firing at high speed.

From here, in essence, the body responds to the frenzy of firing neurons by triggering a greater release of dopamine and glutamate. Dopamine stimulates feelings of pleasure and motivation, while glutamate stimulates cognitive function (think memory and learning). Eventually, the pituitary gland catches wind of all the activity and starts to release more adrenaline. Adrenaline, in turn, causes the body's heart rate to increase, triggers the liver to release more sugar into the bloodstream for energy, tightens muscles, and causes blood vessels to constrict so that more blood can flow into the muscles—preparing the body for fight or flight.

This is why, when you consume more than a moderate amount of caffeine, your hands start to feel a bit colder (due to blood vessel constriction) and your heart rate increases. Though pleasure and cognitive function may be stimulated, caffeine does stress the body.

While there's nothing wrong with a moderate caffeine intake, excessive consumption, especially throughout the day, can keep the body from slowing down and preparing for restful sleep.

Ideal caffeine relationship

Striking a healthy balance with caffeine is possible! It may take some adjusting, but all you need is a little extra awareness and then some practice. Here are some signs of a healthy relationship with caffeine:

- Though you enjoy drinking caffeine, your body doesn't necessarily depend on it.

- You can skip coffee or tea for a day and not suffer a headache or other detox symptoms.

- You intuitively stop consuming caffeine before becoming jittery, shaky, or distracted.

- You drink it only in the morning and prefer water, sparkling water, or herbal tea during the rest of the day.

Caffeine consumption best practices

First, it's important to note that you are the *only one* who can determine whether caffeine is right for you! I'm not here to say that it is, and I'm not here to say that it isn't. If you suspect that your caffeine intake needs adjusting, I recommend that you take a focused look at how the timing, amount, and source impact your day. To track your observations and make informed adjustments, document your findings in your Daily Project Journal by taking note of the following:

- Amount and type of caffeine and time it was consumed.

- Proximity of consumption to a meal: was it consumed before, during, or after eating?

- How your body feels during, just after, and two hours after consumption: relaxed, euphoric, jittery, shaky, focused, distracted, etc.

Make adjustments to your caffeine intake, playing with the amount, timing, and type, until you settle on a routine that speaks to the ideal caffeine relationship.

Ideal timing: My general rule is to consume caffeine only in the morning hours, or the first half of your day if you work an alternative schedule. If you feel that you may be especially sensitive to caffeine, I recommend consuming it only with or after a meal. After noon (or after your midday meal), try to avoid all caffeine.

Ideal amount: Again, as a general rule, most people should try to stay under 200 milligrams of caffeine a day. Definitely try not to exceed 300 milligrams. Three hundred milligrams of caffeine is equivalent to approximately 16 ounces (a medium or "grande") of hot dark roast drip coffee, one serving of store-bought cold-brew coffee, or four shots of espresso. To paint a picture of how much caffeine is in different beverages, here are some *approximate* amounts of caffeine (in milligrams) per serving:

Ideal sources:
- Store-bought cold-brew coffee: 270 mg / 4 oz concentrate
- Boiled or percolated coffee: 200 mg / 8 oz
- Blond-roast drip coffee: 180 mg / 8 oz
- Dark-roast drip coffee: 145 mg / 8 oz
- French-pressed coffee: 108 mg / 8 oz
- Espresso: 75 mg / 1 oz
- Decaf coffee: 15 mg / 8 oz
- Oolong tea: 65 mg / 8 oz
- Chai tea: 50 mg / 8 oz
- Black tea: 47 mg / 8 oz
- White tea: 40 mg / 8 oz
- Matcha tea: 34 mg / 1 g dried
- Green tea: 25 mg / 8 oz
- Decaffeinated black tea: 12 mg / 8 oz

Not ideal sources:
- Coffee in excess (3+ cups a day)
- Tea in excess (3+ cups a day)
- Soda (regular or diet)
- Energy drinks or shots
- Caffeine supplements

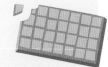

WHAT ABOUT CHOCOLATE?

Chocolate contains trace amounts of caffeine, but the primary stimulant present is a compound called theobromine. Theobromine, a compound with a structure resembling that of caffeine, has a similar effect on the body. Therefore, I recommend that you consume chocolate mindfully and try to avoid enjoying a considerable amount in the evening hours, especially if you're trying to nail down a healthy sleep pattern.

Are there any exceptions to these rules? Of course there are! One key to establishing a true balance is to understand that exceptions are a part of the equation. The occasional bite of dark chocolate after dinner, a warm chocolate soufflé on a special occasion, and an afternoon decaf coffee or iced green tea while you're out with friends are all absolutely reasonable exceptions—but they're just that: exceptions. Staying mindful of your decisions and overall wellness goals will help you keep indulgent exceptions from becoming the new rule. This is how to realistically put the *have your cake and eat it too* concept into practice.

hydration

Ah, the fountain of youth. Does it really exist? So many of us believe in our hearts that there has to be a way to slow the aging process. While lovely spa procedures, luscious face creams, and anti-aging superfoods (like berries and leafy greens) can all help us feel great, the true fountain of youth is much more accessible. In fact, you can probably find it right in your very own home.

Water!

I know that *you know* that our bodies are made mostly of water. But, for the sake of fun science talk, let's review some specifics. Newborn babies are made up of approximately 75 percent water. That's a lot! In fact, that's the highest percentage we see in our lifetime. By one year of age, that number drops to about 65 percent. As we continue to age, our percentage of bodily water composition steadily decreases. Adult women are composed of approximately 55 percent water and men approximately 60 percent water. Men have a slightly higher concentration than women because men typically have a higher muscle mass and women a higher fat mass, and fat cells contain less water than muscle cells.

By the time we hit our senior years, our bodily water content drops even further, landing us at nearly 50 percent. Therefore, you could conceivably argue that a major component of aging is the drying of our bodies. While aging is a completely natural process, we absolutely have the power to speed it up or slow it down based on how well hydrated we keep our bodies.

Let's review some more fun facts! It's important to note that the water in the body is not evenly distributed. Let's review some averages: blood is approximately 80 percent water, muscle 76 percent, brain 75 percent, intestines 75 percent, liver 68 percent, bone 20 percent, and fatty tissue just 10 percent. Of course these percentages vary by person, age, and physical fitness level.

What's the moral of this story? To keep your brain, digestion, and muscles in optimal condition, you need to stay hydrated. In fact, there's a chance that your Daily Water Need is much higher than you might think.

hydrated body versus dehydrated body

One of the first signs, albeit a slightly sneaky one, that you're dehydrated is a feeling of unexplained tiredness. It's entirely possible, especially in the warmer months or if you've just taken up a new fitness routine that makes you work up a sweat, that you're not taking in enough water—causing you to feel fatigued. If you are meeting your Daily Sleep Number each night, eating well, and exercising but still seeing exhaustion creep in, the answer could be as simple as an extra glass of water.

Here are some other signs of a dehydrated body:

- Headaches
- Exhaustion
- Premature aging
- Difficulty recovering from illness
- Difficulty recovering from workouts (soreness lasts longer than three days)
- Difficulty maintaining focus and concentration

And here are some signs of a hydrated body:

- Clear head
- Even energy
- Manageable body weight
- Supple skin
- Speedy recovery from intense workouts

It's important to note that when you replace soda and other mixed beverages with water, in addition to omitting the sweeteners, caffeine, and other chemicals, you're also omitting the sodium. While you don't need all of the sodium that is present in a soda, you do need some of it, and it's important to incorporate both potassium and salt into our hydration plan.

Here are some signs of a body that's hydrated but needs more electrolytes:

- Dizziness or light-headedness
- Feeling "washed out"

Above all, if your symptoms are severe, be sure to visit your physician. These are general notes and not a substitute for medical advice.

your daily water need (DWN)

The age-old recommendation of eight glasses of water a day is not only outdated, it's outrageous. How could eight glasses of water provide sufficient hydration for both a 135-pound female and a 200-pound male? This sweeping generalization is off—way off. Worry not, however! I have good news for you. Determining your optimal water intake starts with a really simple equation. Perfect it from there with some personalized, strategic thinking.

sources of hydration

Some sources of hydration are better than others. While most "beverages" have a high water content, I do not consider them sources of hydration. Here are some ins and outs:

Sources of hydration:	NOT sources of hydration:
Water	Sweetened sparkling water
Sparkling water or mineral water	Soda (regular or diet)
Naturally caffeine-free herbal tea	Coffee (regular or decaffeinated)
	Tea (caffeinated or decaffeinated)
	Smoothies
	Fruit juice

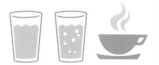

So how much water should you drink? Here's an equation to get you started:

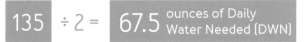

$$\text{BODY WEIGHT} \div 2 = \text{ounces of Daily Water Needed (DWN)}$$

For example, a 135-pound female's equation would look like this:

$$135 \div 2 = 67.5 \text{ ounces of Daily Water Needed (DWN)}$$

Note that if you've been chronically dehydrated for a long time, consuming this much water can feel like serious work. Do your best to reach your number and pace yourself, if need be.

Now, what if you have a job that keeps you out in the sun all day? Or what if you spend at least an hour a day in a rigorous, sweaty workout? Below is a modified calculation that you can use to fine-tune your DWN on a day-by-day basis.

First, calculate how many of the following apply:

- For every 20 minutes you sweat in a workout
- For every two hours you spend in the sun
- For every hour you spend in 90°F+ heat
- For each day you spend with a cold
- For an indulgent meal that included a food outside the scope of the Perfect You Plan

DWN x 1.1	DWN x 1.15	DWN x 1.2	DWN x 1.25	DWN x 1.3
If you chose one of the above, multiply your DWN by 1.1.	If you chose two of the above, multiply by 1.15.	If you chose three of the above, multiply by 1.2.	If you chose four of the above, multiply by 1.25.	If you chose all five of the above, multiply by 1.3.

These calculations aside, remember that when determining your DWN, you should always trust your intuition. If you're still thirsty, drink more water!

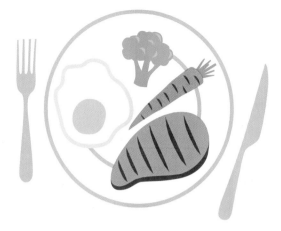

PILLAR #3:

FOOD

I sit firmly in the camp that proudly equates knowledge with power. It's true because it's proven. I've witnessed countless awe-inspiring transformations of serial dieters turned healthy lifestylers, all of whom generally credit their success to just two things: a new knowledge base and a commitment to apply it. While the first two pillars related to mindset, sleep, and hydration have given you a pertinent knowledge base on those subjects, now it's time to explore a topic we can really sink our teeth into: food.

Food is a miles-wide, miles-deep topic, and truthfully I want to cover it all—every last nutritional nuance, recipe method, and nerdy biochemistry scientific fact that I can think of. This particular subject represents my life's work and passion. I've spent a decade devouring nutrition science research the same way many people devour the latest Netflix hit. I want to know it all, and my appetite for information is unquenchable.

Now, while it may be fun to learn every last, evolving detail related to nutrition science, my years spent working with clients and educating large groups has taught me that condensing said details into five concise topics makes for more efficient learning and a more lasting impression. These five topics may not cover every nuance (I'd need about a thousand additional pages for that), but they do cover most of what will empower you to make a permanent lifestyle overhaul. Remember that knowledge, especially easy to remember knowledge, is power.

So what are my top five topics? I'm going to break it down into:

1. Digestion

2. Foods that sabotage

3. Foods that heal

4. Metabolism and weight loss versus fat loss

5. Food for fitness

digestion

Digestion is like one giant assembly line that works to transform a recognizable plate of food into tiny particles that the body can put to good use. Chewing and churning work to mechanically increase the surface area of the food so that enzymes can make contact and chemically digest the available nutrients. Some nutrients are used by the body to help build more body, some are broken down for energy, and some are passed through. Because it's a long process, let's summarize digestion into three main phases: cephalic, gastric, and intestinal digestion.

I think one of the best ways to inspire enthusiasm for the digestive system is to take a Ms. Frizzle–style trip through the body. Let's embark, using my fictional friend Carrie as an example.

To set the stage for this epic trip, we're going to follow the path of a well-balanced dinner made up of a piece of steak from a pastured, grass-fed cow, an organic sweet potato with a little sour cream and sea salt, and some kale sautéed in ghee and lemon juice.

Looking at her plate of food, our subject Carrie realizes how hungry she is. The steak, having been sprinkled with garlic, salt, and pepper and then perfectly seared on the grill, is glistening. The modestly sized and perfectly cooked sweet potato is sliced open and topped with a little Paleo sour cream (page 341) and some crunchy sea salt. Even the healthy serving of sautéed kale, about the same size as the steak and sweet potato combined, looks amazing. She takes in the smells and sights, closes her eyes, and mentally high-fives her kitchen diva–self for having concocted such an incredible meal. Picking up her fork and knife, she prepares to cut into the steak.

Now, Ms. Frizzle–style, let's see what happens!

phase #1: cephalic digestion

This first phase sets the stage for physical digestion. It occurs in the brain, from the moment food is thought about to just before it's swallowed. Let's see how this plays out with Carrie.

Even before Carrie takes her first bite, her body is preparing for this meal. After not having eaten for four hours, hunger strikes—a totally healthy feeling made possible by a hormone known as ghrelin. Ghrelin, which lives mostly in the stomach and the brain, tells Carrie when her blood glucose (blood sugar) and muscle glycogen stores have started to drop and it's time to eat again. Just the thought of food and the meal she plans to prepare signals her brain to communicate "food will happen soon!" to the rest of her body. Her stomach starts to produce more gastric juices and her mouth more saliva.

The smells she registers of the delicious meal sitting in front of her are made possible by airborne odor molecules coming off the food. These molecules travel through the nose and stimulate a distinct combination of sensory receptors that then communicate with the brain, where a spatial map of the odor is formed. This spatial map hangs out in the sensory cortex, where it waits to join up with taste, sight, and texture maps for a more complete picture. The plate sitting in front of a hungry Carrie causes her body to go into a thorough digestion warm-up. More gastric juices containing special enzymes, including saliva, are released to help her break down the food she's about to eat.

SALIVA FUN FACT: *The average adult human produces almost 1.5 liters (6 cups) of saliva a day!*

Finally, Carrie cuts into her medium-rare steak and takes her first bite. Much like how spatial maps of smells are formed, the taste of her steak starts to create a picture of its own after food molecules connect with taste buds.

The steak starts its digestive journey by being broken down into smaller pieces by Carrie's healthy set of teeth; this is known as *mechanical digestion.* While some macronutrients (like carbohydrates) begin their chemical digestion in the mouth due to the presence of carbohydrate-digesting enzymes in saliva (salivary amylase), proteins aren't broken down until they enter the small intestine. At this instant, Carrie's job is to enjoy and chew the steak as well as she can so that those protein-digesting enzymes will have more surface area on which to interact later.

When she's ready, Carrie swallows the steak so that it moves through the esophagus, en route to the stomach and the next phase of digestion.

phase #2: gastric digestion

This phase is where the majority of chemical digestion begins. It occurs in the stomach and the beginning of small intestine, where the food is bathed in digestive enzymes and stomach acids.

Let's pick up where we left off with Carrie's meal: The steak travels down the esophagus and then enters the stomach, which has been preparing for this moment! It's full of hydrochloric acid (meant to dissolve the large food particles into smaller particles), water (the universal solvent), and a bath of enzymes (meant to further chemically break down polymers into monomers). While the stomach can hold two to four liters at a time, Carrie is doing a good job of eating slowly so that she can digest efficiently and not overwhelm her body.

Though hydrochloric acid (HCl) has an incredibly low pH of one (more acidic than battery acid!), the stomach protects itself and keeps the fluid contained with a thick mucus lining. To keep up with the mechanical digestion of food, a web of strong muscles surrounding the stomach keeps this incredible organ in constant motion, almost like a cement mixer truck.

The main job of Carrie's stomach is to continue the work of deconstructing the food. Though the HCl does a great job of transforming her piece of steak into individual proteins (polymers), the body can't make productive use of this material until those proteins are broken down further into individual amino acids. This reaction is made possible by an awesome protein-digesting enzyme called pepsin.

After spending two to three hours in the stomach, the food is finally ready to move on to the next stage of digestion: the intestinal, or absorptive, phase.

NUTRIENT TRANSFORMATION FROM POLYMERS TO MONOMER	
POLYMER	MONOMER
CARBOHYDRATES ⟶ (chemical digestion begins in mouth)	SUGARS
PROTEINS ⟶ (chemical digestion begins in stomach	AMINO ACIDS
LIPIDS ⟶ (chemical digestion begins in small intestine)	FATTY ACIDS

Polymer is an umbrella term for the three macronutrients that all food is made up of: carbohydrates, proteins, and lipids (fats). To make the macronutrients in polymers available to the body, the digestive system transforms polymers into monomers—that is, into sugars, amino acids, and fatty acids. This digestive process happens at different places along the alimentary canal, as shown in the chart.

phase #3: intestinal digestion

The third and final stage of digestion happens in the intestines, and it is where the most exciting action happens! The journey begins with a three-part trek through the small intestine before finally entering the large intestines. Throughout this intestinal phase, special enzymes continue their work transforming polymers into monomers, monomers are absorbed by the body, bacteria help break down what the body's enzymes may have missed, water is reabsorbed, and any unusable material is passed through. It's a pretty incredible, efficient system!

Getting back to the adventure of Carrie's meal, the transfer of food material from the stomach into the duodenum (the first part of the small intestine) happens in a finely tuned symphonic effort by numerous different organs. Because the HCl would cause too much damage to any part of her body unprotected by the thick mucosal lining found in the stomach, her pancreas works up a solution. It produces a highly alkaline bath containing bicarbonate ions that can make quick work of neutralizing the acidic stomach contents. This pancreatic bath contains a mix of enzymes that work to further transform complicated, unusable polymers into the simple, building-blocks-of-life monomers her body needs. These enzymes include trypsin and peptidase, which turns proteins into amino acids; lipase, which turns triglycerides into fatty acids and glycerol; amylase, which turns carbohydrates into glucose and fructose; and nuclease, which turns nucleic acids into DNA and RNA.

This first section of the small intestine, the duodenum, is also where the bile produced by the liver, which has been stored in the gallbladder, is released on the food material. The bile is especially crucial for helping Carrie chemically digest the fat she is consuming.

While the duodenum is mostly a place for chemical digestion, once the food material moves into the jejunum (the second part of the small intestine), it's ready for absorption. Very special channels found in the fingerlike projections of the villi and microvilli, located along the lining of the small intestine, act as bodyguards for what may pass from the gut and into the body. These bodyguards look out for amino acids, sugars, fatty acids, nucleotides, vitamins, minerals, and water. They size up each particle before letting them pass into Carrie's body cavity, where they embark on an epic journey and are used as basic fuel for whatever her body needs. Some of these monomers, which are macronutrients' smaller and more usable counterparts, will be used to make more skin, some to repair muscle after a workout, some to make more digestive enzymes, some to make hormones, and some to make body fat, and some are digested for pure energy.

When the food material finally makes its way into the ilium—the third and final section of the small intestine—the special bodyguard channels located there keep a particularly keen eye out for vitamins and minerals. While some chemical digestion and subsequent absorption of other monomers still happens there, it is not as prevalent.

Things start to slow down a bit when the food material moves from the small intestine into the large intestine. The large intestine is the primary home for nearly a trillion different beneficial gut bacteria. This is where the bacteria, which have a symbiotic relationship with Carrie, their host, work to consume and break down any remaining usable food particles. Though the bacteria are wonderfully helpful in creating more monomers that are then available for absorption, they can also produce gas.

The bacteria found in Carrie's gut have an established, almost prehistoric, system of checks and balances. They all work together so that they flourish and they keep their host, Carrie, as healthy as possible. The roles of these bacteria range from further digestion of food, as just covered, to immune system support and protection from disease. While Carrie's gut flora may not contain the

> **SMALL AND LARGE INTESTINE FUN FACT:**
> *Though the small intestine outstretches the large intestine by four times in length (20 feet versus 5 feet), its diameter is one-third that of the large (1 inch versus 3 inches).*

awesome and wide range of 400 different species she was born with (due to medications and toxins encountered in our modern world), she still has almost more bacteria than cells in her entire body, according to Chris Kresser in his book *Gut Health*.

While the food material hangs out in the large intestine, the bacteria work their way through it, digesting it further. The body does its best to reabsorb water and assimilate any remaining nutrients (especially vitamins B and K and some fatty acids) through those special channels found in the villi and microvilli. When they finally reach the end of the journey, any unused food particles prepare to exit the body.

In this study, Carrie's body worked an incredible feat deconstructing the steak, sweet potato, and sautéed kale into a wealth of amino acids, sugars, fatty acids, nucleotides, vitamins, minerals, and water. Her body will now use these building blocks to keep her healthy, energized, renewed, and ready for the next adventure.

ALIMENTARY CANAL FACT: *Though we tend to think of the intestines as being inside the body, the alimentary canal, which connects the mouth, esophagus, stomach, intestines, and anus, is (in a practical sense) the outside environment. Foods and liquids consumed don't actually enter the body until they pass through the gut lining and move into the bloodstream. If you happen to consume a parasite or other potentially damaging subject, your body will guard against absorbing it until it has passed through your system and finally exits. Though gut bacteria are essential to our health, they technically live outside the body.*

a digestive system gone haywire

We just learned about healthy digestion by taking a Ms. Frizzle–style trip with Carrie's awesome steak dinner. We learned that parts of the alimentary canal, specifically the lining of the stomach, small intestine, and large intestine, act as a gatekeeper for which nutrients are allowed into the bloodstream. In a healthy system, only healthy monomers (such as fatty acids, sugars, and amino acids), vitamins, minerals, and water can make their way through the tight junctions that make up the gut lining.

Unfortunately, effortlessly healthy systems in this modern world are hard to come by. We live in a world that's inundated with toxins, some known and some unknown. Whether by choice (like when we consume alcohol) or not by choice (like when we don't know about water contamination), toxins find their way into our digestive system and have the ability to cause damage. The good news is that this damage is reversible; the bad news is that the damage is easy to come by.

It goes without saying that taking a swig of bleach is sure to cause bodily harm. It's intuitive, in this example, that if the bleach manages to make it past the vomit reflexes of the stomach, it will cause damage to the gut lining. It's easy to envision the toxic chemical eating away at the delicate villi and microvilli–covered lining of the small intestine, damaging the special channels and bodyguards that are meant to police which molecules find their way into the body. With these bodyguards removed, it's easy to understand that some of this toxic bleach could find its way into the bloodstream. At this point, we'd really start to feel sick and our gallant immune system would organize an attack, which would result in a tremendous amount of inflammation and pain while the body waged war against the toxin.

Now, this is obviously an extreme example, but it's not too far from the point I'm trying to make in this chapter. Certain foods in this modern world contain highly processed or poor-quality ingredients that have an abrasive, damaging impact on the gut lining. Some toxins and properties found in everyday foods have a bull-in-a-china-shop impact on the delicate cells of the digestive system. They cause damage, rip holes, and flow freely (though unwanted) into the bloodstream. Because these large food particles and toxins are unrecognizable to the body, the immune system (accurately) interprets their presence as an invasion.

From here, the body's immune response causes inflammation, which can contribute to a number of other issues (see "What's in It for Me?" on page 18). The now-damaged gut, also known as "leaky gut" or "intestinal permeability," has two new problems:

1. It's now "leaking" large food particles, toxins, and potentially harmful bacteria into the bloodstream.

2. Due to the damage inflicted on the villi and microvilli, it may have a hard time absorbing certain nutrients, especially vitamins and minerals, which can lead to deficiencies.

Is it possible to heal a leaky gut? Absolutely! The 28-Day Fed & Fit Project is designed to help heal the gut. Know that completely healing a damaged gut will take longer than twenty-eight days, which is why I recommend avoiding the most egregious of the sabotaging foods for as long as possible.

So am I going to have to eat this way forever in order to be healthy? How on earth can I police every single bite?

It's impractical to think that pursuing a 100 percent squeaky-clean lifestyle is going to be a walk in the park. While I do believe that it's possible to buckle down and get through a twenty-eight-day period of really healthy living, eventually we have to go back to society. There will be birthday dinners, cocktail parties with passed appetizers, and Grandma's pumpkin pie. How are we to approach these situations? Will we have to start over every time we encounter one of these sabotaging foods? Probably not.

It's likely that a healed gut can endure and heal faster from infrequent exposures to small amounts of sabotaging foods (like the highly processed ingredients found in fast food). This is great news! The other great news is that science and practical experience are finally meeting up, lifting the veil on chronic disease and getting to the bottom of the most direct route to true, lasting health. Where's this home base, buck-stops-here foundation of health?

"All disease begins in the gut."
—HIPPOCRATES

Hippocrates, via an educated guess, was onto something, and while we're still working through the complicated science of the human body, we're getting closer to proving his declaration.

It's not outlandish to hold on to the belief that all health, and consequently all disease, stem from the gut. The gut is where, if you really think about it, the majority of our interaction with the outside world occurs. It is where we assimilate nutrients, fight disease (80 to 90 percent of the immune system is present there), and interact with our habitable crew of nearly one trillion bacteria, and it is where our health can most directly be impacted. Above all, it's important to remember that reducing bodily inflammation is the name of this healthy lifestyle game, and your ticket to success is to swap out sabotaging foods for healing foods. In one way or another, the different food groups discussed in the next section promote inflammation in the body and therefore contribute to chronic pain, disease, and weight gain.

foods that sabotage

What makes food, food? Well, for starters, let's see what *Merriam-Webster's Dictionary* has to say!

Food

noun \ füd\

1a: material consisting essentially of protein, carbohydrate, and fat used in the body of an organism to sustain growth, repair, and vital processes and to furnish energy; also: such food together with supplementary substances (as minerals, vitamins, and condiments) b: inorganic substances absorbed by plants in gaseous form or in water solution

2: nutriment in solid form

3: something that nourishes, sustains, or supplies *<food for thought>*

I think it's important to talk about what qualifies as food because it helps set the stage for talking about how not all foods are created (or treated) equal. For the purpose of this book, I'd like to redefine food as the following:

Food is a material consumed for enjoyment, nourishment, or both and is composed of healthy and/or harmful substances that are either assimilated by the body or eventually passed through after digestion.

So I argue that if it's meant to be eaten, then it qualifies as food! This means that soda pop is a food. Zero-calorie sweeteners are a food. Potato chips, collard greens, Cool Whip, ketchup, chicken breast, carrot sticks, and string cheese are all food. This is a nice big umbrella that essentially covers anything you could find on a family reunion potluck table—but it doesn't mean that our bodies interpret all foods the same way.

Instead of vilifying not-ideal food choices as "bad foods," I prefer to discuss them as foods that may sabotage health more than they support health. I'm breaking these foods up into six main groups: grains, fats, dairy, sugars, legumes, and artificial ingredients. We're going to look at why these ingredients are included on the "Foods That Sabotage" list.

note

Some mostly healing foods fall into the "Foods That Sabotage" category for certain people. For example, a person battling an autoimmune disease would probably feel best when avoiding nightshades, eggs, nuts, and seeds, while a person following a low-FODMAP plan to battle irritable bowel syndrome (IBS) would feel best when avoiding garlic, onions, and coconut. These lists are meant as a starting place. From here, you can expand your personal list of sabotage foods.

grains that sabotage

Holy moly, you mean all grains? But I thought whole grains were a healthy choice! What about all of the fiber?

For starters, let's discuss which grains we're referring to! I think it's important to note that not all grains sabotage equally. So I've listed them in order of most obstructive to health (marked by ***) to potentially least obstructive to health (marked by *):

*** Wheat	** Amaranth (a pseudograin)
*** Barley	** Quinoa (a pseudograin)
*** Rye	** Brown rice
*** Buckwheat (a gluten-free pseudograin, but contains an almost equally harmful lectin)	** Conventional and GMO corn
** Oats	* Organic and non-GMO corn
** Sorghum	* White (or "polished") rice
** Millet	

The most important thing to remember is that all grains contain highly abrasive proteins known as lectins. It's worth mentioning that *all plants* contain lectins! They are concentrated in the seeds and are used to protect against predators. Grains, which are seeds, have this high concentration of lectins, and when consumed, these proteins cause damage to our guts, as discussed at the end of the previous section.

Gluten is one kind of lectin, known as a prolamin, that is especially damaging. Wheat, barley, and rye all contain the incredibly damaging gluten protein, while the rest of the grains in this list contain a lectin that's slightly less harmful. All grains also contain protease inhibitors, which are linked to cellular damage that contributes to a leaky gut, and all pseudo-grains contain a high concentration of saponins, a soaplike structure that binds with cellular cholesterol and creates even more holes in the gut lining.

fats that sabotage

The following fats are listed in order of most obstructive to health (***) to least (*).

*** Hydrogenated vegetable oil
** Canola oil
** Vegetable oil
** Impure or rancid olive oil
* Sesame oil (toasted or untoasted)
* Peanut oil

The danger associated with these fats has less to do with their destructive nature in the gut and more to do with the fact that they promote an unhealthy balance of omega-3 fatty acids to omega-6 fatty acids. Both fatty acids are considered "essential," as the body needs them but cannot produce them. While our bodies may need both types, we also need them to be in balance with one another. Omega-6 fatty acids are inflammatory by nature (which is actually necessary in moderation since inflammation is a tool of the immune system), while omega-3s are anti-inflammatory by nature. A delicate balance, ideally around 3:1 (omega-6 to omega-3), is necessary to keep inflammation at bay. While a version of omega-3 fatty acids (ALA) can be found in some seeds, the omega-3s the body truly needs (EPA and DHA) are found only in pasture-raised eggs and poultry, grass-fed meat and dairy, fish, and game meat.

While the body does need omega-6 fatty acids, the oils above are essentially an abuse of the system. These oils contain so much omega-6 that a diet that includes them in addition to conventional meat, eggs, and dairy could have an omega-6 to omega-3 ratio of as high as 40:1. This, combined with intestinal permeability (leaky gut), can promote constant inflammation in the body.

dairy products that sabotage

The following dairy products are listed in order of most obstructive to health (**) to least (*):

> ** Conventionally raised cow dairy (milk, yogurt, cheese, butter, whey)
>
> * Grass-fed cow dairy (milk, yogurt, cheese, butter, whey)
>
> * Grass-fed goat dairy (milk, yogurt, cheese, butter, whey)
>
> * Grass-fed sheep dairy (milk, yogurt, cheese, butter, whey)

As you can see, I don't list any type of dairy as being most obstructive to health (***). The potential damaging impact of dairy is highly individualized and doesn't stop at whether or not a person is lactose intolerant (meaning that they lack the lactase enzyme that helps digest the dairy sugar lactose). It's important to note that dairy has a tendency to spike insulin, is a highly allergenic food (to a large majority of the population), contains protease inhibitors that likely aggravate or contribute to a leaky gut, and introduce other-species hormones (like bovine hormones) to our human systems that may be linked to certain cancers.

While all these reasons sound like logical support for omitting all dairy (which I do recommend for the 28-Day Fed & Fit Project), dairy from healthy sources can prove healthful. Dairy from grass-fed animals is a great source of conjugated linoleic acids and other fat-soluble vitamins. The landscape gets even grayer when we start to discuss raw dairy, which contains the enzymes needed to digest it—making it a better choice for people who are lactose intolerant. Furthermore, goat and sheep dairy products are believed to be less allergenic than dairy products from cows.

sugars that sabotage

The following sugars are listed in order of most obstructive to health (***) to least (*).

> *** Acesulfame potassium (Sunett, Sweet One)
>
> *** Aspartame (Equal, NutraSweet)
>
> *** Neotame
>
> *** Saccharin (SugarTwin, Sweet'N Low)
>
> *** Sucralose (Splenda)
>
> *** Advantame
>
> ** Xylitol
>
> ** Sorbitol
>
> ** All other sugar alcohols
>
> ** High-fructose corn syrup
>
> ** Corn syrup
>
> ** White sugar
>
> ** Confectioners' sugar
>
> ** Cane sugar
>
> ** Turbinado sugar
>
> ** Brown sugar
>
> ** Brown rice syrup
>
> ** Agave nectar (mostly fructose)
>
> * Stevia
>
> * Granulated maple sugar
>
> * Coconut sugar
>
> * Molasses
>
> * Maple syrup
>
> * Honey
>
> * Date sugar

I think it's important to break up this explanation into three categories: artificial sweeteners, sugar alcohols and highly processed sugars, and natural sweeteners. While not all of the sweeteners in this list are available for purchase in retail stores, some show up in the ingredient lists of packaged foods.

Zero-calorie artificial sweeteners contain chemicals that can be poisonous to the human body. I do not recommend consuming them in any amount.

Sugar alcohols, though derived from natural sources, can be aggravating to certain people. I recommend avoiding them if possible.

Processed sugars, most derived from sugarcane, are definitely better choices than artificial sweeteners and, to be honest, have much the same nutritional impact on our bodies as completely natural sweeteners. I have categorized them as mid-level sabotagers (**) because ultimately the *amount* of sugar that we consume poses the real danger. For example, a single serving of a food made with white sugar (like a reasonably sized grain-free cookie) will likely pose a minor threat to health, whereas several servings (three or more) can trigger a blood sugar imbalance.

Most natural and processed sweeteners are roughly half glucose and half fructose. While the body can make immediate use of glucose for energy, fructose must first be converted to blood glucose (if still needed), glycogen (up to a point), and fat for storage. Triglycerides are a byproduct of the conversion of excess glucose and all fructose into glycogen or fat. While this process is completely normal, health problems can arise when it takes place in excess. I have the natural sweeteners marked as slightly better (indicated with *) because they are either more difficult to come by, more expensive, or both and therefore are more difficult to consume in excess. Enjoying one or two servings a day of these natural sweeteners—no more than 1 tablespoon each—is less likely to derail health efforts than consuming their more processed counterparts.

Though potentially less harmful to health, I recommend that you avoid even natural sugars throughout the 28-Day Fed & Fit Project and instead turn to lower-sugar fruits and starchy carbohydrates to help satisfy your need for glucose.

legumes that sabotage

The following legumes are listed in order of most obstructive to health (***) to least (*):

*** Soybeans (and all soy products)	** Beans (all, including garbanzo beans)	** Lentils ** Lupins * Peanuts

Similar to grains, legumes contain lectins and protease inhibitors. Lectins, as we now know, are extremely damaging to the gut lining and may promote intestinal permeability. I have listed peanuts as less dangerous because most people are less likely to eat the same volume of peanuts as they would of beans, and therefore they are likely to take in fewer lectins.

Also note that while all soy products contain lectins, soybeans are one of the most highly genetically modified foods in our world today and contain a compound known as phytoestrogen. It's believed that the body misinterprets phytoestrogen as an actual estrogen compound, which understandably causes confusion and potentially disrupts a healthy hormone balance.

Legumes, like pseudo-grains (buckwheat, amaranth, and quinoa), are also high in saponins. Saponins have a soaplike structure that helps combine fat and water. They're understood to bind with cholesterol molecules found in cell membranes, which then creates a hole, contributing to leaky gut.

note

Though fresh green beans and peas are legumes, they are included in the scope of the 28-Day Fed & Fit Project because they contain more healing nutrients than damaging ones. Carob and tamarind, both technically legumes, are two other exceptions.

artificial ingredients that sabotage

The following artificial ingredients are listed in order of most obstructive to health (***) to least (*).

*** Carrageenan	*** Food colorings (including blue #1, blue #2, citrus red #2, green #3, red #40, red #3, yellow #5, and yellow #6)
*** Hydrolyzed vegetable protein	
*** Monosodium glutamate (MSG; sometimes found under a "natural flavor" label)	** Phosphates, phosphoric acid (meat tenderizer)
*** Textured vegetable protein	** Xanthan gum
*** Transglutaminase	* Guar gum

This list doesn't encompass all of the artificial ingredients that sabotage. Instead, it includes those that are the most prevalent in store-bought foods or that may be used in homemade recipes. While each of these ingredients has its own signature damaging impact on the body, it's important to be aware of their use in foods as preservatives, stabilizers, or colorants. You can essentially equate them to toxic chemicals being ingested. Though potentially less harmful when consumed in moderation on a healthy stomach, they could lead to myriad health complications when consumed regularly on a stomach that's not yet healed.

foods that heal

Now that we're on the same page about how certain foods contribute to a damaged gut and subsequently a chronically inflamed body, it's time to talk about the good news!

The good news is that while food may be part of the problem, it's also part of the solution. When healing food is combined with a healthy outlook, proper rest, and plenty of water, the body can and will heal. That's the neatest part of this entire adventure! Our bodies are made to heal. That's what they do, all day, every day. They are constantly working to reconstruct cells, reorganize, and combat the rough world we live in. Although regeneration and healing tend to slow down as we age, we can remove some healing roadblocks by omitting health-sabotaging foods and replacing them with health-supporting foods.

Before we get into the specific categories of healing foods, I'd like to talk briefly about the importance of a colorful, varied plate. It's apparent that foods come in all shapes and sizes. It's easy to recognize that broccoli is different from cauliflower (though they're in the same family) and that eggs are different from chicken breast (though they originate from the same animal). As much as food differs to the naked eye, it also differs on a molecular level. While similar, broccoli's roster of nutrients differs from that of cauliflower, and eggs offer up a completely different concentration of fatty acids than chicken breast. Wonderfully complex and incredibly needy, human beings really require a little of everything (nutrient-wise), and as such, we do best when we eat a little of everything. Falling into a routine of eating the same foods over and over again is both likely and, when comprised of the Paleo-friendly foods outlined in this section, perfectly healthy, but we do our bodies best when we try to mix it up and keep things fresh and different.

So, while the following all qualify as healing foods, remember that supplying the body with all of the building blocks required for health and wellness requires an array of not just the three key macronutrients, but also individual micronutrients, such as vitamins and minerals. The good news is that many of these micronutrients are represented by color, texture, shape, and source. So do your best to cycle through the three macronutrient categories and their subcomponents as often as possible and change up the color, texture, shape, and source of what you're eating. If you do, you're sure to get a wealth of chewable nutrition!

across the macronutrients

By now we understand that macronutrients are the proteins, carbohydrates, and fats present in the food we eat. These are the large building blocks that, through the process of digestion, are broken down into their monomer counterparts, which are then used by the body for fuel and rebuilding. Almost everything we consume contains its own unique array of these three structures. While it's easy to think of the macronutrients represented by a simple plate of steak (protein), sweet potato (carbohydrate), and pat of butter (fat), individual foods aren't that simple. Each individual food contains a majority of one macronutrient and a minority of one or both of the others. The steak contains some protein (majority) and fat (minority), the sweet potato contains some carbohydrate (majority) and protein (minority), and the butter contains protein (minority), carbohydrate (minority), and fat (majority). While I do think it's important to note their presence, the minor nutrients have a relatively minor impact on the body—so there's no great need to be overly concerned about them. This is why the foods listed in this chapter are organized by their major macronutrient.

Some people prefer to track their nutritional needs by measuring the exact macronutrients they need each day (usually by weight). When it comes to counting or tracking macronutrients, I tend to fall on the supportive but unobtrusive side. I support anyone who pursues this method, as seen in this book by the approximate macronutrient information provided for each recipe, but I don't offer specific advice about how to build your own numbers. You see, macronutrient needs can vary greatly from person to person. The numbers will change based on whether you're male or female, as well as your age, height, weight, fitness level, goals, and overall metabolic constitution (fast metabolism versus slow metabolism).

Another way to measure your body's specific macronutrient needs is to take an intuitive, versus calculated, approach. This intuitive approach starts with a program, like the 28-Day Fed & Fit Project, and ends with a series of lessons learned about what exactly your body needs and when. Intuitive eating allows you to interpret when you're hungry for protein, when your body needs more fat, when you need more carbohydrates, when you're simply thirsty, when you need a big meal, and when you need a small meal. This intuitive approach is the one that I personally use and recommend to my clients for lasting healthy lifestyle success.

Efforts to establish a healthy lifestyle are much more effective when healthy, responsibly sourced foods are a priority. On the lists that follow, I've broken out the healthier, more healing foods into their macronutrient categories. These macronutrient categories are not meant to inspire macro-calculations, but rather an awareness of the nutrition a food has to offer. I encourage you to browse the proteins, carbohydrates, and fats so you arrive at the understanding that there are endless possibilities for delicious and nutritious meals. Healthy foods that allow the body to heal are far from boring!

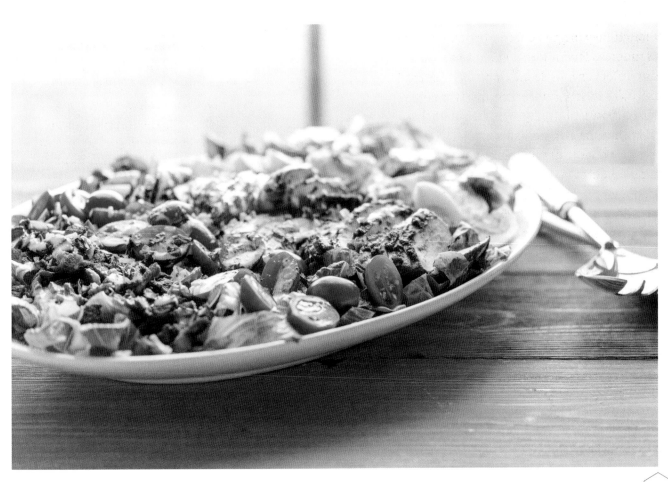

proteins

Sources

The following list of proteins is organized in order of most (***) to least (*) beneficial sources. Note that you can achieve wellness by choosing from the least beneficial (*) proteins on this list! Upgrade wherever possible, but remember that excluding the foods from the sabotage list is more important than seeking perfection.

note

Note that these recommendations are based on striking a balance between ideal nutrition and lowest environmental impact. The pendulum between whether to choose wild or farm-raised swings over time, so I recommend that you monitor the EDF Seafood Selector (http://seafood.edf.org/) for regular updates.

*** 100% grass-fed beef and other red meats

*** Pasture-raised eggs, chicken, and other poultry

*** Pasture-raised pork and pork products

*** Game meat

*** Gelatin from grass-fed beef or pastured pork

*** Collagen peptides from grass-fed beef

*** Wild Alaskan salmon (frozen or canned)

*** Wild-caught albacore tuna (U.S. and Canada)

*** Bay scallops (farmed)

*** Clams (farmed)

*** Black sea bass (trap-caught, handline)

*** Pacific or California halibut (hook/line)

*** Spiny lobster (U.S.)

*** Crawfish (U.S.)

*** Dover sole

*** Catfish (U.S.)

*** Oysters (wild or farmed)

*** Giant freshwater prawns (U.S. and Canada)

*** Northern shrimp (U.S. and Canada)

*** Mahi mahi (U.S. troll/pole)

*** Pacific sardines (U.S. and Canada)

*** Rainbow trout (farmed)

*** Snow or stone crab (U.S.)

*** Tilapia (U.S.)

** Organic, hormone-free, and antibiotic-free beef and other red meats

** Cage-free or omega-3-enriched eggs

** Organic, air-chilled chicken and other poultry

** Organic pork and pork products

** Organic whey from grass-fed dairy cows (with no more than two ingredients)

** U.S. white or brown shrimp (farmed or wild)

** Yellowfin tuna (U.S. Atlantic troll/pole, Western Central Pacific handline)

** Anchovies (canned)

** Sea scallops (mid-Atlantic U.S. and Canada)

** Clams (wild)

** European sea bass (farmed)

** Summer flounder

** Blue or Dungeness crab

* Beef and other red meats

* Eggs

* Chicken and other poultry

* Pork and pork products

* Whey protein (with no more than two ingredients)

* Canned light, white, or albacore tuna (U.S. or imported)

* Farm-raised salmon

* Atlantic halibut

* Spiny lobster (imported)

* Crawfish (imported)

* Giant tiger prawns

* Blue shrimp

* Atlantic or farmed salmon

* Red or blue king crab (imported)

How They Heal

We understand that the body digests proteins into their amino acid monomer counterparts. What I haven't discussed is that out of twenty essential amino acids, there are nine that the body cannot produce. Therefore, we need to make sure that we take in these essential amino acids via our diet! They are especially prevalent in the foods listed above. They're necessary for building and rebuilding muscle tissues, forming collagen, developing organ tissue, and manufacturing enzymes.

In addition to amino acids, proteins carry an array of fatty acids (DHA, EPA, CLA), nucleotides, vitamins (A, B12, D, and K2), minerals (like zinc), selenium, creatine, and taurine. Fish and other marine life (such as shellfish) are among the most nutrient-dense foods on Earth when it comes to DHA and EPA omega-3 fatty acids, iodine, and vitamin D. Organ meats from healthy animals, including tongue, liver, and heart, are also among the most nutritious foods available.

starchy carbohydrates

Sources

Let's get one thing straight: carbohydrates are a very important part of a healthy diet. Just because grains and legumes (which are generally thought of as dietary carbs) are on the sabotage list does not mean that the 28-Day Fed & Fit Project is meant to be low-carb. There are plenty of other healthy carbohydrate sources derived from plants, mostly roots, that will help keep our plates balanced and our bodies happy.

The following is a pretty comprehensive list of the in-scope carbohydrates, with the healthiest options marked by ***. The foods marked by ** and * are still healthy choices but may contain pesticides that are harmful to health.

*** Organic sweet, boiling, fingerling, new, russet, and Yukon Gold potatoes

*** Organic yams

*** Organic winter squash, such as acorn, buttercup, butternut, carnival, delicata, kabocha, pumpkin, and spaghetti

*** Organic beets

*** Organic parsnips

*** Organic carrots

*** Organic green, snap, and snow peas

*** Organic plantains

** Conventional sweet potatoes

** Conventional yams

* Conventional fingerling, new, russet, and Yukon Gold potatoes

* Conventional winter squash, such as acorn, buttercup, butternut, carnival, delicata, kabocha, pumpkin, and spaghetti

* Conventional beets

* Conventional parsnips

* Conventional carrots

* Conventional green, snap, and snow peas

* Conventional plantains

How They Heal

Finding replacements for the starchy foods found on the sabotage list is a top, but often underrated, priority of this lifestyle adjustment. Human beings desperately need carbohydrates. When we remove grains, legumes, and sugars from our plates, we must find adequate carbohydrate replacements. While nonstarchy vegetables can provide a wide range of nutrients and fiber, we must look to starchy vegetables as our main source of glycogen. Have fun and experiment with the starchy vegetables listed below! There's a wide range that is sure to keep your palate entertained.

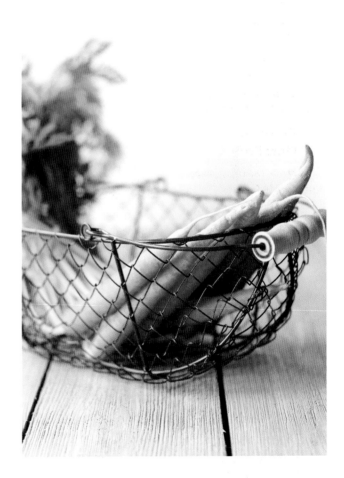

nonstarchy carbohydrates

Sources

- *** Organic leafy greens (kale, collards, Swiss chard, spinach, turnip)
- *** Organic lettuce (romaine, butterhead (Bibb), iceberg)
- *** Organic bok choy
- *** Organic broccolini
- *** Organic Brussels sprouts
- *** Organic cabbage (napa, green, and red)
- *** Organic celery
- *** Organic green beans
- *** Organic large peppers (bell, poblano, chili, hatch)
- *** Organic radicchio
- *** Organic cucumbers
- *** Organic eggplant
- *** Organic tomatillos
- *** Organic tomatoes
- *** Organic zucchini
- *** Organic yellow squash
- *** Organic artichokes
- *** Organic broccoli
- *** Organic cauliflower
- *** Organic okra
- *** Organic onions

- *** Organic asparagus
- *** Organic fennel bulb
- *** Organic leeks
- *** Organic jicama
- *** Organic turnips
- *** Organic radishes
- *** Organic sea vegetables
- *** Organic bamboo shoots
- *** Organic sprouts
- *** Organic daikon
- *** Organic kohlrabi
- *** Organic mushrooms
- *** Organic turnips
- *** Organic rhubarb
- ** Hearts of palm (canned)
- ** Artichoke hearts (canned or jarred), drained
- ** Conventional asparagus
- ** Conventional cabbage (napa, green, and red)
- ** Conventional cauliflower
- ** Conventional eggplant
- ** Conventional onions

- * Conventional leafy greens (kale, collards, Swiss chard, spinach, turnip)
- * Conventional lettuce (romaine, butterhead (Bibb), iceberg)
- * Conventional bok choy
- * Conventional broccolini
- * Conventional Brussels sprouts
- * Conventional cabbage (napa, green, and red)
- * Conventional celery
- * Conventional green beans
- * Conventional large peppers (bell, poblano, chili, hatch)
- * Conventional radicchio
- * Conventional cucumbers
- * Conventional eggplant
- * Conventional tomatillos
- * Conventional tomatoes
- * Conventional zucchini
- * Conventional yellow squash

- * Conventional artichokes
- * Conventional broccoli
- * Conventional cauliflower
- * Conventional okra
- * Conventional onions
- * Conventional asparagus
- * Conventional fennel bulb
- * Conventional leeks
- * Conventional jicama
- * Conventional turnips
- * Conventional radishes
- * Conventional sea vegetables
- * Conventional bamboo shoots
- * Conventional sprouts
- * Conventional daikon
- * Conventional kohlrabi
- * Conventional mushrooms
- * Conventional turnips
- * Conventional rhubarb

How They Heal

I have a true, unabashed love for nonstarchy vegetables. Leafy greens, crunchy peppers, delicious seaweed, and versatile eggplant are some of my favorites. While each vegetable packs its own unique formula of micronutrients, know that when you eat a variety of colorful vegetables, you're likely getting a balanced spread of vitamins (A, C, K), calcium (sometimes even more than milk!), fiber (both soluble and insoluble), flavonoids, polyphenols, and carotenoids.

While the occasional raw vegetable serving can be beneficial, I recommend eating mostly well-cooked vegetables (especially from the cruciferous family) to minimize potential discomfort and maximize nutrient intake.

fruits

Sources

- *** Organic dates
- *** Organic raspberries
- *** Organic blueberries
- *** Organic cherries
- *** Organic strawberries
- *** Organic blackberries
- *** Organic grapes
- *** Organic cranberries
- *** Organic currants
- *** Organic gooseberries
- *** Organic lingonberries
- *** Organic clementines
- *** Organic navel oranges
- *** Organic blood oranges
- *** Organic tangerines
- *** Organic grapefruit
- *** Organic limes
- *** Organic key limes
- *** Organic kumquats
- *** Organic lemons
- *** Organic mandarin oranges
- *** Organic Meyer lemons
- *** Organic pomelos
- *** Organic tangelos
- *** Organic pomegranates
- ** Conventional grapefruit
- * Conventional dates
- * Conventional raspberries
- * Conventional blueberries
- * Conventional cherries
- * Conventional strawberries
- * Conventional blackberries
- * Conventional grapes
- * Conventional cranberries
- * Conventional currants
- * Conventional elderberries
- * Conventional gooseberries
- * Conventional lingonberries
- * Conventional clementines
- * Conventional navel oranges
- ** Conventional blood oranges
- * Conventional tangerines
- * Conventional limes
- * Conventional key limes
- * Conventional kumquats
- * Conventional lemons
- * Conventional mandarin oranges
- * Conventional Meyer lemons
- * Conventional pomelos
- * Conventional tangelos
- * Conventional pomegranates

How They Heal

Just like their starchy and nonstarchy carbohydrate counterparts, fruits are healing to the body because they are broken down into usable sugars, fibers, vitamins, and minerals. These nutrients are then transported to places all over the body, where they're used for a variety of metabolic reactions. Similar to the sugars on the sabotage list, amount matters. Too much fruit, especially a fruit that's high in sugar, can raise blood sugar too much.

After years of study and practice, I've drawn a carefully calculated line in the world of fruits for the purpose of the 28-Day Fed & Fit Project. To summarize, the in-scope fruits include all citrus and almost all berries, but almost all other fruits are out. I include berries because they pack less sugar (fructose) than their sweeter counterparts (think: mangoes). Berries also tend to have more fiber per serving and allow us to enjoy what feels like more food. I include citrus fruits because of their high concentration of other vitamins, and the acidity present makes us less likely to overeat them. Note that this list speaks to *whole* fruits; their fruit juice counterparts are not considered in scope.

Though technically drupes (stone fruits), dates are included as the one sweetener available while on the Project. The vitamins, minerals, and fiber present in dates make them a great choice for use in an occasional treat.

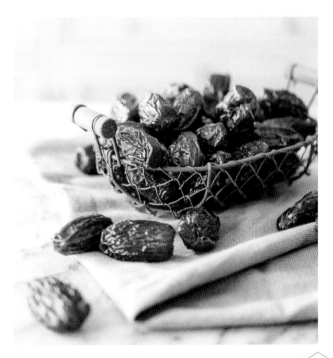

fats

Sources

The following list includes fats that are great for cooking, adding flavor to foods, and adding to a meal as a bonus source of this key macronutrient (such as nuts, seeds, and avocados). I encourage you to use the fats that you're most drawn to, but remember that the best fats for cooking at high temperatures are typically solid at room temperature, such as ghee, tallow, lard, and coconut oil. Fats that are liquid at room temperature, such as olive oil and avocado oil, are best for unheated uses.

*** Ghee from 100% grass-fed cows	** Almonds
*** Butter from 100% grass-fed cows	** Almond butter
*** Tallow from 100% grass-fed cows	** Cashews
	** Cashew butter
*** Lard from pasture-raised pigs	** Coconut butter
*** Full-fat coconut milk (canned)	** Sunflower seeds
	** Sunflower seed butter
*** Coconut oil	** Pecans
*** Avocado fruit or oil	** Pecan butter
*** Extra-virgin olive oil	** Pine nuts
*** MCT oil	** Pumpkin seeds
*** Palm oil/shortening	** Chia seeds
*** Unsweetened shredded coconut or coconut flakes	** Flax seeds
	** Sesame seeds
	** Tahini
	** Olives

How They Heal

Nourishing fats that span the categories of saturated, monounsaturated, and polyunsaturated are available in a wide variety of delicious forms. It's important to note the healing power of saturated fats (which are usually solid at room temperature) from healthy sources, especially as it pertains to brain health. Monounsaturated fats (which are usually liquid at room temperature) are also wonderfully beneficial because they contain oleic acid, which is great for the heart. Polyunsaturated fats (which are liquid at room temperature but can solidify when chilled) can help combat inflammation, high cholesterol, and an imbalanced omega-6 to omega-3 profile.

As with all foods, moderation is key. Enjoy healthy fats that work for your body and taste preferences, but remember to keep your intake within reason. In other words, don't go nuts on the nuts.

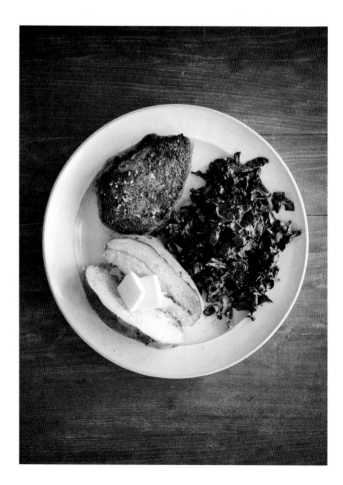

metabolism and weight loss versus fat loss

Metabolism is a word that's thrown around a great deal in the health and fitness arena, but the meaning behind it is often lost. Metabolism doesn't necessarily speak just to how fast a person burns body fat (often referred to as a "fast metabolism") or to how someone's metabolism started to slow down "after I turned 40." While metabolism is related to energy production and expenditure, it encompasses so much more.

Here's my definition:

Metabolism, as it pertains to the human body, encompasses the entire span of chemical reactions that both break down nutrients and create new material that the body can then put to use; this includes (but is not limited to) cellular energy production and consumption, building of new body cells, hormone development, and enzyme production.

So what does this mean? Is the 28-Day Fed & Fit Project going to boost your metabolism? The truth of the matter is that changing your constitution is extremely difficult—some would argue impossible. There are no magical diets, workouts, or nutritional supplements that will turn you into a healthy, energetic, vibrant, fat-burning machine for the rest of your life. You can, however, work to remove nutrient, toxic chemical, stress, and dehydration-related roadblocks that keep your metabolism from functioning at its best.

The metabolism I'm referring to is the energy that you feel every day. Having a healthy metabolism doesn't necessarily mean that you're actively burning body fat. A healthy metabolism can simply mean that you have ample energy throughout your day, your muscles easily recover from workouts and have fuel for each new workout, your sleep is restorative, and your mind is sharp. You see, *metabolism* is a broad term that covers so much more than just the rate at which the body burns energy.

how does the calorie count?

This is a big hairy topic, and I'm going to do my best not to chase any rabbits down their obsessive, hair-splitting holes. Let's start off by explaining what a calorie represents:

A calorie is a standard measure that quantifies the amount of energy a food will produce in the human body.

Carbohydrates and proteins contain approximately four calories per gram, while fats contain approximately nine calories per gram. But is the energy calculation of food really that simple? Absolutely not. Think of a fatty cut of meat from a grass-fed, grass-finished cow versus a lean breast from a pasture-raised chicken. While the steak is made up mostly of the macronutrient protein, it contains more fat (and therefore more calories) than the chicken. But that doesn't make the steak a bad choice. This fattier cut of meat also contains a wealth of nourishing micronutrients that the chicken may be lacking.

Once again, it all comes down to moderation. If you're looking for a new approach, I propose approximate portion control as opposed to calorie counting. In my experience, calorie counting leads most people to eat the foods that offer the most volume with the fewest calories (like egg whites instead of whole eggs). But fattier, more calorically dense foods are often the richest source of healthy nutrients.

While calories do count to an extent, there's more value in seeking nutrients and, at the same time, staying mindful of hunger and satiety. This kind of awareness is what we're working toward with the Project and is the ultimate hallmark of the Perfect You Plan.

weight loss versus fat loss

So much more than body fat goes into the number we see when we step on a scale. We've got bones, muscles, organs, blood and other bodily fluids, *and* body fat to account for! In fact, of all the material in the body, body fat weighs the least when compared volume-for-volume against other tissue. Many, if not most, people pursue new and different diets or lifestyles because they're looking to lose weight. There's nothing wrong with this sentiment, but I think it's important to distinguish between losing *weight* and losing *fat*. One is relatively simple, and the other requires that we take healing into account while we restrict.

How to Lose Weight

Losing weight is relatively simple, believe it or not. All you need to do is rack up a calorie deficit (most folks opt for filling but nutritionally vapid food options like artificially sweetened fat-free yogurt) against expenditures by daily activity. The age-old equation of calories-in-versus-calories-out *is* applicable, but it's not that simple.

While you can and will experience weight loss with a calorie deficit, it's possible to take it so far that the body will interpret it as prolonged starvation. As a result, the body will slow down basic internal energy expenditures (for example, you may start to feel especially sleepy) so that it doesn't burn through all of its fat and muscle reserves too quickly. While this metabolic disposition is easy to reverse by consuming more calories, it may take a while for the metabolism to speed up again—causing an upswing in weight and body fat. Hence the familiar pendulum swing from extreme weight loss (due to an extreme diet) to almost immediate weight gain once the dieting is over.

How to Lose Body Fat—and Keep It Off

Losing body fat may seem more complicated, but I argue that it's actually more fun than simply losing weight. The way to lose body fat is (yes) to eat less than you expend in energy, but also to make sure that the deficit isn't so great that it causes the body's basal metabolic rate (BMR) to slow down. Exercise helps keep this rate up, so be sure to make fitness a priority! And remember that *you don't have to go hungry to have a calorie deficit and lose weight.* Be sure to take in a variety of proteins, starchy and nonstarchy vegetables, healthy fats, and fruits to provide your body with a wide array of micronutrients and help you stay vibrant and healthy.

The simple key to losing body fat is to consume less food than your body needs for energy, which causes your body to tap into fat stores for energy between meals. A healthy spread of proteins, carbohydrates, and fats at regular meals throughout the day will help your body understand that you're not starving, and regular doses of healthy foods will keep your blood sugar at a stable level and your glycogen stores replenished. Regular exercise will cause your body to consume the glycogen stores in your muscles, which tells your liver to convert fat stores into energy while blood sugar is lower between meals. By not eating more than your body uses, you will not contribute to additional fat stores.

How do you know if you're consuming too few calories? If you're getting adequate rest, getting adequate hydration, and eating nutrient-dense vibrant foods but after seven days you still feel like you have no energy, you likely need to eat more.

Also keep in mind that when you first pursue a Paleo lifestyle, such as the one outlined in this book, your body will likely go through a detoxifying phase during which it may shed water as inflammation begins to drop. Water weighs quite a lot and will cause the number on the scale to dip. This loss of water weight will plateau as soon as your body has shed the excess baggage.

Constant starvation and too-extreme calorie restriction can slow your basal metabolic rate, causing you to burn fewer calories.

Nutrient-dense foods provide your body with the micronutrients (like vitamins and minerals) you need to stay healthy and metabolically vibrant.

I recommend that you avoid the scale, as it's not a true indicator of health or progress toward fat-loss goals.

snacks:
do they sabotage or support?

Snacks are a relatively touchy subject in the world of nutrition because there are two main schools of thought:

- that snacks support a "faster metabolism"
- that snacks impede a natural metabolism

I tend to fall in the latter group. As discussed in the Sleep section, when the body is in its most natural state, it abides by a predictable, healthy circadian rhythm. Training your body to know when it's going to be presented with nutrients and when it's going to have a break from digestion is just as important to metabolic health as a regular sleep schedule.

Constant snacking keeps hunger and satiety hormones from ever truly fulfilling their responsibilities, and the practice provides no rest for the digestive system. It essentially puts the body in a constant state of low-level stress caused by frequent eating.

I argue that the feeling of hunger between meals is natural—healthy, even. Let's go back to our beloved case study, Carrie, for a moment:

When Carrie finishes her lunch of leftover beef stew (page 208) at about 12:30, leptin (along with a variety of other post-meal-related hormones) signifies satiety, telling her that she's no longer hungry. Her body then gets to work digesting and assimilating the nutrients that she just consumed. Throughout the afternoon, Carrie sips on sparkling water and caffeine-free herbal tea and does a great job of avoiding the temptation to indulge in the plate of cookies in the office break room.

By 5:00 p.m., Carrie is packing up her workspace and driving home. Though not famished, her main hunger hormone, ghrelin, is released by her liver, and she starts to think about dinner. On her way home, she gets stuck in traffic, which ends up adding a whopping forty-five minutes to her commute.

By the time Carrie gets home, she's hungry, but still not starving. Her body is relatively metabolically nimble, and a minor spike in cortisol and glucagon tell her body to start drawing on glycogen and body fat for energy. Carrie calmly prepares her dinner and sits down to eat. She eats no more than she would have if the meal had been at the usual time, and she feels the same amount of satiety when she's finished.

The important takeaway here is that Carrie didn't need a mid-afternoon snack to keep her metabolism "primed," so to speak. Her body is well equipped to get from one meal to the next, even if the period between the two is longer than expected. Making the adjustment may take practice and a little patience, but I strongly recommend making snacks the exception, not the rule.

Save for one major exception: food for fitness! With regard to pre- and post-workouts, snacks, or mini meals, have a distinct purpose and a direct metabolic use. Though not always necessary (see pages 58 and 59 for further explanation), mini meals can be quite advantageous to a person wanting to get the most out of his or her exercise efforts.

food for fitness

Because we're going to cover a wealth of fun scientific information in the fourth and final pillar, Fitness, I'd like to take this time to briefly discuss ideal nutrient types and timing as they relate to efforts exerted in a workout.

pre-workout

In some ways, you can think of any meal after your last workout and before your next workout as a pre-workout meal. Whatever you take in is going to be used as fuel for your body in some regard! However, for the sake of this discussion, I'm going to cover the small meals that best help prepare the body for a workout.

Aside from carbohydrate loading before an endurance event, most pre-workout meals (or snacks) really need only a little fat and a little protein. Any carbohydrates (or sugars) present won't hurt, but they won't be of much immediate use.

Sample pre-workout meal templates

First-Thing-in-the-Morning Workout

Option A: *Fasting. If you can get through your workout with even energy and don't feel dizzy, you can absolutely roll out of bed and right into your sweat session. Fasting workouts, depending on your individual symptoms, can be perfectly healthy.*

Option B: *A small piece of* *protein and a small piece of fat.*

Mid-Morning Workout
None; your breakfast counts as a pre-workout meal.

Pre-Lunch Workout

Option A: *None, especially if you had a nice big breakfast and don't feel hungry.*

Option B: *A small piece of protein and a small piece of fat.*

Mid-Afternoon Workout
None; your lunch counts as a pre-workout meal.

Before-Dinner Workout

Option A: *None, especially if you had a nice big lunch and don't feel hungry.*

Option B: *A small piece of protein and a small piece of fat.*

Post-Dinner Workout
None; your dinner counts as a pre-workout meal.

Sample pre-workout snacks (mix and match with your favorite proteins and fats!)

- *1 hard-boiled egg with a small dollop of homemade mayo made with avocado oil (page 349)*

- *2 to 3 ounces of deli meat and a small handful of nuts*

- *A small handful of leftover poultry, pork, or red meat with a small dollop of homemade ranch dressing (page 338)*

- *1 homemade protein bar (page 306)*

- *Any other combination of protein and fat within the scope that you enjoy!*

WHAT ABOUT CARB-LOADING?

I get this question a lot from endurance athletes, and I think it bears a dedicated answer. For the most part, carbohydrate loading is an activity that should be reserved for a minimum of two days out. While carbohydrates taken in the day before and the day of an athletic event can contribute to blood glucose and some muscle glycogen, if you want to make sure that your muscles have a healthy bank of energy stored up (in the form of glycogen), it's best to get a two-day head start. If you're looking to run a half marathon on Sunday morning, for example, I recommend enjoying a giant baked sweet potato for dinner on Friday.

post-workout

There are three important things to take in for post-workout nutrition: water (with electrolytes if needed; see "Hydration" on pages 36 and 37), starchy vegetables (for glucose and eventual glycogen replenishment), and protein (to provide plenty of readily available amino acids for repairing muscle damage). Choose any starchy vegetable from the list of healing foods presented earlier in this chapter. The protein, though the options are endless, can be more easily put to use by the body if it's partially broken down (think: slow cooker shredded chicken, pot roast, whey protein powder, or collagen peptides).

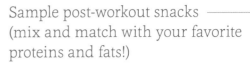
Sample post-workout snacks (mix and match with your favorite proteins and fats!)

- *2 to 3 ounces of shredded chicken and half a sweet potato*
- *2 to 3 ounces of deli meat and 1 cup of carrot sticks*
- *1 scoop of protein powder blended with half a plantain*
- *Any other combination of protein and carbohydrate within the scope that you enjoy!*

Sample post-workout meal templates ———

First-Thing-in-the-Morning Workout

Option A: *Breakfast! Make sure that it includes a healthy starch and protein.*

Option B: *A small serving of protein and healthy starch.*

Mid-Morning Workout

A small serving of protein and healthy starch.

Pre-Lunch Workout

Option A: *Lunch! Make sure that it includes a healthy starch and protein.*

Option B: *A small serving of protein and healthy starch.*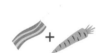

Mid-Afternoon Workout

A small serving of protein and healthy starch.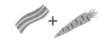

Before-Dinner Workout

Option A: *Dinner! Make sure that it includes a healthy starch and protein.*

Option B: *A small serving of protein and healthy starch.*

Post-Dinner Workout

A small serving of protein and healthy starch.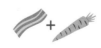

nutrient timing

Isn't there a really narrow window that I need to hit to make the most of my pre- and post-workout nutrition?

This is another one of the most-asked questions I get related to workout nourishment. My answer is yes and no.

Why Yes—If you're an elite athlete or really looking to fine-tune your athletic efforts with nutrition and meal timing, it's good to consider that the body is more efficient in converting glucose to glycogen and up-taking that glycogen in the muscles within approximately one hour after an exerted physical activity.

Why No—If you're not an elite athlete but are looking both to make the most out of your workout and to establish a new healthy lifestyle, nutrient timing may not be something you need to worry about. As long as you're eating three healthy, balanced meals each day, you're going to see progress and feel amazing. If the thought of organizing dedicated pre- and post-workout mini meals feels overwhelming or even keeps you from working out altogether, then I say forget about it. Just find an activity you enjoy and eat healthy foods. Progress comes in all kinds of simple and complex formats. Choose the one that fits *you* best.

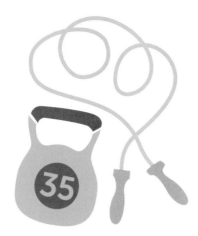

PILLAR #4:

FITNESS

Fitness is the last piece of the puzzle—or, rather, the last pillar of this rock-solid healthy lifestyle foundation that we're building together. We're about to have some real fun! I hope you don't expect Juli and me to tell you that you simply need to get out there and sweat for an hour each day to achieve ideal physical fitness. We've had some experience with purely cardio-centric workout routines, and we know that they tend to result in untimely mental and physical burnout.

Instead of the overused "exercise more" mantra, we've chosen to draw from our years of experience in transitioning monotonous, surface-deep exercise routines into fun, active lifestyles. When you view physical fitness as a means to happiness rather than exercise as a means to physical fitness, you're much more likely to choose and then incorporate activities you love into a long-term healthy lifestyle. "Exercise more" evolves into "Consistently exercise more like *you*."

Juli's talent for writing entertaining muscle group–focused workouts combined with my passion for mobility results in a balanced, challenging, and fun approach to exercise. We're here to say that it is possible to design a fitness routine that you absolutely love. Your Ideal Fitness Fit (IFF), once you design it, will become the tempo of your life. It's marked by the reflective walk between the car and the grocery store, the before-sunrise yoga class, the strength-training class at the end of the workday, and the at-home workout you save for when the kids go down for a nap. When you take your IFF and combine it with the right mindset, a customized sleep schedule, a smart hydration strategy, and a healing meal plan, the result is a balanced, healthy lifestyle. You will start to realize that while you are working toward your larger end goals, the journey is the true adventure. The journey is the part that offers you fulfillment and keeps you motivated.

If you find your current fitness routine daunting, punishing, or just plain miserable, now is the time to make some changes.

the science of exercise

Let's go back to the truism that knowledge is power. Though learning about the basic science of the body may seem tedious, we argue that the more you know about what happens on a cellular level, the more empowered you are to make healthy decisions. If you understand how your body moves, processes nutrients, and recovers after a workout, then you're better equipped to make more informed, nourishing decisions with regard to fueling your body pre-workout, recovering post-workout, and building a mixed fitness routine that truly helps you feel your best. And the more you know about what's actually going on inside your body, the less likely you are to feel as if you're falling victim to an unexplained symptom, whether it be a positive one, like a burst of energy or a sudden fitness breakthrough, or a negative one, like a lack of energy or difficulty achieving fitness goals.

What we want you to take away from this review of the science is that how you feel—the ultimate measure of success—is directly affected not only by a healthy mindset, sufficient rest and hydration, a healing diet, and efforts to exercise, but also by your body's chemistry, which in turn is entirely dependent on how you treat your body.

Because the science of exercise is a broad topic, we're going to zero in on just a few pieces: breath and the distribution of oxygen, the creation of energy, muscle glycogen stores, fat stores, and what happens when we strength train, speed train, endurance train, and stretch. To accomplish all this, let's take a Ms. Frizzle–style trip through the body!

what happens when we move our bodies?

You could almost argue that anytime we move our bodies, we're exercising. When the diaphragm (the large muscle that sits under the lungs) expands, it causes low pressure in the lungs. As a result, the lungs fill with air (that is, we take a breath). Though air is made up of approximately 80 percent nitrogen and only 20 percent oxygen, we're really in it only for the oxygen (O_2). Thanks to well-moistened microscopic beds of lung tissue and capillaries, the oxygen we breathe in is infused into the blood and readied for transport across the body. The powerful heart pumps the oxygenated blood through a series of large and small arteries for the purpose of delivering precious oxygen to muscle tissues. Once the oxygen is deposited, the blood picks up carbon dioxide (CO_2) and transports it back to the heart through a series of large and small veins. CO_2 is deposited in the tiny moist lung capillary beds for exhalation, and then the process starts all over again!

The oxygen that is delivered to our muscles is (essentially) digested via a series of chemical reactions known collectively as *cellular respiration*. Though a great number of small but significant steps, reactions, and by-products are involved (one of them being CO_2), the end goal of cellular respiration is to produce the energy currency of the body—adenosine triphosphate, or ATP for short. To keep things extremely simple, O_2 reacts with glucose to form this precious energy compound. Our muscles can then consume (or "cash in") ATP as needed. We're able to walk through the grocery store, clean the house, and drive a car with ease thanks to blood glucose (the body's preferred energy source), muscle and liver glycogen (its secondary energy source), body fat (the backup energy source), normal oxygen intake, and signals from our muscles to our brains to keep making and delivering ATP for readily available energy.

energy and exercise

Some people exercise because they want to compete at an elite level, some because they're battling chronic disease, some because they want to lose body fat, and some because they just want to feel healthier. Regardless of current health or motive, all bodies metabolize energy similarly. There are three main sources of energy for the body: blood glucose, muscle and liver glycogen, and fat reserves. The body always relies on blood glucose first for energy, then it uses muscle and liver glycogen, and finally it taps into fat reserves. While energy stores and the rate at which they're metabolized will differ between an elite athlete and a person trying to lose body fat, the chemical processes are almost identical. Certain training exercises (like strength, speed, and endurance training) have an impact not only on muscle development but also on the rate at which energy is consumed.

This basic scientific overview equips each and every athlete, whether beginner or pro, with the knowledge of where energy comes from, how it's used, and how different training exercises have a unique impact on overall conditioning.

Where does blood glucose come from?

Terrific question! The food we eat is broken down into six main groups: proteins, carbohydrates, fats, minerals, vitamins, and water. Carbohydrates are broken down into their most basic state: glucose, also known as sugar. Glucose flows into the bloodstream and floats around until the body decides what to do with it. It can be used immediately for cellular respiration (the production of ATP), slightly modified and put into short-term storage as glycogen in the muscles and liver, or significantly modified and put into long-term storage as fat. Throughout the day, most bodies maintain an even amount of blood sugar for immediate use. When that energy runs out (possibly because we haven't eaten in a while), it turns to glycogen.

Where does glycogen come from?

The rise in blood glucose after eating triggers the pancreas to release the enzyme insulin. Insulin acts as the key to "unlock" our muscles (and liver tissue) so that the glucose can be collected and then stored for energy. Glucose is transformed into its short-term storage form, glycogen, through a process called *glycogenesis*. Twenty percent of the body's glycogen is found in the liver, and the remaining 80 percent is found in the muscles. Just a short reaction away from being transformed back into glucose, glycogen is readily available as fuel for cellular respiration (the production of ATP).

Where does body fat come from?

If, after insulin has completed its job of refilling the muscle and liver glycogen stores, there is still excess blood sugar present, it will get to work facilitating the transformation of that excess glucose into body fat via a process called *lipogenesis*. This fat, a long-term storage of energy, is the backup source to blood sugar and muscle glycogen. In the absence of blood sugar, body fat can be used for energy if needed.

What happens when we strength train?

Strength training (aka weight training) is essentially the process of skeletal muscles contracting against pressure for multiple repetitions. Think about doing a medium-weight back squat for ten consecutive reps. The leg and back muscles (plus some other important stabilizing muscles) work together to hold the joints in place while contracting against the leveraged bones to move the weight of the body and bar. Going from the bottom to the top of a squat requires the large muscles in the legs to contract. These relatively slow but challenging movements nurture the health of the skeletal structure and metabolism. When performed properly, the weight and sustained resistance promote stronger bones, healthier joints, and muscles more readily able to make use of insulin (meaning that they're more sensitive to insulin). The intense effort causes tiny muscle tears that, once rebuilt through proper nutrition, rest, and hydration, heal up stronger and more metabolically efficient than before.

What happens when we speed train?

To keep things simple, let's discuss speed training in terms of cardio impact and fast-twitch muscle fiber development.

Every muscle contains both fast- and slow-twitch fibers. Speed training, which encompasses activities like high-intensity interval training (HIIT), sprints, Tabata (squats, sit-ups, push-ups, etc.), and other explosive movements, is made possible by our fast-twitch fibers. Fast-twitch muscle fibers work exactly the way they sound—they allow for a quick, intense muscular response to a stimulus or demand. Fast-twitch fibers, as opposed to their slow-twitch cousins, get larger in response to weight and speed training. These fibers use and then quickly deplete energy stores. Speed training is typically performed under anaerobic conditions, where the body is moving faster than the breath can supply oxygen to muscle tissues. Heavy breathing and difficulty sustaining a conversation are hallmarks of anaerobic exercise.

What happens when we endurance train?

Endurance training, for the sake of this explanation, involves working at or below approximately 60 percent of capacity for at least 20 minutes. Your breathing may be more intense, but it's not overly labored, and you can still communicate easily. Both everyday movements and intentional endurance workouts make use of our slow-twitch muscle fibers. These muscle fibers, while they move more slowly and have a less explosive response to stimulus, typically operate under aerobic conditions and are more efficient at continually creating energy.

What happens when we stretch?

Strength, speed, and endurance training are all activities of contraction. Strength training works to contract against excess pressure, speed training against tempo, and endurance training against time. Exercise as a result of constant contractions can result in shorter muscle groups and increasingly limited range of motion. Long muscles and an increased range of motion are beneficial for total strength and overall joint health—thus the importance of stretching, or mobility training. When we stretch or work through mobility and flexibility exercises, we actively force muscles to elongate and realign so that they're able to heal properly.

the importance of a mixed fitness program

What we're after isn't just to help you get fit! We're here to offer up an all-encompassing view of the key physical fitness components that will empower you to maintain a *lifetime* of active wellness. Establishing a balanced and varied fitness program that combines strength, speed, and endurance training with mobility is critical for the optimal long-term health with a reduced risk of injury.

Quality coaching and years of practice not to be taken for granted, the true secret weapon in my (Cassy's) sustained athletic success is my focus on flexibility and scheduled rest. I have been able to participate in CrossFit (an efficient "mixed fitness program" in and of itself) for the last eight-plus years without major injury because I take two things very seriously: mobility and moderation. I make it a point to pay attention to my body, and I do not allow myself to compete past healthy limits. I also make it a point to integrate regular yoga classes, stretching, and daily post-workout mobility to keep my body healthy and nimble.

the savvy seven

We've boiled down the components that make up a healthy, balanced fitness regimen to seven savvy pursuits. They include the four we've already discussed plus three more: rest, fun, and movement.

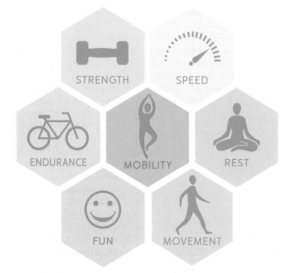

Keep your mind's eye on all seven of these components *most of the time.* Make sure that you're intentionally touching each one at least twice throughout the week. This means two mobility sessions, two strength-training sessions, two endurance-training activities, two speed-training activities, *at least* two activities that you consider to be fun, and at least two days of rest a week. For "movement," we encourage you to make a conscious effort to move more each and every day. Ideas on how to make your days more active are listed on the opposite page.

Note that most sports, fitness classes, and other physical fitness practices span several of the Savvy Seven. While you can tackle each component independently by doing a mix of focused strength training sessions, speed training sessions, endurance training sessions, and mobility sessions, other, more efficient solutions can prove just as effective. For example, Olympic lifting offers both strength and speed, and a 90-minute yoga class can offer both mobility and endurance. Aside from the four different kinds of training, remember to schedule rest days and do your best to incorporate fun into as many activities as possible.

Movement, the last piece of the puzzle, is a daily pursuit that involves staying as active as you can. Healthy people don't just eat well and exercise; they also take an active approach to life! In your effort to live Fed & Fit, you will likely unearth your own personal brand of daily movement and opportunities to stay active between workouts.

Before you create your own signature healthy habits, here are some suggestions to get you started:

- Take the stairs.
- Park your car in the spot farthest from the door.
- Walk to lunch.
- Go for a walk after dinner.
- Go for a walk after breakfast.
- Take your conference calls on the go (put on a pair of wireless headphones and strap on your tennis shoes).

- Don't try to take all your groceries inside on one trip—spread it out!
- Foam roll while you watch TV.
- If you have a sedentary job, stop every hour on the hour and take a five-minute walk around the building, go up and down the stairs, or knock out ten quick air squats by your desk.
- If possible, transition to a standing desk.

workouts

Now that we've covered the importance of a mixed fitness program combined with intentional daily movement, rest, and keeping it fun, let's discuss some options. Some fitness programs naturally hit on all Savvy Seven, while others require a little creative thinking. If you're looking for a program that covers all the bases, follow the at-home workouts outlined in our 28-Day Food & Fitness Plan (pages 86 to 97). If you'd like to combine gym fitness classes with workouts from the 28-Day Plan, you can do that, too! Remember, what's important is that you're moving, strength training, speed training, endurance training, stretching, and resting. Let's put our creative hats on and design the fitness template of your dreams.

home workout routine (the 28-day food & fitness plan)

All you need to get started on a workout routine are a little space and a willingness to sweat! Bodyweight workouts are a great way to strategically leverage your own weight in an effort to tone, build muscle, reduce inflammation, and shed body fat. The workouts provided in the 28-Day Food & Fitness Plan can be completed in under 30 minutes and without any equipment!

If you want to use the 28-Day Plan but also love group classes, ask a few friends to join you! Countless lives have been changed because a few like-minded people gathered around common goals and a desire to develop new healthy habits.

What do you do when the Project ends? You have so many options! You can repeat the 28-Day Plan as many times as you like, or you can use it as an opportunity to fine-tune your routine: explore the fitness areas that interest you and work to incorporate those into your weekly routine.

note

If you have a home workout video or other program that you enjoy using, keep using it! Just pay attention to how many of the Savvy Seven components it hits, and be sure to incorporate any missing components into your routine each week.

group class hero

We love group fitness classes. We love the fun, the variety, the sense of community, and the fact that we just have to show up and do as we're told. Attending a class is a nice healthy break from the day and allows us to feel even more connected to our community! That being said, some group fitness classes are more well rounded than others.

A DISCLAIMER ABOUT GROUP CLASSES AND TRAINERS:
Not all affiliates, trainers, programming, and coaching teams are created equal. It's up to you to be a savvy consumer. Interview current clients and inquire about the coaches' certifications, education, and goals for their clients. (Hint: You want a coach who says that he or she wants athletes to be challenged but also healthy and injury-free.)

Let's review:

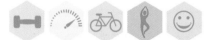

CrossFit—*One of the most efficient group class options out there. With balanced, responsible programming, CrossFit hits most of the Savvy Seven: strength, speed, endurance, mobility, and fun.*

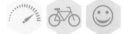

Kickboxing—*Great for getting in an hour of speed, endurance, and fun.*

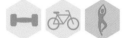

Athletic yoga—*Great for endurance, strength, and mobility. Examples of athletic yoga are Ashtanga, strong vinyasa, Bikram, hot yoga, and yoga for athletes.*

Restorative yoga—*A great way to incorporate a healthy mobility practice into your weekly routine. Examples of restorative yoga are gentle hatha, slow flow, slow vinyasa, Anusara, and Iyengar yoga.*

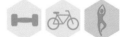

Spinning—*A good source of speed and endurance training.*

Pilates—*Resistance (strength) training, moderate endurance, and some mobility.*

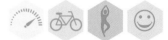

Dance—*Depending on the intensity, dance classes such as modern, jazz, ballet, tango, swing, and ballroom can span speed, endurance, mobility, and a good deal of fun.*

Zumba—*Enjoy some light endurance (sustained cardio) and fun.*

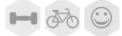

Barre—*Strength, moderate endurance, and fun!*

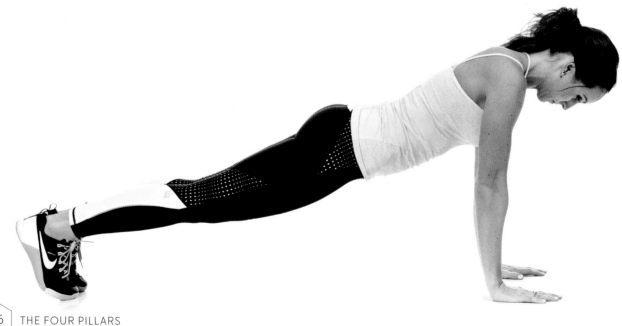

she's going the distance

If your IFF falls more into the category of true endurance, we salute you! We also caution you, in the interest of the longevity of your career as an endurance athlete, to intentionally incorporate the following into your routine:

Strength training—*Are we starting to sound like a broken record? Strength training is so important. You'll be able to push farther, tap into deeper levels of energy, and (most important) protect your joints with conditioned muscles. Find what works best for your schedule, but we recommend that you strength-train each muscle group (arms, shoulders, core, butt, and legs) at least once a week, ideally under the direction of a qualified coach.*

Speed training—*Putting a focus on developing your fast-twitch muscle fibers can help protect against injury. Though your mileage may be in the double digits during a marathon or on the last leg of a triathlon, you're better prepared to avoid an injury-causing misstep if your muscles' fast-twitch fibers are ready to step in. Weekly sprints or other quick-burst high-intensity training can do wonders for preventing injury and improving your overall performance.*

Mobility—*Endurance athletes know the importance of stretching, but we'd like to up the ante a bit. If you're putting in 20-plus miles a week on foot or 60-plus miles a week on a bike, it's crucial that you dedicate 30 to 90 minutes a week to careful stretching and mobility.*

Rest—*Rest is crucial for all athletes, including endurance athletes. A well-conditioned endurance athlete may not often feel sore or exhausted, but that doesn't make rest any less important. Giving muscles a full day to repair and replenish themselves every three or four days will greatly improve your progress and recovery time.*

I want it all

Heck yes, you do! In fact, I (Cassy) identify with that sentiment. I love a mixed fitness program that spans home workouts, group classes, and the occasional endurance event. If this resonates with you, know that there's a formula here, too!

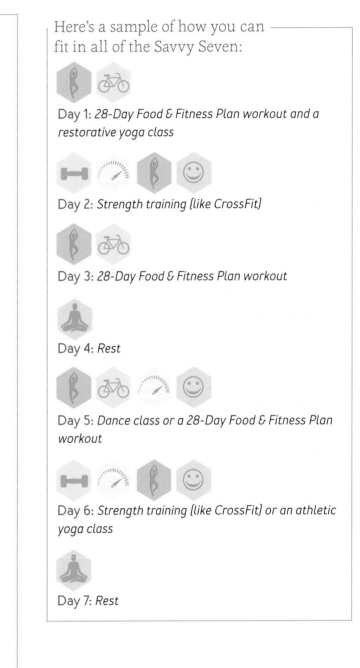

Here's a sample of how you can fit in all of the Savvy Seven:

Day 1: *28-Day Food & Fitness Plan workout and a restorative yoga class*

Day 2: *Strength training (like CrossFit)*

Day 3: *28-Day Food & Fitness Plan workout*

Day 4: *Rest*

Day 5: *Dance class or a 28-Day Food & Fitness Plan workout*

Day 6: *Strength training (like CrossFit) or an athletic yoga class*

Day 7: *Rest*

a note about rest

In the 28-Day Fed & Fit Project, we recommend that you get two full days of rest a week. On rest days, our bodies have time to replenish muscle glycogen levels, rebuild, and detoxify. Periods of rest help us avoid burnout and injury while allowing us to make the most of the five days a week we are sweating it out. When it comes to intense exercise, more is *not* better.

That being said, there are some exceptions to the rule, and it all comes down to personal preference. If, after paying close attention to your energy levels and how quickly you recover from your workouts, you decide that one rest day a week offers you sufficient recovery time, that's completely okay. It's also completely okay to take up to three days off a week. At the end of the day, it's important that you listen to your body and give it both the work and the rest that it needs.

taking time off

Sometimes it's important to stop working out altogether. If you are experiencing any of the following conditions, complete rest is usually the best option:

- Acute pain
- Adrenal fatigue
- Chronic pain
- Cold or flu
- Extreme exhaustion

When it comes to deciding whether to forgo working out, please remember that of the priorities listed in this book, *sleep precedes fitness*. Getting more sleep is more beneficial to your well-being than the workout.

That said, if your symptoms are mild, you can try incorporating healing body movements, such as restorative yoga. A mild cold, minor muscle aches, and a manageable level of stress are all symptoms that could possibly benefit from mild stretching or a mobility-focused workout.

your ideal fitness fit (IFF)

So what to make of all this? At the end of the day, the best fitness solution for you is one that you design, based on the information presented in this pillar and your personal preferences. When your fitness routine is tailored to your needs and tastes, it is more likely to become a lasting and enjoyable part of your lifestyle and lead to positive results. Though your goals and abilities may evolve over time, your weekly Ideal Fitness Fit (IFF) routine should:

| Touch on each of the Savvy Seven. | Keep you excited and motivated. | Be personally feasible in terms of cost, location, and schedule. | Result in the healthiest, happiest you. |

Designing and scheduling a weekly routine that accomplishes all of the above may seem like a daunting task at first, but with a little effort and experience, you can absolutely get there.

To find your IFF, we encourage you to work through the following steps:

1. Write down the following training types across the top of a piece of paper: strength, speed, endurance, and mobility. Think of all the fitness pursuits that fall under each of these training types. Create a written list of pursuits for each training type.

2. Find two different-colored highlighters or pens. Use one color to circle the fitness pursuits that sound like the most fun and the other color to circle the fitness pursuits that are the most practical (think: cost, location, and schedule). If a pursuit is practical as well as fun, circle it twice, using both colors.

3. On a separate sheet of paper, write down any fitness pursuits that you circled twice and that span two or more training types. If you can build a complete fitness plan around these pursuits, this is a good place to stop! You're ready to move on to Step 4. If you don't have enough double-circled pursuits to build a complete fitness plan, then expand your list by including the items you circled that are the most practical.

4. Put this new plan into action. Break out your planner and start scheduling these workouts! This could involve getting set up at a gym, reserving class times, or setting reminders on your phone for when it's time to do your home workout. The thought behind this step: if it's not scheduled, it isn't going to happen.

5. Remember that you can always go back to the drawing board. If you become interested in a new sport, we encourage you to chase that passion! Your IFF will constantly evolve, and it's your job to make changes if boredom sets in.

Above all, remember that the Fed & Fit Project, for the initial 28 days and beyond, is about *progress*, not perfection. Working in this material every day and making an effort to be consistent are what matter most. If a week goes by and you haven't touched on each of the Savvy Seven, or if you haven't made it through a single mobility exercise in over a month, don't fret. If having a balanced fitness program is a priority, write it into next week's calendar and continue to apply yourself until the material starts to feel intuitive.

You've got this!

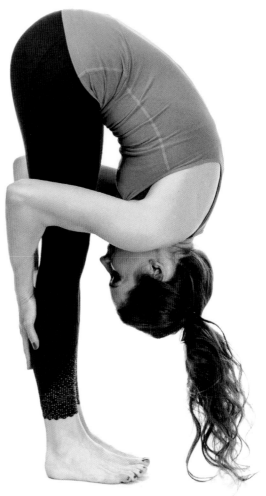

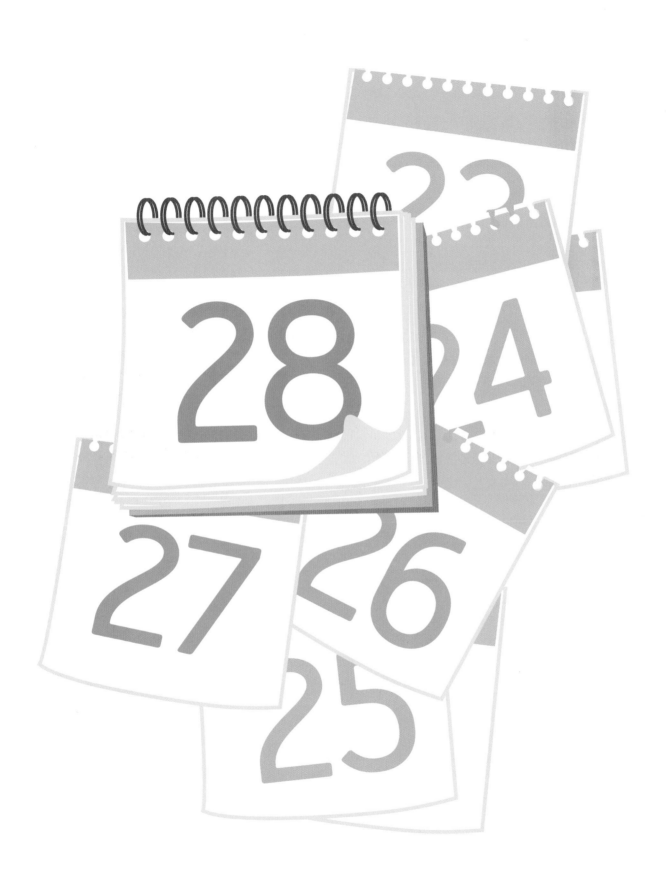

THE 28-DAY PROJECT

This is it! This is where the rubber meets the road. We're going to talk sleep plans, hydration plans, food, fitness, and journaling. I'm going to give you a practical overview of the 28-Day Food & Fitness Plan as it relates to everything I've covered in the book so far.

Remember, this Project is meant to be a feel-good reset and a solid foothold from which you can start to build your own healthy lifestyle, referred to here as the Perfect You Plan.

the project in a nutshell

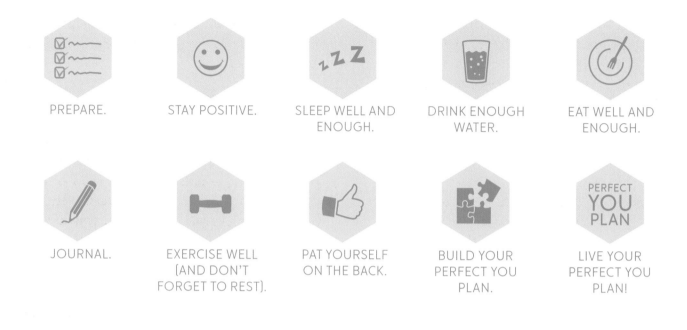

PREPARE.

STAY POSITIVE.

SLEEP WELL AND ENOUGH.

DRINK ENOUGH WATER.

EAT WELL AND ENOUGH.

JOURNAL.

EXERCISE WELL (AND DON'T FORGET TO REST).

PAT YOURSELF ON THE BACK.

BUILD YOUR PERFECT YOU PLAN.

LIVE YOUR PERFECT YOU PLAN!

the project in a slightly larger, more informative nutshell

First off, let's talk about Projecters. Who's a Projecter? You are! You're in the material, working to establish a healthy baseline and wholesome habits. A Projecter is anyone who is committed to learning how to build his or her own Perfect You Plan.

Prepare. For starters, you need to think about how you plan to prepare. Preparing for the Project can include reading about the Four Pillars (pages 20 to 69); making all of the necessary pantry, refrigerator, and freezer swaps (pages 114 to 116); recruiting a friend; finding a community (the Project Online is a great option!); and creating an accountability system. Other ways to prepare include deciding how you're going to journal, zeroing in on the meal plan you will follow, and creating a fitness plan. Remember that you can edit as you go, but it's a good idea to at least be familiar with the material before you start.

Stay Positive. It's imperative that you keep your chin up. You may experience some ups and downs during these 28 days, but everything is going to be A-OK. Lean on your community (learn about finding a community in Pillar #1: Mindset) and do your best to see opportunities, not obstacles. For example, if you miss a workout because you had to stay late at the office, use that as an opportunity to schedule a fun new makeup workout (maybe a yoga class?) on your rest day. If you get a terrible night's sleep, use that as an opportunity to strategically journal how the lack of sleep affected your food choices and your overall outlook. At the end of the Project, you may be left with a lesson learned about sleep deprivation that demystifies why you crave sweets after too few hours in bed.

Sleep Well and Enough. This is critical! I cover the whys extensively in Pillar #2: Rest & Hydration, but remember that it's important to establish your Daily Sleep Number (DSN) first. Work through the exercise outlined on page 32 to find your DSN, then try to hit that number every night of the Project! Lean on the tips I've included there for getting a better night's sleep. Also note that there will be occasions when getting a full night's sleep is impossible. I completely understand. Just do your best and remember to journal your progress.

Drink Enough Water. Like sleep, hydration is imperative! In fact, of all the pillars and activities involved in the Project, this one is the lowest of the low-hanging fruit. You can use the calculation on page 37 to establish your Daily Water Need (DWN). From there, it's simply a matter of filling up and drinking up! Do your best to hit your DWN each and every day, but remember: the Project is about progress, not perfection. Don't fret if you fall short one day.

Eat Well & Enough. Rule #1: Don't go actually hungry. While you're detoxing from the sugar-loaded and artificial ingredient–loaded foods found in the Standard American Diet, you may think that you're hungry when you're not. Do your best to distinguish true hunger pangs from symptoms of withdrawal. Lean on the healing foods identified in this book and make sure that you're getting enough nourishment from your three main meals!

Exercise Well (and Don't Forget to Rest). While rest, hydration, and proper nutrition will get you close to feeling your best, exercise will help you hit the ball out of the park. Do your best to work through the material on page 69 so that you can establish your Ideal Fitness Fit (IFF). Before the Project begins, schedule these workouts at home or your gym, find a partner, and set up your space. If you need equipment, get your equipment! Eliminate as many obstacles as possible before you start.

Journal. Journaling is the heart and soul of the Project. I go into more details on the whys, hows, and whens on pages 104 and 105, but remember that the lessons learned that you record in your journal are what will enable you to upsell your 28-day commitment into a lasting healthy lifestyle. Don't skip this step!

Pat Yourself on the Back. You are *awesome.* So darn awesome! Look at you. You're making a commitment to better yourself. You're bettering yourself for yourself, of course, but also for your family and every other person you encounter. This is really big. I'm so proud of you for taking this enormous step, and you should be enormously proud of yourself. Remember that even if things don't go exactly as planned, we're all about progress here!

Build Your Perfect You Plan. This is the pot of gold at the end of the rainbow. I've got more details on what the Perfect You Plan is and how to build it on pages 108 and 109, but remember that this plan summarizes all of the lessons you're going to learn over the next 28 days. This is the summary of best practices for *you!* It includes your DSN, your DWN, your IFF (tired of acronyms yet?), and your favorite healthy foods. It includes the healthiest practices that you love—which means that they'll be easier to maintain in the future.

Live your Perfect You Plan! You got this! Now go out there and live it. At the end of the 28-Day Project, you will feel *great!* Use that positive momentum to find and live out your real-life template. Show yourself some grace as you adjust to the real world again (it's unlikely that you'll get it right out of the gate) and stay nimble. You will continue to refine and adjust your PYP for years, but staying on the cutting edge of happy and healthy is the fun part.

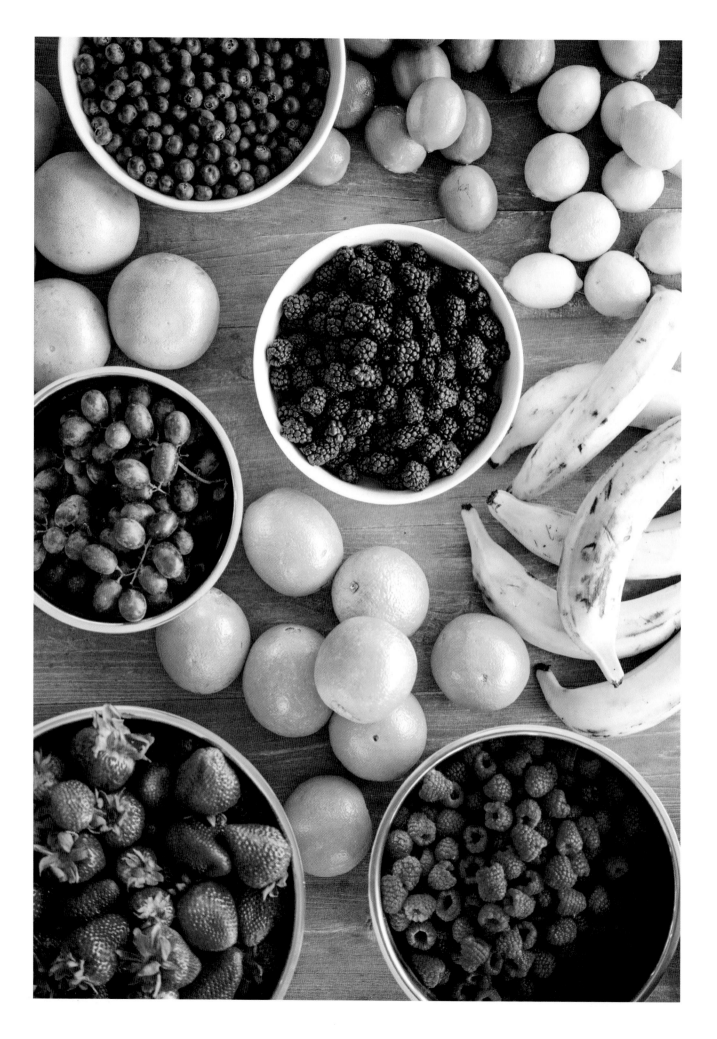

the scoop on the scope

I refer to all of the healing, anti-inflammatory foods that are included in the Project as "in scope" and all of the sabotaging, inflammatory foods that are discouraged in the Project as "out of scope." You'll find complete lists of these foods on the following pages, but in the meantime, let's discuss some distinctions.

Paleo

The Paleo template excludes all dairy, grains, artificial ingredients, legumes, and refined sugars. It's important to note that Paleo is broader than what I've outlined for the 28-Day Fed & Fit Project. While the scope of the traditional Paleo template is debated some, I've done my best to provide an overview on the following chart for comparison.

The Project

The Project is the most exclusive of the templates outlined in the scope, but for good reason! As discussed in Pillar #3: Food, the Project accounts for berries, citrus, bananas, and plantains as the only fruits and excludes all dairy, sweeteners (save for dates), gluten-free grains, and pseudo-grains. I've designed the plan this way so that we're left with the foods that are the most healing and benign to our health. Although you may be able to tolerate some out-of-scope foods, the intention of these 28 days is to get you feeling your best quickly.

The Perfect You Plan

The Perfect You Plan is the most open template. This is the one that you'll build after you've completed the 28-Day Project. If you find that you tolerate dairy, then include dairy! If you find that you tolerate gluten-free grains, then include those as well! I talk about how to customize your plan on pages 108 and 109, but remember that anything is possible. No two people will have the same food tolerance spectrum, so don't be afraid to individualize the plan as much as you like.

A NOTE ABOUT BANANAS

When it comes to bananas as a fruit source on the Project, it's important to remember that the ideal serving size is half a banana. Because it's easier to portion pre-chopped and then frozen bananas as opposed to eating only half of a fresh banana, I encourage you to freeze your bananas for ideal portion sizing during the Project.

note

For more information about portion sizes, losing body fat, and general metabolism science, check out Pillar #3: Food, beginning on page 38.

food scope

	PALEO		THE PROJECT		PERFECT YOU PLAN	
	IN	OUT	IN	OUT	IN	OUT
PROTEIN	all grass-fed red meat all fish & seafood all free-range pork & poultry cage-free, pastured eggs	commercially raised, antibiotic- & hormone-injected, & grain-fed meats	all grass-fed red meat all fish & seafood all free-range pork & poultry cage-free, pastured eggs	commercially raised, antibiotic- & hormone-injected, & grain-fed meats	all responsibly raised proteins that work with your taste and budget	any protein that does not promote your true health
DAIRY	ghee	milk butter cheese kefir yogurt	butter from grass-fed cows ghee	milk conventional butter cheese kefir yogurt	any dairy that agrees with your body, ideally organic & grass-fed	any dairy that causes digestive or skin problems
CRUNCHY VEG	all leafy greens all crunchy vegetables		all leafy greens all crunchy vegetables		all leafy greens all crunchy vegetables that work for your body	any vegetable that causes digestive problems
STARCHY VEG	all potatoes all squash all tubers all other root vegetables		all potatoes all squash all tubers all other root vegetables		all starchy vegetables that work for your body	any starchy vegetable that causes digestive problems
LEGUMES	green beans	all beans peanuts	green beans	all beans peanuts	green beans (if tolerated) peanuts (if tolerated) beans (if tolerated)	any legume that causes digestive problems
GRAINS		wheat barley rye oatmeal rice (brown & white) corn all other grains		wheat barley rye oatmeal rice (brown & white) corn all other grains	rice (if tolerated) non-GMO corn (if tolerated) gluten-free oatmeal (if tolerated) gluten-free breads (if tolerated)	wheat barley rye any gluten-containing bread
FRUIT	all fruits		all berries: blueberries raspberries, strawberries all citrus: lemons, limes, grapefruit, oranges cherries, grapes, bananas, plantains	all other fruits, including apples, mangoes, pineapple, & stone fruits	all fruits that work for your body	any fruit that causes diegstive problems
FATS	avocado (all forms) coconut (all forms) nuts & seeds olives (all forms) palm oil palm shortening	canola oil vegetable oil vegetable shortening	avocado (all forms) coconut oil & milk nuts & seeds olives (all forms) palm oil palm shortening	canola oil vegetable oil vegetable shortening	all natural, healthy, unprocessed fats that work for your body	any healthy fat that causes diegstive problems unhealthy fats (canola oil, vegetable oil, vegetable shortening)

	PALEO		THE PROJECT		PERFECT YOU PLAN	
	IN	OUT	IN	OUT	IN	OUT
FLOURS	nut & seed flours coconut flour cassava flour arrowroot starch tapioca starch	flours made from grains		flours made from grains nut & seed flours coconut flour cassava flour tapioca starch arrowroot starch	any gluten-free flour that supports a healthy body & relationship to food	flours containing gluten GMO flours any gluten-free flour that does not support a healthy body & relationship to food
SUGARS	agave coconut sugar date sugar honey maple sugar maple syrup molasses stevia	refined sugars brown sugar powdered sugar artificial sweeteners	dates	refined sugars artifical sweeteners natural sweeteners	any natural or processed sugar (ideally organic) that supports a healthy body & relationship to food	artificial sweeteners any natural or processed sugar (organic or conventional) that does not support a healthy body & relationship to food
DRINKS	100% fruit juice coffee tea sparkling water	soda (diet or regular)	coffee tea unflavored sparkling water	soda (diet or regular) flavored sparkling water 100% fruit juice	any natural coffee, tea, sparkling water, and occasional fruit juice that supports a healthy body & relationship to food	soda (diet or regular) any natural coffee, any tea, sparkling water, or fruit juice that does not support a healthy body & relationship to food
ALCOHOL	clear liquors champagne hard cider red wine	beer brown liquors		all alcohol	any wine, beer, cider, or liquor that doesn't jeopardize a healthy body & relationship to food	any wine, beer, cider, or liquor that jeopardizes a healthy body & relationship to food
OTHER	vanilla extract other natural flavor extracts sea salt seaweed algae	MSG artificial food colorings artificial ingredients	vanilla extract other natural flavor extracts sea salt seaweed algae	MSG artificial food colorings artificial ingredients	natural flavor extracts sea salt seaweed algae	MSG artificial food colorings that don't support a healthy body artificial ingredients that don't support a healthy body & relationship to food
SUPPLEMENTS	collagen peptides gelatin	any supplement containing sugar, dairy, non-natural sweeteners, food dyes, or other unnatural ingredients	grass-fed whey protein (no more than 2 ingredients) collagen peptides gelatin vitamins, minerals, & medications prescribed by a physician natural multivitamins as needed	pre-mixed pre- & post-workout complex protein powders caffeine supplements energy supplements	grass-fed whey protein (no more than 2 ingredients) collagen peptides gelatin vitamins, minerals, & medications prescribed by a physician natural multivitamins as needed	pre-mixed pre- & post-workout complex protein powders caffeine supplements energy supplements

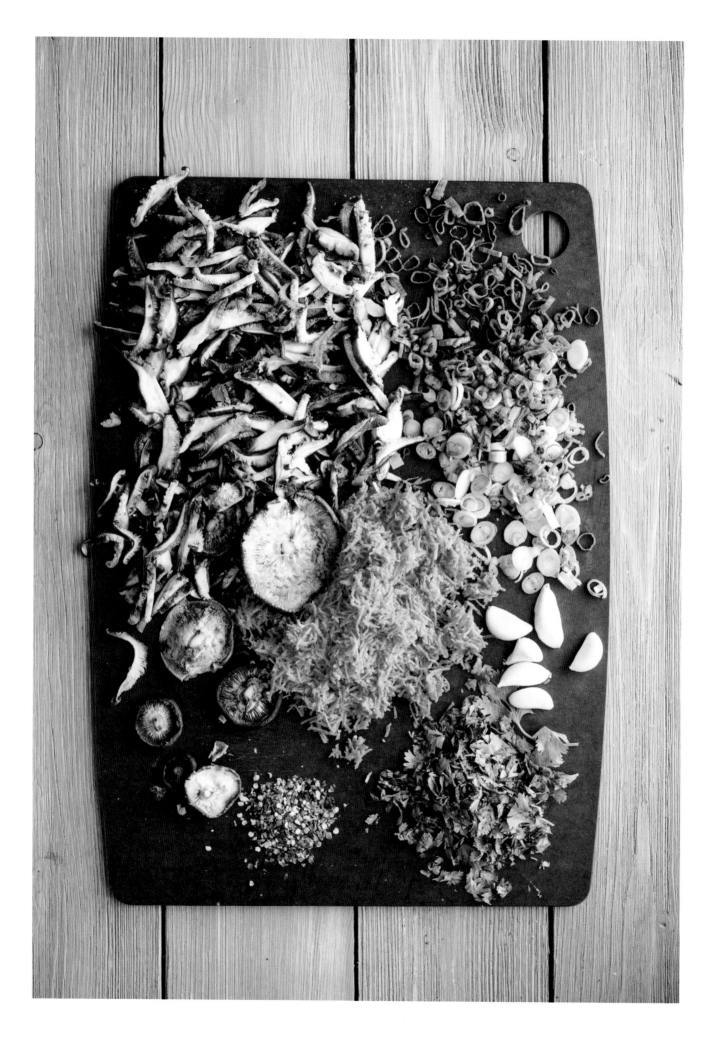

your portion compass

Let's get you up to speed on this new (actually not that new) topic of conversation.

Do portion sizes really matter? I thought that as long as I ate healthy, nourishing, whole, real foods that fall within the Paleo template, I don't need to track serving sizes. Now you're saying otherwise?

A subjective view on the history: I believe that in order to get the majority of the population to overcome their obsessive calorie-counting habit (which largely stems from the belief that fat is bad), we (the nutritionists, coaches, and other healthcare professionals who advocate for a "real food" lifestyle), have been telling people to make the leap from:

COUNT CALORIES   TO   JUST EAT REAL FOOD

But I'd like to take this one step further. While the "just eat real food" mantra can help you achieve freedom from dietary dogma, it's not guaranteed to help you achieve all your health goals. The thing is, size does matter. *Portions matter.*

If you have specific health and fitness goals, there are ways to fine-tune the Paleo lifestyle to support your efforts. While an obsessive "the fewer calories, the better" approach can actually counteract efforts to maintain a healthy body and mind, staying mindful of major food groups and appropriate portions for *your* body can be wonderfully enlightening and empowering . . . at least for a short time.

Here's the thing: I'm not suggesting that you count or measure your food for eternity. Rather, in order to heal your relationship with food, I suggest that you make the effort to learn what your body truly needs. Track, journal, and learn *from yourself.* After four weeks of learning as much as you can about your body, healthy intuitive eating that (almost magically) supports your long-term health goals should become habit.

So how much should I eat?

That's a fantastic question. The best answer I can give you is intentionally ambiguous. You see, each person is unique—with unique needs. What works for one person will not work for the next. That being said, I'm going to give you a rough go-by as it pertains to the Fed & Fit Project, the 28-Day Food & Fitness Plan, and the recipes in this book. In an effort to keep things as straightforward as possible, I've broken up portion needs into just two categories: male and female.

The amounts listed in the chart on the following pages are guidelines, and my perspective is that people wanting to lose weight will lose weight by following these numbers; people wanting to maintain weight will maintain; and people wanting to gain healthy body mass will gain. This portion compass is a great starting point while you work to fine-tune the plan for your body's unique needs, but you do not have to use it while on the Project. It is meant as a resource for those of you who are looking for portion guidance.

If you're looking for portion information for a food that is in scope but is not listed in the chart, simply find a similar food in the chart and use its portion recommendation.

FOODS WITH NO PORTION SIZE LIMITS

All herbs (fresh or dried)	Lemongrass	Vinegar
Capers	Mustard	Wasabi
Chives	Onions (raw)	Caffeine-free herbal tea
Garlic	Scallions	Unflavored sparkling water
Ginger	Shallots	
Horseradish	Turmeric	Water

note

For more information about portion sizes, losing body fat, and general metabolism science, check out Pillar #3: Food, beginning on page 38.

	Count	Volume (cup)	Weight	Calories	Protein (g)	Fat (g)	Carbs (g)
UNPREPARED PROTEINS							
WHOLE EGGS	2–3 large eggs		150 g / 5.3 ounces	213	18	15	0
CHICKEN BREASTS	1 small breast half		140 g / 5 ounces	155	30	0	0
CHICKEN THIGHS	2 thighs		138 g / 4.9 ounces	164	28	6	0
CHICKEN WINGS	6 wings		126 g / 4.5 ounces	279	22.5	18	0
GROUND CHICKEN	5 ounces		140 g / 5 ounces	200	25	10	0
TURKEY BREAST	⅛ whole breast		112 g / 4 ounces	116	20	0	4
GROUND TURKEY	5 ounces		140 g / 5 ounces	210	25	10	0
QUAIL	1 quail		109 g / 3.8 ounces	209	21	13	0
BEEF CHUCK (LEAN)	5 ounces		140 g / 5 ounces	340	25	25	0
BEEF FLANK STEAK	5 ounces		140 g / 5 ounces	190	29.4	7	0
BEEF LIVER	4 ounces		112 g / 4 ounces	152	24	4	4
BEEF RIB EYE	4 ounces		112 g / 4 ounces	308	20	24	0
BEEF SIRLOIN	5 ounces		140 g / 5 ounces	200	30	10	0
BEEF TENDERLOIN	4 ounces		112 g / 4 ounces	276	20	20	0
BEEF TONGUE	5 ounces		140 g / 5 ounces	315	20	25	5
GROUND BEEF	5 ounces		140 g / 5 ounces	300	25	20	0
GROUND BUFFALO	5 ounces		140 g / 5 ounces	310	25	20	0
PORK CHOPS	1 medium chop		158 g / 5.6 ounces	194	34	7	0
PORK TENDERLOIN	¼ tenderloin		134 g / 4.7 ounces	146	27	4	0
GROUND PORK	5 ounces		140 g / 5 ounces	370	25	30	0
LAMB CHOPS	5 ounces		140 g / 5 ounces	290	25	20	0
BRATWURST	1½ links		99 g / 3.5 ounces	294	12	25.5	2
BREAKFAST SAUSAGE	4 ounces		112 g / 4 ounces	336	16	30	0
CHORIZO	4 ounces		112 g / 4 ounces	516	28	44	2
ITALIAN SAUSAGE	1½ links		126 g / 4.5 ounces	188	21	11	3
VENISON / OTHER GAME MEAT	5 ounces		140 g / 5 ounces	155	30	5	0
COD	5 ounces		140 g / 5 ounces	115	25	0	0
GROUPER	5 ounces		140 g / 5 ounces	130	25	0	0
HALIBUT	5 ounces		140 g / 5 ounces	155	30	5	0
SALMON	5 ounces		140 g / 5 ounces	200	30	10	0
SEA BASS	5 ounces		140 g / 5 ounces	135	25	5	0
SNAPPER	5 ounces		140 g / 5 ounces	140	30	0	0
TILAPIA	5 ounces		140 g / 5 ounces	135	30	0	0
TUNA	5 ounces		140 g / 5 ounces	155	35	0	0
WHITEFISH	5 ounces		140 g / 5 ounces	190	25	10	0
CANNED CRAB MEAT	1 (5-ounce) can		140 g / 5 ounces	115	25	1	0
CANNED SALMON	1 (5-ounce) can		140 g / 5 ounces	225	40	10	0
CANNED TUNA	1 (5-ounce) can		140 g / 5 ounces	180	35	5	0
SARDINES (PACKED IN WATER)	1 (4.4-ounce) tin		140 g / 5 ounces	183	32.5	5	0
COLLAGEN PEPTIDES	2 scoops	3 heaping tablespoons	20 g / .7 ounces	72	18	0	0
GELATIN	1 tablespoon		7.5 g / .26 ounces	25	6	0	0
GRASS-FED WHEY PROTEIN	1 scoop	about 2 tablespoons	26 g / 0.9 ounces	110	21	1.5	2
CRUNCHY VEGETABLES							
ARUGULA, RAW	3 large handfuls	2 packed cups	40 g / 1.4 ounces	12	1.2	0.4	1.6
ARTICHOKES	2 artichokes		256 g / 9 ounces	120	8.4	0.4	26
ARTICHOKE HEARTS (CANNED OR JARRED), DRAINED		½ cup	85 g / 3 ounces	40	3	0	8
ASPARAGUS	½ bundle	1½ cups	201 g / 7.1 ounces	41	4.4	0.3	7.5
BAMBOO SHOOTS		½ cup	76 g / 2.7 ounces	21	2	0.2	4
BOK CHOY, COOKED		½ cup	85 g / 3 ounces	10	1.35	0.15	1.5
BROCCOLI, RAW	1 small head	1½ heaping cups	137 g / 4.8 ounces	46	3.9	0.5	9
BROCCOLINI, RAW	½ bundle	1 cup	88 g / 3.1 ounces	30	2.4	0	5.8
BRUSSELS SPROUTS, COOKED	⅓ bag	1 cup	156 g / 5.5 ounces	56	4	0	12
CABBAGE	¼ head	1 cup	89 g / 3.1 ounces	22	1.1	0.1	5
NAPA CABBAGE, COOKED	¼ head	1 cup	109 g / 3.8 ounces	13	1	0	2

MEN

	Count	Volume (cup)	Weight	Calories	Protein (g)	Fat (g)	Carbs (g)
UNPREPARED PROTEINS							
WHOLE EGGS	3–4 large eggs		200 g / 7 ounces	284	24	20	0
CHICKEN BREASTS	1½ small breast halves		210 g / 7.5 ounces	233	45	0	0
CHICKEN THIGHS	3 thighs		207 g / 7.3 ounces	246	42	9	0
CHICKEN WINGS	10 wings		210 g / 7.5 ounces	465	37.5	30	0
GROUND CHICKEN	8 ounces		224 g / 8 ounces	320	40	16	0
TURKEY BREAST	⅕ whole breast		168 g / 6 ounces	174	30	0	6
GROUND TURKEY	8 ounces		224 g / 8 ounces	336	40	16	0
QUAIL	2 quail		218 g / 7.7 ounces	418	42	26	0
BEEF CHUCK (LEAN)	8 ounces		224 g / 8 ounces	544	40	40	0
BEEF FLANK STEAK	8 ounces		224 g / 8 ounces	299	46.2	11	0
BEEF LIVER	6 ounces		168 g / 6 ounces	228	36	6	6
BEEF RIB EYE	6 ounces		168 g / 6 ounces	462	30	36	0
BEEF SIRLOIN	8 ounces		224 g / 8 ounces	320	48	16	0
BEEF TENDERLOIN	6 ounces		168 g / 6 ounces	414	30	30	0
BEEF TONGUE	8 ounces		224 g / 8 ounces	504	32	40	8
GROUND BEEF	8 ounces		224 g / 8 ounces	480	40	32	0
GROUND BUFFALO	8 ounces		224 g / 8 ounces	496	40	32	0
PORK CHOPS	1½ medium chops		237 g / 8.4 ounces	291	51	11	0
PORK TENDERLOIN	⅓ tenderloin		179 g / 6.3 ounces	195	36	5.7	0
GROUND PORK	8 ounces		224 g / 8 ounces	592	40	48	0
LAMB CHOPS	8 ounces		224 g / 8 ounces	464	40	32	0
BRATWURST	2 links		133 g / 4.7 ounces	392	16	34	2.6
BREAKFAST SAUSAGE	6 ounces		168 g / 6 ounces	511	24.5	45.5	0
CHORIZO	6 ounces		168 g / 6 ounces	774	42	66	3
ITALIAN SAUSAGE	2 links		168 g / 6 ounces	250	28	14	4
VENISON / OTHER GAME MEAT	8 ounces		224 g / 8 ounces	248	48	8	0
COD	8 ounces		224 g / 8 ounces	184	40	0	0
GROUPER	8 ounces		224 g / 8 ounces	208	40	0	0
HALIBUT	8 ounces		224 g / 8 ounces	248	48	8	0
SALMON	8 ounces		224 g / 8 ounces	320	48	16	0
SEA BASS	8 ounces		224 g / 8 ounces	216	40	8	0
SNAPPER	8 ounces		224 g / 8 ounces	224	48	0	0
TILAPIA	8 ounces		224 g / 8 ounces	216	48	0	0
TUNA	8 ounces		224 g / 8 ounces	248	56	0	0
WHITEFISH	8 ounces		224 g / 8 ounces	304	40	16	0
CANNED CRAB MEAT	1½ (5-ounce) cans		210 g / 7.5 ounces	172.5	37.5	1.5	0
CANNED SALMON	1½ (5-ounce) cans		210 g / 7.5 ounces	338	60	14	0
CANNED TUNA	1½ (5-ounce) cans		210 g / 7.5 ounces	270	52.5	7	0
SARDINES (PACKED IN WATER)	1½ (4.4-ounce) tins		210 g / 7.5 ounces	274	48	7.5	0
COLLAGEN PEPTIDES	2½ scoops	about ¼ cup	26 g / .9 ounces	96	24	0	0
GELATIN	1½ tablespoons		10.5 g / .37 ounces	37.5	9	0	0
GRASS-FED WHEY PROTEIN	1½ scoops	about 3 tablespoons	39 g / 1.4 ounces	165	31.5	2.3	3
CRUNCHY VEGETABLES							
ARUGULA, RAW	3 large handfuls	2 packed cups	40 g / 1.4 ounces	12	1.2	0.4	1.6
ARTICHOKES	2 artichokes		256 g / 9 ounces	120	8.4	0.4	26
ARTICHOKE HEARTS (CANNED OR JARRED), DRAINED		¾ cup	113 g / 4 ounces	53	4	0	11
ASPARAGUS	½ bundle	1½ cups	201 g / 7.1 ounces	41	4.4	0.3	7.5
BAMBOO SHOOTS		½ cup	76 g / 2.7 ounces	21	2	0.2	4
BOK CHOY, COOKED		½ cup	85 g / 3 ounces	10	1.35	0.15	1.5
BROCCOLI, RAW	1 small head	1½ heaping cups	137 g / 4.8 ounces	46	3.9	0.5	9
BROCCOLINI, RAW	½ bundle	1 cup	88 g / 3.1 ounces	30	2.4	0	5.8
BRUSSELS SPROUTS, COOKED	⅓ bag	1 cup	156 g / 5.5 ounces	56	4	0	12
CABBAGE	¼ head	1 cup	89 g / 3.1 ounces	22	1.1	0.1	5
NAPA CABBAGE, COOKED	¼ head	1 cup	109 g / 3.8 ounces	13	1	0	2

	Count	Volume (cup)	Weight	Calories	Protein (g)	Fat (g)	Carbs (g)
CRUNCHY VEGETABLES							
CAULIFLOWER, RAW	½ head	1½ heaping cups	160 g / 5.6 ounces	41	3	0.4	7.5
CELERY	4 stalks	1½ cups	150 g / 5.3 ounces	24	1.2	0.4	4.8
COLLARDS, RAW	3 large handfuls	2 packed cups	72 g / 2.5 ounces	22	2.2	0.4	4
COLLARDS, COOKED		½ cup	95 g / 3.4 ounces	31	2.5	0.7	5.5
CUCUMBER	⅓ cucumber	1 cup	104 g / 3.7 ounces	16	0.6	0.2	3.8
DAIKON	½ (7-inch) radish	1 cup	169 g / 6 ounces	30	1	0.1	7
EGGPLANT		1 cup	82 g / 2.9 ounces	20	0.8	0.1	4.8
FENNEL	⅓ bulb	1 cup	87.5 g / 3.1 ounces	27	1.1	0.2	6
GREEN BEANS	1 large handful	1 cup	100 g / 3.5 ounces	31	1.8	0.2	7
HEARTS OF PALM (CANNED)		½ cup	73 g / 2.6 ounces	20	2	0.5	3.5
JICAMA	½ medium jicama	2 cups	260 g / 9.2 ounces	100	1.8	0.2	22
KALE, RAW	3 large handfuls	2 packed cups	134 g / 4.7 ounces	66	5.8	1.2	12
KALE, COOKED		½ cup	65 g / 2.3 ounces	18	1.25	0.25	3.5
KOHLRABI	1–2 bulbs	1 cup	135 g / 4.8 ounces	37	2.3	0.1	8
LEEKS	1 leek	1 cup	89 g / 3.1 ounces	54	1.3	0.3	13
BUTTER (BIBB) LETTUCE	3 large handfuls	2 packed cups	110 g / 3.9 ounces	14	2	0	2
ICEBERG LETTUCE	3 large handfuls	2 packed cups	144 g / 5.1 ounces	20	1.2	0.2	4.2
ROMAINE LETTUCE	3 large handfuls	2 packed cups	94 g / 3.3 ounces	16	1.2	0.2	3
MUSHROOMS		1 cup	54 g / 1.9 ounces	21	0.8	0.3	3.7
OKRA, RAW	10 pods	1½ cups	150 g / 5.3 ounces	50	3	0.3	10.5
LARGE PEPPERS (BELL, POBLANO, HATCH), RAW	1 pepper	1 cup	150 g / 5.3 ounces	30	1.3	0.3	7
LARGE PEPPERS (BELL, POBLANO, HATCH), COOKED	2 peppers	1½ cups	202 g / 7.1 ounces	57	1.8	0.4	14
RADICCHIO	3 large handfuls	2 packed cups	80 g / 2.8 ounces	18	1.2	0.2	3.6
RADISHES	1 bunch	1 cup	116 g / 4.1 ounces	18	0.8	0.1	3.9
RHUBARB	3 stalks	1 cup	123 g / 4.3 ounces	26	1	0	6
SEA VEGETABLES, FRESH		⅔ cup prepared	100 g / 3.5 ounces	60	5	1	5
SEA VEGETABLES, DRIED (NO OIL)			5 g / .18 ounces	20	2	0	2
SPINACH, RAW	3 large handfuls	2 packed cups	60 g / 2.1 ounces	14	1.8	0.2	2.2
SPINACH, COOKED		½ cup	90 g / 3.2 ounces	20.5	2.5	0.25	3.5
SPROUTS	1 small handful	½ cup	17 g / 0.6 ounces	4	0.7	0.1	0.4
SWISS CHARD, RAW	3 large handfuls	2 packed cups	72 g / 2.5 ounces	14	1.2	0.2	2.6
SWISS CHARD, COOKED		½ cup	87.5 g / 3.1 ounces	17.5	1.65	0	3.5
TOMATILLOS		1 cup	132 g / 4.7 ounces	42	1.2	1.4	7.8
TOMATOES		1 cup	180 g / 6.3 ounces	32	1.6	0.4	7
TURNIPS	2 medium turnips	2 cups	260 g / 9.2 ounces	72	2.4	0.2	16
TURNIP GREENS	3 large handfuls	2 packed cups	110 g / 3.9 ounces	36	2	0	8
YELLOW SQUASH	1–2 squash	2 cups	126 g / 4.5 ounces	38	2.8	0.4	7.6
ZUCCHINI, RAW	1–2 zucchini	2 cups	148 g / 5.2 ounces	42	3	0.8	7.8
STARCHY VEGETABLES							
BEETS	2 small beets	1½ cups cubed	204 g / 7.2 ounces	89	3.3	0.3	20
CARROTS	3 medium carrots	1½ cups chopped	192 g / 6.8 ounces	80	1.8	0.5	18
GREEN PEAS		¾ cup	110 g / 3.9 ounces	89	6	0.5	16
PARSNIPS	3 medium parsnips	1½ cups chopped	200 g / 7.1 ounces	150	2.4	0.6	36
PLANTAINS, RAW	½ plantain	⅓ cup	50 g / 1.8 ounces	60	0.6	0.1	17
PLANTAIN CHIPS	20 chips		28 g / 1 ounce	140	1	6.5	20
FINGERLING POTATOES	1 handful	1 cup cubed	170 g / 6 ounces	140	2	0	30
NEW POTATOES	1 handful	1 cup cubed	150 g / 5.3 ounces	104	2.6	0.2	24
RUSSET POTATOES	1 small potato	1 cup cubed	150 g / 5.3 ounces	120	3.2	0.2	28
YUKON GOLD POTATOES	1 small potato	¾ cup cubed	112 g / 4 ounces	77	1.9	0.1	18
PUMPKIN (BAKING)	¼ pumpkin	1½ cups	174 g / 6.1 ounces	45	1.8	0.2	12
SNAP PEAS		1 cup	62 g / 2.2 ounces	26	1.8	0.1	4.8
SNOW PEAS		1 cup	62 g / 2.2 ounces	26	1.8	0.1	4.8
ACORN SQUASH	¼ squash	1 cup cubed	140 g / 5 ounces	56	1.1	0.1	15
BUTTERCUP SQUASH	¼ squash	1 cup cubed	113 g / 4 ounces	40	1.3	0	9.3

	Count	Volume (cup)	Weight	Calories	Protein (g)	Fat (g)	Carbs (g)
CRUNCHY VEGETABLES							
CAULIFLOWER, RAW	½ head	1½ heaping cups	160 g / 5.6 ounces	41	3	0.4	7.5
CELERY	4 stalks	1½ cups	150 g / 5.3 ounces	24	1.2	0.4	4.8
COLLARDS, RAW	3 large handfuls	2 packed cups	72 g / 2.5 ounces	22	2.2	0.4	4
COLLARDS, COOKED		½ cup	95 g / 3.4 ounces	31	2.5	0.7	5.5
CUCUMBER	⅓ cucumber	1 cup	104 g / 3.7 ounces	16	0.6	0.2	3.8
DAIKON	½ (7-inch) radish	1 cup	169 g / 6 ounces	30	1	0.1	7
EGGPLANT		1 cup	82 g / 2.9 ounces	20	0.8	0.1	4.8
FENNEL	⅓ bulb	1 cup	87.5 g / 3.1 ounces	27	1.1	0.2	6
GREEN BEANS	1 large handful	1 cup	100 g / 3.5 ounces	31	1.8	0.2	7
HEARTS OF PALM (CANNED)		½ cup	73 g / 2.6 ounces	20	2	0.5	3.5
JICAMA	½ medium jicama	2 cups	260 g / 9.2 ounces	100	1.8	0.2	22
KALE, RAW	3 large handfuls	2 packed cups	134 g / 4.7 ounces	66	5.8	1.2	12
KALE, COOKED		½ cup	65 g / 2.3 ounces	18	1.25	0.25	3.5
KOHLRABI	1–2 bulbs	1 cup	135 g / 4.8 ounces	37	2.3	0.1	8
LEEKS	1 leek	1 cup	89 g / 3.1 ounces	54	1.3	0.3	13
BUTTER (BIBB) LETTUCE	3 large handfuls	2 packed cups	110 g / 3.9 ounces	14	2	0	2
ICEBERG LETTUCE	3 large handfuls	2 packed cups	144 g / 5.1 ounces	20	1.2	0.2	4.2
ROMAINE LETTUCE	3 large handfuls	2 packed cups	94 g / 3.3 ounces	16	1.2	0.2	3
MUSHROOMS		1 cup	54 g / 1.9 ounces	21	0.8	0.3	3.7
OKRA, RAW	10 pods	1½ cups	150 g / 5.3 ounces	50	3	0.3	10.5
LARGE PEPPERS [BELL, POBLANO, HATCH], RAW	1 pepper	1 cup	150 g / 5.3 ounces	30	1.3	0.3	7
LARGE PEPPERS [BELL, POBLANO, HATCH], COOKED	2 peppers	1½ cups	202 g / 7.1 ounces	57	1.8	0.4	14
RADICCHIO	3 large handfuls	2 packed cups	80 g / 2.8 ounces	18	1.2	0.2	3.6
RADISHES	1 bunch	1 cup	116 g / 4.1 ounces	18	0.8	0.1	3.9
RHUBARB	3 stalks	1 cup	123 g / 4.3 ounces	26	1	0	6
SEA VEGETABLES, FRESH		⅔ cup prepared	100 g / 3.5 ounces	60	5	1	5
SEA VEGETABLES, DRIED (NO OIL)			5 g / .18 ounces	20	2	0	2
SPINACH, RAW	3 large handfuls	2 packed cups	60 g / 2.1 ounces	14	1.8	0.2	2.2
SPINACH, COOKED		½ cup	90 g / 3.2 ounces	20.5	2.5	0.25	3.5
SPROUTS	1 small handful	½ cup	17 g / 0.6 ounces	4	0.7	0.1	0.4
SWISS CHARD, RAW	3 large handfuls	2 packed cups	72 g / 2.5 ounces	14	1.2	0.2	2.6
SWISS CHARD, COOKED		½ cup	87.5 g / 3.1 ounces	17.5	1.65	0	3.5
TOMATILLOS		1 cup	132 g / 4.7 ounces	42	1.2	1.4	7.8
TOMATOES		1 cup	180 g / 6.3 ounces	32	1.6	0.4	7
TURNIPS	2 medium turnips	2 cups	260 g / 9.2 ounces	72	2.4	0.2	16
TURNIP GREENS	3 large handfuls	2 packed cups	110 g / 3.9 ounces	36	2	0	8
YELLOW SQUASH	1–2 squash	2 cups	126 g / 4.5 ounces	38	2.8	0.4	7.6
ZUCCHINI, RAW	1–2 zucchini	2 cups	148 g / 5.2 ounces	42	3	0.8	7.8
STARCHY VEGETABLES							
BEETS	3 small beets	2 cups cubed	272 g / 9.6 ounces	118	4.4	0.4	26
CARROTS	4 medium carrots	2 cups chopped	256 g / 9 ounces	106	2.4	0.6	24
GREEN PEAS		1 cup	145 g / 5.1 ounces	118	8	0.6	21
PARSNIPS	4 medium parsnips	2 cups chopped	166 g / 5.9 ounces	200	3.2	0.8	48
PLANTAINS, RAW	¾ plantain	½ cup	74 g / 2.6 ounces	90	1	0.25	24
PLANTAIN CHIPS	30 chips		42 g / 1.5 ounce	210	1.5	9.8	30
FINGERLING POTATOES	1 large handful	1½ cups cubed	255 g / 9 ounces	210	6	0	45
NEW POTATOES	1 large handful	1½ cups cubed	225 g / 7.9 ounces	156	3.9	0.3	36
RUSSET POTATOES	1 medium potato	1½ cups cubed	225 g / 7.9 ounces	180	4.8	0.3	42
YUKON GOLD POTATOES	1 small-medium potato	1 cup cubed	150 g / 5.3 ounces	104	2.6	0.2	24
PUMPKIN (BAKING)	⅓ pumpkin	2 cups	232 g / 8.2 ounces	60	2.4	0.2	16
SNAP PEAS		1½ cups	93 g / 3.3 ounces	39	2.7	0.2	7.2
SNOW PEAS		1½ cups	93 g / 3.3 ounces	39	2.7	0.2	7.2
ACORN SQUASH	⅓ squash	1½ cups cubed	210 g / 7.5 ounces	84	1.7	0.2	22
BUTTERCUP SQUASH	⅓ squash	1½ cups cubed	168 g / 6 ounces	60	2	0	14

	Count	Volume (cup)	Weight	Calories	Protein (g)	Fat (g)	Carbs (g)
STARCHY VEGETABLES							
BUTTERNUT SQUASH		1½ cups cubed	210 g / 7.4 ounces	95	2.1	0.2	24
CARNIVAL SQUASH	¼ squash	1 cup cubed	113 g / 4 ounces	40	1.3	0	9.3
DELICATA SQUASH	about ½ squash	1½ cups cubed	168 g / 6 ounces	60	2	0	14
KABOCHA SQUASH		1 cup	140 g / 5 ounces	80	1	0	7
SPAGHETTI SQUASH		1½ cups	150 g / 5.3 ounces	46	0.9	0.9	11
SWEET POTATOES	1 small sweet potato	1 cup cubed	133 g / 4.7 ounces	114	2.1	0.1	27
YAMS	½ large yam	¾ cup cubed	113 g / 4 ounces	133	1.7	0.2	32
FATS							
AVOCADOS	¼ medium avocado	¼ cup	38 g / 1.3 ounces	60	0.8	5.5	3.3
UNSWEETENED SHREDDED COCONUT		2 tablespoons	10 g / .35 ounces	73	6.6	0.6	2.7
ALMONDS	12 almonds	2 tablespoons	14 g / .5 ounces	82	3	7	3
ALMOND BUTTER		1 tablespoon	16 g / .56 ounces	105	3	9	3.5
CASHEWS	12 cashews	2 tablespoons	14 g / .5 ounces	79	2.5	6	4.5
CASHEW BUTTER		1 tablespoon	16 g / .56 ounces	90	3	7	5
CHIA SEEDS		2 tablespoons	24 g / .85 ounces	120	6	6	10
FLAX SEEDS		1 tablespoon	7.5 g / .26 ounces	45	1.5	3.5	2
PUMPKIN SEEDS		2 tablespoons	8 g / .3 ounces	36	1.5	1.5	4.3
SESAME SEEDS		1 tablespoon	9 g / .32 ounces	52	1.6	4.5	2.1
SUNFLOWER SEEDS		2 tablespoons	17 g / 0.6 ounces	102	3.6	9	3.5
SUNFLOWER SEED BUTTER		1 tablespoon	16 g / .56 ounces	110	3	10	2.5
TAHINI		1 tablespoon	16 g / .56 ounces	89	2.6	8	3.2
BUTTER		1 tablespoon	14 g / .5 ounces	100	0	12	0
GHEE		1 tablespoon	14 g / .5 ounces	120	0	14	0
COCONUT OIL		1 tablespoon	14 g / .5 ounces	120	0	14	0
MCT OIL		1 tablespoon	14 g / .5 ounces	120	0	14	0
OLIVES	depends on the olive	¼ cup	34 g / 1.2 ounces	40	0.4	3.6	2
OLIVE OIL		1 tablespoon	14 g / .5 ounces	120	0	14	0
FRUITS							
BANANAS	½ large banana	½ cup chopped	136 g / 4.8 ounces	60	0	0	15
BLACKBERRIES		1 cup	144 g / 5.1 ounces	62	2	0.7	14
BLOOD ORANGES	1 orange		240 g / 8.5 ounces	105	0	0	24
BLUEBERRIES		¾ cup	148 g / 5.2 ounces	85	1.1	0.5	21
CHERRIES		½ cup pitted	78 g / 2.8 ounces	39	0.8	0.25	9.5
CLEMENTINES	1 clementine		74 g / 2.6 ounces	35	0.6	0.1	9
CRANBERRIES		1 cup	100 g / 3.5 ounces	46	0.4	0.1	12
CURRANTS		1 cup	113 g / 4 ounces	63	1.6	0.2	15
DATES	2 pitted dates	2 tablespoons	14 g / .5 ounces	20	0.2	0	5
ELDERBERRIES		½ cup	145 g / 5.1 ounces	106	1	0.7	27
GOOSEBERRIES		1 cup	150 g / 5.3 ounces	66	1.3	0.9	15
GRAPEFRUIT	½ grapefruit		123 g / 4.3 ounces	52	0.9	0.2	13
GRAPES		½ cup	46 g / 1.6 ounces	31	0.3	0.2	8
KEY LIMES	4 limes, juiced		88 g / 3.1 ounces	22	0.5	0.1	8
KUMQUATS	5 kumquats		95 g / 3.4 ounces	65	2	1	15
LEMONS	2 lemons, juiced		94 g / 3.3 ounces	24	0.6	0.2	8
LIMES	2 limes, juiced		88 g / 3.1 ounces	22	0.5	0.1	8
MANDARIN ORANGES	1 orange		88 g / 3.1 ounces	47	1	0	12
MEYER LEMONS	2 lemons, juiced		94 g / 3.3 ounces	24	0.6	0.2	8
NAVEL ORANGES	1 small orange		140 g / 5 ounces	69	1.3	0.2	18
POMEGRANATES		¼ cup	44 g / 1.6 ounces	36	0.8	0.5	8
POMELOS	½ pomelo		304 g / 10.7 ounces	116	2.3	0.1	30
RASPBERRIES		1 cup	123 g / 4.3 ounces	65	1.5	0.8	15
STRAWBERRIES		1 cup sliced	166 g / 5.9 ounces	54	1.1	0.5	13
TANGELOS	1 tangelo		109 g / 3.8 ounces	70	1	1	13
TANGERINES	1 tangerine		88 g / 3.1 ounces	47	0.7	0.3	12

	Count	Volume (cup)	Weight	Calories	Protein (g)	Fat (g)	Carbs (g)
STARCHY VEGETABLES							
BUTTERNUT SQUASH		2 cups cubed	280 g / 9.9 ounces	126	2.8	0.2	32
CARNIVAL SQUASH	⅓ squash	1½ cups cubed	168 g / 6 ounces	60	2	0	14
DELICATA SQUASH	about ⅔ squash	2 cups cubed	224 / 8 ounces	80	2.6	0	18.6
KABOCHA SQUASH		1½ cups	210 g / 7.5 ounces	120	1.5	0	11
SPAGHETTI SQUASH		1¾ cups	175 g / 6.2 ounces	54	1.1	1.1	13
SWEET POTATOES	1 medium sweet potato	1.5 cups cubed	200 g / 7 ounces	171	3.2	0.2	41
YAMS	¾ large yam	1 cup cubed	150 g / 5.3 ounces	177	2.3	0.3	42
FATS							
AVOCADOS	⅓ avocado	⅓ cup	50 g / 1.8 ounces	80	1	7.3	4.3
UNSWEETENED SHREDDED COCONUT		3 tablespoons	15 g / .53 ounces	110	1	10	4
ALMONDS	18 almonds	3 tablespoons	21 g / .74 ounces	122	4.5	10.5	4.5
ALMOND BUTTER		2 tablespoons	32 g / 1.1 ounces	210	6	18	7
CASHEWS	18 cashews	3 tablespoons	21 g / .74 ounces	118	3.8	9	6.8
CASHEW BUTTER		2 tablespoons	32 g / 1.1 ounces	180	6	14	10
CHIA SEEDS		3 tablespoons	36 g / 1.3 ounces	180	9	9	15
FLAX SEEDS		2 tablespoons	15 g / .53 ounces	90	3	7	4
PUMPKIN SEEDS		3 tablespoons	12 g / .4 ounces	54	2.3	2.3	6.4
SESAME SEEDS		2 tablespoons	18 g / .63 ounces	104	3.2	9	4.2
SUNFLOWER SEEDS		3 tablespoons	26 g / .9 ounces	154	5.8	13.6	5.3
SUNFLOWER SEED BUTTER		2 tablespoons	32 g / 1.1 ounces	220	6	20	5
TAHINI		2 tablespoons	32 g / 1.1 ounces	178	5.2	16	6.4
BUTTER		2 tablespoons	28 g / 1 ounce	200	0	24	0
GHEE		2 tablespoons	28 g / 1 ounce	240	0	28	0
COCONUT OIL		2 tablespoons	28 g / 1 ounce	240	0	28	0
MCT OIL		2 tablespoons	28 g / 1 ounce	240	0	28	0
OLIVES	depends on the olive	⅓ cup	42 g / 1.5 ounce	50	0.5	4.5	2.5
OLIVE OIL		2 tablespoons	28 g / 1 ounce	240	0	28	0
FRUITS							
BLACKBERRIES		1 cup	144 g / 5.1 ounces	62	2	0.7	14
BLOOD ORANGES	1 orange		240 g / 8.5 ounces	105	0	0	24
BLUEBERRIES		¾ cup	148 g / 5.2 ounces	85	1.1	0.5	21
CHERRIES		½ cup pitted	78 g / 2.8 ounces	39	0.8	0.25	9.5
CLEMENTINES	1 clementine		74 g / 2.6 ounces	35	0.6	0.1	9
CRANBERRIES		1 cup	100 g / 3.5 ounces	46	0.4	0.1	12
CURRANTS		1 cup	113 g / 4 ounces	63	1.6	0.2	15
DATES	3 pitted dates	3 tablespoons	21 g / .74 ounces	60	0.6	0	15
ELDERBERRIES		½ cup	145 g / 5.1 ounces	106	1	0.7	27
GOOSEBERRIES		1 cup	150 g / 5.3 ounces	66	1.3	0.9	15
GRAPEFRUIT	½ grapefruit		123 g / 4.3 ounces	52	0.9	0.2	13
GRAPES		½ cup	46 g / 1.6 ounces	31	0.3	0.2	8
KEY LIMES	4 limes, juiced		88 g / 3.1 ounces	22	0.5	0.1	8
KUMQUATS	7 kumquats		95 g / 3.4 ounces	65	2	1	15
LEMONS	2 lemons, juiced		94 g / 3.3 ounces	24	0.6	0.2	8
LIMES	2 limes, juiced		88 g / 3.1 ounces	22	0.5	0.1	8
MANDARIN ORANGES	1 orange		88 g / 3.1 ounces	47	1	0	12
MEYER LEMONS	2 lemons, juiced		94 g / 3.3 ounces	24	0.6	0.2	8
NAVEL ORANGES	1 small orange		140 g / 5 ounces	69	1.3	0.2	18
POMEGRANATES		⅓ cup	58 g / 2 ounces	48	1	0.7	10.7
POMELOS	½ pomelo		304 g / 10.7 ounces	116	2.3	0.1	30
RASPBERRIES		1 cup	123 g / 4.3 ounces	65	1.5	0.8	15
STRAWBERRIES		1 cup sliced	166 g / 5.9 ounces	54	1.1	0.5	13
TANGELOS	1 tangelo		109 g / 3.8 ounces	70	1	1	13
TANGERINES	1 tangerine		88 g / 3.1 ounces	47	0.7	0.3	12
BANANAS	½ large banana	½ cup chopped	136 g / 4.8 ounces	60	0	0	15

the 28-day food & fitness plan

This is where the Four Pillars come together into an actionable plan! Food guidance is offered in the form of a detailed meal plan, fitness is covered by a comprehensive workout regimen, sleep and water intake are tracked daily, and mindset is actively incorporated via the journal. Note that the meal and fitness plans provided should be considered *an* option, not the *only* option. If you prefer to design your own 28-day food and fitness plans, you'll find a DIY template on page 103.

meal plan: use this one!

Using the recipes in this book, I've designed a 28-day meal plan that abides by the scope and approximate portion sizes of the Project. This meal plan is designed for two people who don't mind eating leftovers from dinner for lunch the next day. Shopping lists are included in this book (see pages 98 to 102) as well as in the Fed & Fit app.

Note that several recipes involve subrecipes. For example, the Chile Relleno Enchilada Casserole on day 28 calls for ½ batch of Paleo Sour Cream.

While the ingredients needed for these subrecipes are included in the shopping lists, you will need to account for the extra time it takes to make them while you're scheduling your meal prep efforts.

Some meals in this 28-day plan will make more than one day's leftovers for two people. In this case, I highly recommend freezing the extras so that you'll have healthy food at the ready after the Project concludes! I discuss the steps to freezing large meals into individual portions on page 118.

build your own meal plan

While you can absolutely follow the meal plan that I've designed for the Project, you can also build your own! Here's the daily template that I follow to build the perfect plate:

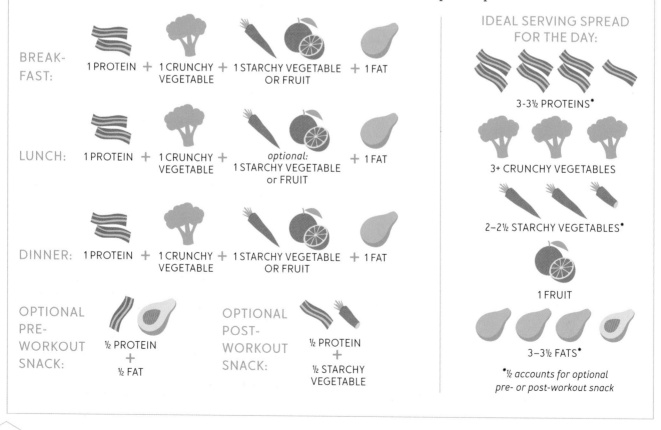

a couple sample days of eating on the project

EMILY *likes to work out at 5:30 a.m. She feels good during her workout without eating anything beforehand, so she chooses not to have a pre-workout snack (opting instead for a fasting workout). When she gets home, she fixes herself a big breakfast that also accounts for her post-workout snack (that is, she makes sure to include a starchy vegetable). Her breakfast includes a protein, a crunchy vegetable, a starchy vegetable, and a fat. She then gets ready for the day, packs her lunch, and drives to work. For lunch, Emily pulls out a meal made up of protein, crunchy vegetables, and fat. She opts out of a fruit or starchy vegetable; she doesn't feel she needs it, as her energy level is still high. She enjoys water and a cup of hot herbal tea in the afternoon and then drives home. For dinner, Emily has a protein, a crunchy vegetable, a starchy vegetable, and half a fat. She then has a dessert that combines the remaining half serving of fat and a fruit.*

WINSTON *leaves for work at 7:00 a.m. His mornings tend to feel a little rushed, so he likes to eat breakfast on the go, usually on his way to work. His breakfast includes a protein, a crunchy vegetable, a fruit, and a fat. For lunch, he enjoys a premade meal made up of protein, crunchy vegetables, and fat. He enjoys sparkling water in the afternoon and then leaves work by 6:00 p.m. Winston heads straight to the gym. Because it has been almost six hours since lunch, he eats a quick pre-workout snack to optimize his energy level. His snack consists of half a protein and half a fat. He drinks water on the way home and eats dinner when he gets there. Dinner consists of a protein, a crunchy vegetable, a starchy vegetable, and half a fat. He enjoys a dessert of fruit and his remaining half portion of fat.*

	WHAT EMILY ATE:	WHAT WINSTON ATE:
BREAKFAST:	[Post-workout] 3 eggs (1 protein) cooked in 1 teaspoon butter (⅓ fat) 1 cup steamed broccoli (1 crunchy vegetable) ½ plantain (1 starchy vegetable) cooked in 2 teaspoons butter (⅔ fat) *Consumed but little nutritional impact:* coffee, water, sea salt, and other natural seasonings	2 scoops protein powder (1 protein) 1½ cups frozen spinach (1 crunchy vegetable) ¾ cup frozen blueberries (1 fruit) 3 tablespoons coconut milk (1 fat) *Consumed but little nutritional impact:* 1 cup coffee and water
LUNCH:	1 grilled chicken breast half (1 protein) 2 cups chopped spinach plus ½ cup cherry tomatoes (1+ crunchy vegetable) 2 tablespoons Paleo ranch dressing (1 fat) *Consumed but little nutritional impact:* water and extra dried dill	8 ounces smoked salmon (1 protein) 2 cups chopped spinach plus ½ cup cherry tomatoes (1+ crunchy vegetable) 2 tablespoons Paleo ranch dressing (1 fat) *Consumed but little nutritional impact:* water and extra dried dill
AFTERNOON:	*Consumed but little nutritional impact:* 2 cups caffeine-free peppermint tea	1 hard-boiled egg (¼ protein) and a small handful of almonds (½ fat) *Consumed but little nutritional impact:* sparkling water and water
DINNER:	4 ounces pulled pork (1 protein) stuffed in a small baked potato (1 starchy vegetable) 1 cup steamed chopped kale (1 crunchy vegetable) topped with 1 tablespoon Paleo Buffalo sauce (½ fat) 1 cup fresh raspberries (1 fruit) topped with 1 tablespoon coconut milk (½ fat portion) *Consumed but little nutritional impact:* sea salt and water	6 ounces shredded chicken (1 protein) 1 cup basic cauliflower rice (1 crunchy vegetable) ½ cup hash browns (1 starchy vegetable) topped with 1 tablespoon 3-Ingredient Ranch (½ fat) and a handful of chopped cilantro ½ frozen banana (1 fruit) with 1 tablespoon unsweetened almond butter (½ fat) and cinnamon
EVENING:	*Consumed but little nutritional impact:* 1 mug of warm lemon ginger herbal tea	*Consumed but little nutritional impact:* 1 mug of warm lemon ginger herbal tea

remember, no snacking

As you may recall from Pillar #3: Food, I advise against snacking. Ideally, you should get the majority of your nutrition from three large, balanced meals each day so that your digestive system can rest between meals.

Exceptions to the no-snacking rule:

• Pre-workout snack
See page 58 for examples.

• Post-workout snack
See page 59 for examples.

• Before an event, or if you think your level of hunger will cause you to make unhealthy food choices. *Example #1: before a dinner party when you're unsure of the type of food that will be available. Example #2: if your previous meal was too small and you think that your level of hunger will cause you to overindulge at the next meal.*

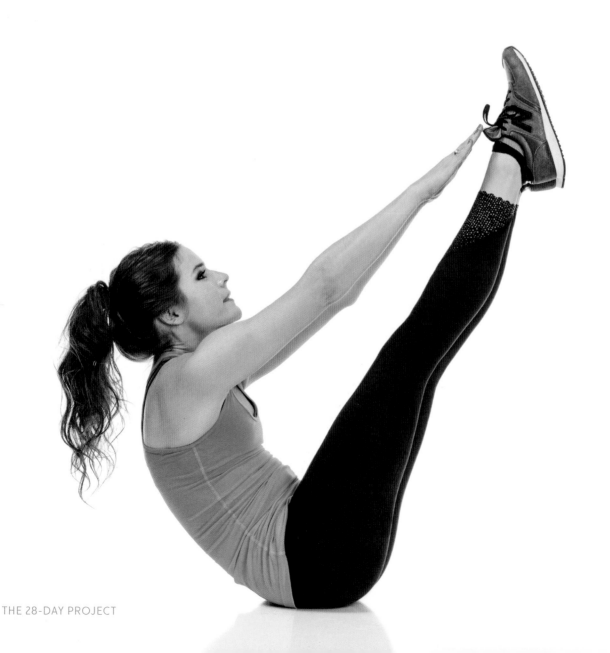

fitness plan: use this one!

Juli Bauer has given us her best here! The 28-day fitness program that she's designed especially for Project participants is great for anyone who's looking to work out alone or with a group at home. These workouts are challenging but doable. Remember that it's okay to modify the movements as you go. Lean on the Fitness Index (beginning on page 351) for details about the warm-up and mobility options and explanations of how to approach the workouts and do the exercises, and have fun with it!

DON'T FORGET YOUR STEPS!
You'll notice in the plan that your goal for each and every day is to hit 10,000 steps, including any steps that you take during your workouts. See page 65 for ideas on how to incorporate more movement into your day.

build your own fitness plan

If you prefer to do things your own way, follow the steps recommended on page 69 to brainstorm, plan, and schedule your IFF (Ideal Fitness Fit). Don't be intimidated by this process! It can be an exciting way to develop a fitness program that you *love.* Jump in with both feet, and don't be afraid to edit your plan as you work your way through the next 28 days.

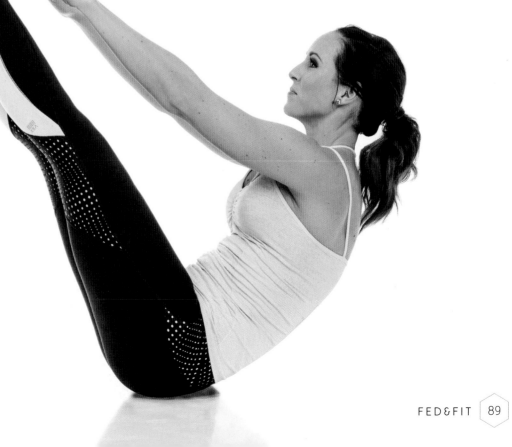

the 28-day food & fitness plan

	① MONDAY	② TUESDAY	③ WEDNESDAY	
BREAKFAST	Sausage & Tomato Frittata (148), in-scope fruit, Simple Hash Browns (134)	leftover Sausage & Tomato Frittata, in-scope fruit, leftover Hash Browns	Cinnamon Sage Sausage Patties (143), Braised Greens (129), Pan-Fried Plantains (145), in-scope fruit	
LUNCH	Cold Cut Roll-Ups x2 (298)	leftover Pork Tenderloin, leftover Parsnip Mash	leftover Garam Masala Beef & Butternut Stew, leftover Roasted Broccoli	
DINNER	Basic Pork Tenderloin (123), Easy Parsnip Mash (135)	Garam Masala Beef & Butternut Stew (208), Roasted Broccoli (129)	Chorizo-Stuffed Mushrooms with Avocado Mayo x2 (188), Tangy New-Fashioned Coleslaw (½ batch) (281)	
DESSERT (if desired)	Roasted Fruit Pops of choice (318)	Roasted Fruit Pops leftover	Lemon Lime Juice Gummies (316)	
PRE-WORKOUT SNACK*	See page 58 for options	See page 58 for options	See page 58 for options	
POST-WORKOUT SNACK*	See page 59 for options	See page 59 for options	See page 59 for options	
WARM-UP	Warm-up A	Warm-up C	Warm-up B	

WORKOUT	A: run/jog for 2 miles (or 20 minutes), then
	
	B: 4 rounds for time:
	  10 jumping squats
	  10 sit-ups
	  10 hand-release push-ups
	
	See page 384 for details
		as far as possible in 15 minutes; 5 reps, 10 reps, 15 reps, 20 reps, 25 reps, etc.:
		  burpees
		  pike push-ups
		  tuck jumps
		
		See page 384 for details
			A: 1-mile run, then
			
			B: 5 rounds of:
			  1 minute: wall sit
			  1 minute: burpees
			  1 minute: mountain climbers
			  1 minute: jumping lunges
			  1 minute: rest
			
			See page 384 for details	

MOBILITY	Mobility A	Mobility C	Mobility A	
TOTAL STEPS	Goal = 10,000	Goal = 10,000	Goal = 10,000	
TOTAL WATER	Results from Water Equation on page 37	Results from Water Equation on page 37	Results from Water Equation on page 37	
TOTAL SLEEP	Results from Sleep Analysis on page 32	Results from Sleep Analysis on page 32	Results from Sleep Analysis on page 32	
JOURNAL	Today's Lessons Learned (template on page 106)	Today's Lessons Learned (template on page 106)	Today's Lessons Learned (template on page 106)	

* = only if needed

4 THURSDAY	5 FRIDAY	6 SATURDAY	7 SUNDAY
leftover Cinnamon Sage Sausage Patties / *leftover* Braised Greens / *leftover* Pan-Fried Plantains / in-scope fruit	150 Anti-Inflammatory Smoothie x2 / Braised Greens / 2–3 eggs per person 129	150 Anti-Inflammatory Smoothie x2 / *leftover* Braised Greens / 2–3 eggs per person 129	146 Plantain Protein Pancakes with Salted Raspberry Jam / Braised Greens 129
leftover Chorizo-Stuffed Mushrooms *with Avocado Mayo* / *leftover* Tangy New-Fashioned Coleslaw	*leftover* Barbacoa with Jicama Tortillas / *leftover* Roasted Citrus Beets	*leftover* Buffalo Ranch Bison Burgers / *leftover* Zesty Okra Fries / *leftover* Mashed Potatoes	*leftover* Oven Baby Back Ribs / *leftover* Baked Potatoes / *leftover* Whole Brussels Bake
214 Barbacoa with Jicama Tortillas / 292 Roasted Citrus Beets	242 Buffalo Ranch Bison Burgers / 283 Zesty Okra Fries / 289 Old-Fashioned Mashed Potatoes	250 Oven Baby Back Ribs / 133 Baked Potatoes / 282 Whole Brussels Bake	226 Creamy Chicken Piccata Casserole / 269 Lemony Bacon Super Greens
leftover Lemon Lime Juice Gummies	314 Puddings of choice	*leftover* Puddings	321 Berries & Cream
See page 58 for options	See page 58 for options	See page 58 for options	See page 58 for options
See page 59 for options	See page 59 for options	See page 59 for options	See page 59 for options
REST or yoga	Warm-up D	Warm-up C	REST or yoga
	A: 3 rounds of: 30 push-ups 30 box jumps (or step-ups) 30 bench dips 2-minute rest, then B: 3 rounds of: 30 ab leg lifts 30 skater jumps 30 dead bugs *See page 384 for details*	3 rounds of 10-9-8-7-6-5-4-3-2-1-rep of: in-and-out jumps walking lunges (each leg) mountain climbers *See page 384 for details*	
	Mobility D	Mobility B	
Goal = 10,000	Goal = 10,000	Goal = 10,000	Goal = 10,000
Results from Water Equation on page 37	Results from Water Equation on page 37	Results from Water Equation on page 37	Results from Water Equation on page 37
Results from Sleep Analysis on page 32	Results from Sleep Analysis on page 32	Results from Sleep Analysis on page 32	Results from Sleep Analysis on page 32
Today's Lessons Learned (template on page 106)	Today's Lessons Learned (template on page 106)	Today's Lessons Learned (template on page 106)	Today's Lessons Learned (template on page 106)

Note: If your leftovers last longer than the two days listed in this meal plan, just skip any recipes that aren't needed.

the 28-day food & fitness plan

	8 MONDAY	9 TUESDAY	10 WEDNESDAY	
BREAKFAST	leftover Plantain Protein Pancakes / leftover Sautéed Lemon Garlic Spinach	144 Jicama Breakfast Cakes / 2–3 eggs per person & in-scope fruit	leftover Jicama Breakfast Cakes / 2–3 eggs per person & in-scope fruit	
LUNCH	leftover Creamy Chicken Piccata Casserole / leftover Lemony Bacon Super Greens	leftover Vegetable Beef Soup	leftover Loaded White Potatoes: Supreme Pizza	
DINNER	206 A Very Good Vegetable Beef Soup	196 Loaded White Potatoes: Supreme Pizza	254 Rustic Pot Roast	
DESSERT (if desired)	leftover Berries & Cream	318 Roasted Fruit Pops of choice	leftover Roasted Fruit Pops	
PRE-WORKOUT SNACK*	See page 58 for options	See page 58 for options	See page 58 for options	
POST-WORKOUT SNACK*	See page 59 for options	See page 59 for options	See page 59 for options	
WARM-UP	Warm-up A	Warm-up D	Warm-up C	
WORKOUT	run for distance, Bulgarian split squats, pike push-ups, and V-ups for reps (4 rounds total): 800m–20 reps–20 reps–20 reps 600m–15 reps–15 reps–15 reps 400m–10 reps–10 reps–10 reps 200m–5 reps–5 reps–5 reps *See page 384 for details*	A: 10-20-30 reps of: Russian twists legs-up-a-wall toe touches (each leg), then B: 18-minute EMOM (every minute on the minute): 14 jumping squats 7 burpees *See page 385 for details*	A: ladder for 15 minutes: lateral box jumps/jump-overs knees to squats pike push-ups, then B: 5-minute AMRAP (as many rounds as possible): 10 forearm plank to hand planks 10 Supermans 10 V-ups *See page 385 for details*	
MOBILITY	Mobility B	Mobility A	Mobility D	
TOTAL STEPS	Goal = 10,000	Goal = 10,000	Goal = 10,000	
TOTAL WATER	Results from Water Equation on page 37	Results from Water Equation on page 37	Results from Water Equation on page 37	
TOTAL SLEEP	Results from Sleep Analysis on page 32	Results from Sleep Analysis on page 32	Results from Sleep Analysis on page 32	
JOURNAL	Today's Lessons Learned (template on page 106)	Today's Lessons Learned (template on page 106)	Today's Lessons Learned (template on page 106)	

* = only if needed

11 THURSDAY	12 FRIDAY	13 SATURDAY	14 SUNDAY
Purple Protein Smoothie x2 (150) / Sautéed Lemon Garlic Spinach (268)	Purple Protein Smoothie x2 (150) / Sautéed Lemon Garlic Spinach (leftover)	Paleo Diner Breakfast Plate (158)	Paleo Diner Breakfast Plate (leftover)
Rustic Pot Roast (leftover)	Panang Curry (leftover)	Sausage & Cranberry Stuffed Acorn Squash *with Rosemary Orange Cream Sauce* (leftover) / Crispy Brussels Sprouts (leftover)	Curried Beef & Butternut Squash Stuffed Peppers (leftover)
The Panang Curry My Husband Loves (252)	Sausage & Cranberry Stuffed Acorn Squash *with Rosemary Orange Cream Sauce* x2 (200) / Crispy Brussels Sprouts (127)	Curried Beef & Butternut Squash Stuffed Peppers (190)	Roasted Garlic Cottage Pie (230)
Fudgesicles (320)	Fudgesicles (leftover)	Puddings of choice (314)	Puddings (leftover)
See page 58 for options	See page 58 for options	See page 58 for options	See page 58 for options
See page 59 for options	See page 59 for options	See page 59 for options	See page 59 for options
REST or yoga	Warm-up C	Warm-up B	REST or yoga
	30-minute AMRAP (as many rounds as possible): 5 burpees / 20 jumping lunges / 30 Russian twists / 20 tuck jumps *Every 2 minutes, do 5 burpees, then pick up where you left off.* *See page 385 for details*	A: 3 x 400m sprints, rest 1 minute between, then B: 50 reps each as fast as possible, then 1 minute rest: legs-up-a-wall toe touches / high knees / sit-ups, then / 40: 1; 30: 1; 20:1, 10:done *See page 385 for details*	
	Mobility A	Mobility D	
Goal = 10,000	Goal = 10,000	Goal = 10,000	Goal = 10,000
Results from Water Equation on page 37	Results from Water Equation on page 37	Results from Water Equation on page 37	Results from Water Equation on page 37
Results from Sleep Analysis on page 32	Results from Sleep Analysis on page 32	Results from Sleep Analysis on page 32	Results from Sleep Analysis on page 32
Today's Lessons Learned (template on page 106)	Today's Lessons Learned (template on page 106)	Today's Lessons Learned (template on page 106)	Today's Lessons Learned (template on page 106)

Note: If your leftovers last longer than the two days listed in this meal plan, just skip any recipes that aren't needed.

	15 MONDAY	16 TUESDAY	17 WEDNESDAY	
BREAKFAST	Tuscan Chicken Frittata (½ batch) 156 — in-scope fruit	Tuscan Chicken Frittata leftover — in-scope fruit	Green Detox Smoothie x2 150 — 2–3 eggs per person & in-scope fruit	
LUNCH	Cottage Pie leftover	Crispy Baked Chicken Thighs leftover — Cowboy Potatoes leftover — Loaded Cauliflower Mac & Cheese leftover	Kale & Sausage Soup leftover	
DINNER	Crispy Baked Chicken Thighs x2 122 — Cowboy Potatoes 287 — Loaded Cauliflower Mac & Cheese 270	Lemony Kale & Sausage Soup 163	Fork-Tender Balsamic Pork Chops 209 — Browned Butter Butternut Mash 286 — Simple Roasted Cauliflower x2 128	
DESSERT (if desired)	Carrot Orange Juice Gummies 316	Carrot Orange Juice Gummies leftover	Roasted Fruit Pops of choice 318	
PRE-WORKOUT SNACK*	See page 58 for options	See page 58 for options	See page 58 for options	
POST-WORKOUT SNACK*	See page 59 for options	See page 59 for options	See page 59 for options	
WARM-UP	Warm-up B	Warm-up A	Warm-up A	
WORKOUT	A: 5 rounds: 20 tuck jumps 10 hand-release push-ups, then B: 15-minute AMRAP (as many rounds as possible): 12 slow single-leg deadlifts 24 bicycle crunches 36 mountain climbers *See page 385 for details*	A: 50 burpees for time, then B: 3 rounds: 50 flutter kicks 40 alternating walking lunges 30 bench dips *See page 385 for details*	run for distance, burpees, ab leg lifts, and jumping squats for reps: 800m–21 reps–21 reps–21 reps 600m–18 reps–18 reps–18 reps 400m–15 reps–15 reps–15 reps 300m–12 reps–12 reps–12 reps 200m–9 reps–9 reps–9 reps 100m–6 reps–6 reps–6 reps *See page 385 for details*	
MOBILITY	Mobility C	Mobility A	Mobility B	
TOTAL STEPS	Goal = 10,000	Goal = 10,000	Goal = 10,000	
TOTAL WATER	Results from Water Equation on page 37	Results from Water Equation on page 37	Results from Water Equation on page 37	
TOTAL SLEEP	Results from Sleep Analysis on page 32	Results from Sleep Analysis on page 32	Results from Sleep Analysis on page 32	
JOURNAL	Today's Lessons Learned (template on page 106)	Today's Lessons Learned (template on page 106)	Today's Lessons Learned (template on page 106)	

* = only if needed

18 THURSDAY	19 FRIDAY	20 SATURDAY	21 SUNDAY
Green Detox Smoothie x2 **150** / 2–3 eggs per person & in-scope fruit	Bubble & Squeak x2 **140** / in-scope fruit	Bubble & Squeak *leftover* / in-scope fruit	Sweet Potato Breakfast Hash Casserole **154** / in-scope fruit
Balsamic Pork Chops *leftover* / Browned Butter Butternut Mash *leftover* / Roasted Cauliflower *leftover*	Thai Beef Salad *with Zesty Lime Dressing* *leftover*	Taco Squash Boats *leftover* / Root Veggie Hash *leftover*	Caramelized Onion Bacon Bison Meatloaf *with Balsamic Mustard Glaze* *leftover* / Roasted Garlic Cauliflower Mash *leftover*
Thai Beef Salad *with Zesty Lime Dressing* x2 **182**	Taco Squash Boats **203** / Root Veggie Hash **294**	Caramelized Onion Bacon Bison Meatloaf *with Balsamic Mustard Glaze* **246** / Roasted Garlic Cauliflower Mash **277**	Buffalo Chicken Casserole **222**
Roasted Fruit Pops *leftover*	Strawberry Raspberry Jam Gummies **316**	Strawberry Raspberry Jam Gummies *leftover*	Puddings of choice **314**
See page 58 for options	See page 58 for options	See page 58 for options	See page 58 for options
See page 59 for options	See page 59 for options	See page 59 for options	See page 59 for options
REST or yoga	Warm-up D	Warm-up C	REST or yoga

	A: 6 rounds:
	  200m sprint
	  20 push-ups, then
	
	B: as fast as possible:
	  30 burpees
	  30 V-ups
	  30 burpees
		21-15-9-9-15-21 reps of each exercise:
		  in-and-out jumps
		  V-ups
		  burpees	

	See page 386 for details	*See page 386 for details*	
	Mobility C	Mobility D	
Goal = 10,000	Goal = 10,000	Goal = 10,000	Goal = 10,000
Results from Water Equation on page 37	Results from Water Equation on page 37	Results from Water Equation on page 37	Results from Water Equation on page 37
Results from Sleep Analysis on page 32	Results from Sleep Analysis on page 32	Results from Sleep Analysis on page 32	Results from Sleep Analysis on page 32
Today's Lessons Learned (template on page 106)	Today's Lessons Learned (template on page 106)	Today's Lessons Learned (template on page 106)	Today's Lessons Learned (template on page 106)

Note: If your leftovers last longer than the two days listed in this meal plan, just skip any recipes that aren't needed.

the 28-day food & fitness plan

	22 MONDAY	23 TUESDAY	24 WEDNESDAY	
BREAKFAST	Sweet Potato Breakfast Hash Casserole (leftover) — in-scope fruit	Spaghetti Squash & Dill Egg Cups (152) — fresh tomatoes (if in season) & in-scope fruit	Spaghetti Squash & Dill Egg Cups (leftover) — fresh tomatoes (if in season) & in-scope fruit	
LUNCH	Buffalo Chicken Casserole (leftover)	Pan-Seared Steak (leftover) · Roasted Buffalo Cauliflower (leftover) · Cowboy Potatoes (leftover)	Asian-Style Cabbage Rolls (leftover) · Pan-Fried Plantains (leftover)	
DINNER	Pan-Seared Steak x4 (125) · Roasted Buffalo Cauliflower (276) · Cowboy Potatoes (287)	Asian-Style Cabbage Rolls *with Savory Almond Sauce* (238) · Pan-Fried Plantains (145)	Lemon Thyme Chicken & Vegetables (212)	
DESSERT *(if desired)*	Puddings (leftover)	Roasted Fruit Pops of choice (318)	Roasted Fruit Pops (leftover)	
PRE-WORKOUT SNACK*	See page 58 for options	See page 58 for options	See page 58 for options	
POST-WORKOUT SNACK*	See page 59 for options	See page 59 for options	See page 59 for options	
WARM-UP	Warm-up B	Warm-up D	Warm-up A	
WORKOUT	A: 6 x 200m sprints (sprint 200 meters, walk back for rest), then B: 20 seconds on, 10 seconds rest for 4 minutes: air squats (0:00-4:00) push-ups (4:00-8:00) sit-ups (8:00-12:00) *See page 386 for details*	8 rounds for time: 20 skater jumps 10 hand-release push-ups 20 jumping squats 10 V-ups *See page 386 for details*	A: 5-minute AMRAP (as many rounds as possible): 20 jumping lunges 10 pike push-ups B: 7 rounds: 100m sprint 1-minute plank hold *See page 386 for details*	
MOBILITY	Mobility A	Mobility C	Mobility B	
TOTAL STEPS	Goal = 10,000	Goal = 10,000	Goal = 10,000	
TOTAL WATER	Results from Water Equation on page 37	Results from Water Equation on page 37	Results from Water Equation on page 37	
TOTAL SLEEP	Results from Sleep Analysis on page 32	Results from Sleep Analysis on page 32	Results from Sleep Analysis on page 32	
JOURNAL	Today's Lessons Learned (template on page 106)	Today's Lessons Learned (template on page 106)	Today's Lessons Learned (template on page 106)	

* = only if needed

25 THURSDAY	26 FRIDAY	27 SATURDAY	28 SUNDAY
One-Stop-Shop Smoothie x2 (150)	One-Stop-Shop Smoothie x2 (150)	Chorizo & Egg Breakfast Scramble (142) · Oven-Baked Tostones (291) · in-scope fruit	Chorizo & Egg Breakfast Scramble (leftover) · Oven-Baked Tostones (leftover) · in-scope fruit
Lemon Thyme Chicken & Vegetables (leftover)	Turkey & Sweet Potato Casserole (leftover) · Crispy Garlic Green Beans (leftover)	Caramelized Onion Balsamic Beef Burgers (leftover) · Crispy Garlic Steak Fries (leftover) · Cauliflower "Potato" Salad (leftover)	BBQ Cobb Chicken Salad *with Creamy Jalapeño Ranch* (leftover)
Turkey & Sweet Potato Casserole (232) · Crispy Garlic Green Beans (266)	Caramelized Onion Balsamic Beef Burgers x2 (244) · Crispy Garlic Steak Fries (288) · Cauliflower "Potato" Salad (½ batch) (262)	BBQ Cobb Chicken Salad *with Creamy Jalapeño Ranch* (168)	Chile Relleno Enchalada Casserole (224) · Caramelized Carrots (132)
Blueberry Cherry Jam Gummies (316)	Blueberry Cherry Jam Gummies (leftover)	Roasted Fruit Pops of choice (318)	Roasted Fruit Pops (leftover)
See page 58 for options	See page 58 for options	See page 58 for options	See page 58 for options
See page 59 for options	See page 59 for options	See page 59 for options	See page 59 for options
REST or yoga	Warm-up A	Warm-up D	REST or yoga

	3 rounds:
	  12 pistols (each leg)
	  20 sit-ups
	  400m run, then
	
	3 rounds:
	20 jumping squats
	10 V-ups
	400-m run, then
	
	3 rounds:
	12 Bulgarian split squats *(each foot elevated)*
	20 dead bugs
	400m run
	
	See page 386 for details
		A: 6 minutes total (no rest between movements):
		  2 minutes push-ups
		  2 minutes air squats
		  2 minutes sit-ups
		
		B: 5 rounds, with 3-minute clock:
		300m run, then max burpees
		1 minute rest between rounds
		
		See page 386 for details	

	Mobility A	Mobility A	
Goal = 10,000	Goal = 10,000	Goal = 10,000	Goal = 10,000
Results from Water Equation on page 37	Results from Water Equation on page 37	Results from Water Equation on page 37	Results from Water Equation on page 37
Results from Sleep Analysis on page 32	Results from Sleep Analysis on page 32	Results from Sleep Analysis on page 32	Results from Sleep Analysis on page 32
Today's Lessons Learned (template on page 106)	Today's Lessons Learned (template on page 106)	Today's Lessons Learned (template on page 106)	Today's Lessons Learned (template on page 106)

Note: If your leftovers last longer than the two days listed in this meal plan, just skip any recipes that aren't needed.

FRESH PRODUCE

avocados, 2

broccoli, 2 heads

Brussels sprouts, 2 pounds

butternut squash, 1 medium (about 3 pounds)

carrots, 2 medium

collards, 1 bunch

collards, kale, or other braising green of choice, 2 small bunches (about 2 pounds)

garlic, 2 large bulbs

golden beets, 4

green cabbage, ¼ medium head

jalapeño peppers, 2

jicamas, 1 large + ½ small

kale, 1 bunch

kale, collard, or Swiss chard leaves, 6

okra, 1 pound

parsnips, 6 large

portabella mushrooms, 12

purple cabbage, ¼ medium head

purple onions, 2

red beets, 4

red bell peppers, 2

red potatoes, 2 pounds

russet potatoes, 3 medium (about 1 pound)

spaghetti squash, 1 medium (about 5 pounds)

sweet or russet potatoes, 1 pound

tomatoes, 3 or 4 medium

Herbs:

chives, 1 small bunch

cilantro, 2 large bunches

flat-leaf parsley, 1 small bunch

Fruit:

bananas, 2

grapefruit, 1

lemons, 19

limes, 9

oranges, 2

plantains, 4 ripe

raspberries, fresh or frozen, 1 cup

in-scope fruit, 8 servings *(see page 76 for guidance)*

MEAT & BROTH

baby back pork ribs, 4 pounds (1 full rack or 2 half racks)

bacon, 1 pound

beef stew meat, 2 pounds

boneless, skinless chicken thighs, 2 pounds

bulk breakfast sausage or ground pork, 1 pound

chorizo (bulk or link), 2 pounds

chuck roast, 1 (3-pound)

deli roast beef, 4 ounces (about 4 slices)

deli turkey meat, 4 ounces (about 4 slices)

ground bison, 2 pounds

ground pork, 2 pounds

pork tenderloin, 1 (1¼-pound)

beef broth, 6 cups *(If making homemade, you will need 3 pounds beef stock bones with marrow, 2 onions, 2 carrots, 2 cloves garlic, 2 tablespoons apple cider vinegar, and 2 bay leaves.)*

EGGS & BUTTER

eggs, large, 2 dozen + 3

salted butter, 2½ sticks (1¼ cups/10 ounces) *(check recipes for alternatives if dairy-sensitive)*

FATS & OILS

avocado oil, 5¼ ounces (⅔ cup)

bacon fat, 3 tablespoons

extra-virgin olive oil, 4 ounces (½ cup)

FROZEN FOODS

frozen whole strawberries, 1 (20-ounce) bag

SPICES & DRIED HERBS

bay leaves, 3

cayenne pepper, 2 teaspoons

chipotle chili powder, 1 tablespoon

dried dill weed, 1 tablespoon

dried Mexican oregano leaves, 1 tablespoon

fennel seeds, 1½ teaspoons

garam masala, 2 tablespoons

garlic powder, 1 tablespoon + 2½ teaspoons

ginger powder, 1 tablespoon + 1 teaspoon

ground cinnamon, 3¼ teaspoons

ground cloves, ½ teaspoon

ground cumin, 1 tablespoon

onion powder, 1 tablespoon + 1 teaspoon

paprika, 2 teaspoons

rubbed dried sage, 2 tablespoons

turmeric powder, 2 tablespoons + 2 teaspoons

MISCELLANEOUS PANTRY ITEMS

apple cider vinegar, 10 ounces (1¼ cups)

balsamic vinegar, 1 tablespoon

barbecue sauce, 1 cup *[If making homemade, you will need 1 (15-ounce) can strained tomatoes or tomato sauce, 1 (6-ounce) can tomato paste, ½ cup apple cider vinegar, ½ cup coconut aminos, 1 tablespoon chili powder, 1 tablespoon garlic powder, and 1 tablespoon onion powder.]*

capers, 3 tablespoons

coconut aminos, 1 tablespoon

coconut milk, full-fat, 1 (13½-ounce) can + 10 ounces (1¼ cups)

mayonnaise, Paleo-friendly, 32 ounces (4 cups) *[If making homemade, you will need 2 large eggs, 2 lemons, and 24 ounces (3 cups) avocado oil for two batches.]*

mustard, 2 tablespoons

pecans, 1⅓ ounces (⅓ cup)

unflavored protein powder, 2 scoops

vanilla extract, 1 teaspoon

white wine vinegar, 2 tablespoons

OPTIONAL DESSERT INGREDIENTS

For Roasted Fruit Pops *(choice of 5 flavors)*:

extra-virgin olive oil, 1 tablespoon

lemon, 1

and one of the following:

- fresh blueberries, 4 ounces (1 cup)
- fresh cherries, ¾ pound (1 cup stemmed and pitted)
- fresh raspberries, 1 pint (2 cups)
- fresh strawberries, 1 pint (2 cups)
- grapefruits, 2

For Lemon Lime Juice Gummies:

lemons, 3

limes, 3

unflavored gelatin, ¼ cup

For all puddings:

coconut milk, full-fat, 1 (13½-ounce) can

Medjool dates, 2

unflavored gelatin, 2 teaspoons

and

for Vanilla Bean Pudding:
vanilla bean pods, 2

for Chocolate Pudding:
unsweetened cocoa powder, 2 tablespoons + extra for garnish

vanilla extract, 1 teaspoon

for Toasted Coconut Pudding:
unsweetened shredded coconut, 1½ ounces (½ cup) + extra for garnish

vanilla extract, 1 teaspoon

For Berries & Cream:

coconut milk, full-fat, 1 (13½-ounce) can

fresh berries of choice, 1 pint (2 cups)

vanilla extract, ½ teaspoon

notes

FOR DAY 2: *If making homemade beef broth, after using the 6 cups needed for the beef and butternut stew, freeze an 8-cup portion and a 4-cup portion, both for use in week 2 of the Project. Freeze the remainder for later use.*

FOR DAY 3: *The ingredients to make the optional Salsa Verde for serving with the Barbacoa with Jicama Tortillas are not included in the shopping list. If you wish to make it, you will need 1 pound tomatillos, 1 yellow onion, 8 cloves garlic (about 1 bulb), 4 jalapeño peppers, ½ small bunch cilantro, and 4 limes.*

FOR DAY 5: *You will need a total of 1 cup plus 2 tablespoons of homemade Buffalo sauce for the meals during the 28-Day Project. Because the recipe makes just 1 cup, I suggest that you double it and, after using ¼ cup of the sauce to make the Buffalo Ranch Bison Burgers, freeze ¾ cup of the sauce for meal prep during week 3 of the Project and 2 tablespoons (or two ice cubes) for meal prep during week 4. Freeze the remainder for later use.*

FOR DAY 6: *If making homemade BBQ sauce, after using the 1 cup needed for the ribs and setting some aside for serving with the ribs, freeze a ⅓-cup portion for use in week 4 of the Project. Freeze the remainder for use after you've completed the Project.*

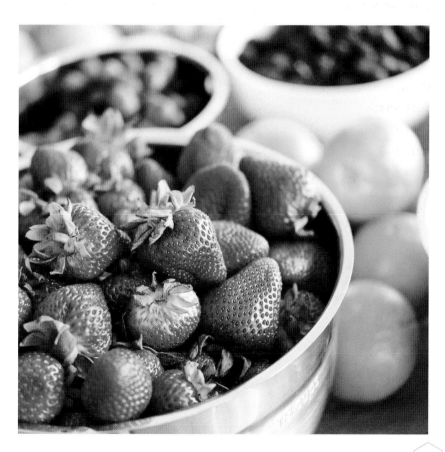

grocery shopping list

FRESH PRODUCE

acorn squash, 2

avocado, 1

Brussels sprouts, 12 ounces

butternut squash, 1 small (about 2 pounds)

carrots, 1¾ pounds

cauliflower, 6 heads

celery, 4 stalks

collards or kale, 1 small bunch (about 1 pound)

garlic, 4 bulbs

green beans, 6 ounces

jicamas, 2 large (about 1¾ pounds)

mushrooms, 8 ounces

parsnips, 1 pound

potatoes, round red-skinned or white-skinned, 1½ pounds (about 4 large)

red bell peppers, 8 large

russet potatoes, 1½ pounds (about 4 small)

spinach, 1 pound (about 6 heaping cups)

white potatoes, 4 medium

yellow onions, 5½

Herbs:

basil, 1 bunch

chives, 1 small bunch

cilantro, 1 small bunch (optional)

flat-leaf parsley, 1 bunch

rosemary, 4 sprigs

thyme, 3 sprigs

Fruit:

berries of choice, 1 pint, or 2 oranges or grapefruits

cranberries, fresh or frozen, 7 ounces (2 cups)

lemons, 4

limes, 6

orange, 1

in-scope fruit, 4 servings *(see page 76 for guidance)*

MEAT & BROTH

bacon, ½ pound

beef stew meat, 2 pounds

boneless chuck roast, 1 (5-pound)

boneless, skinless chicken breasts, 2½ to 3 pounds

bulk Italian sausage or ground pork, ½ pound

ground beef, 4 pounds

hot Italian sausage (bulk or link), 2 pounds

pepperoni, ½ pound

beef broth, 12 cups *(If using homemade, see note on page 99.)*

EGGS & BUTTER

eggs, large, 1 dozen + 10

salted butter, 2¾ sticks (1⅓ cups/11 ounces) *(check recipes for alternatives if dairy-sensitive)*

FATS & OILS

bacon fat, 3 tablespoons

extra-virgin olive oil, 2 ounces (¼ cup)

FROZEN FOODS

frozen blueberries, 18 ounces (3 cups)

frozen crinkle-cut carrots, 16 ounces

frozen green peas, 16 ounces

SPICES & DRIED HERBS

bay leaves, 2

cayenne pepper, ⅛ teaspoon

curry powder, 1 tablespoon

dried ground oregano, ½ teaspoon

dried rosemary leaves, 1 teaspoon

dried thyme leaves, 1 teaspoon

garlic powder, ¼ teaspoon

ground coriander, ½ teaspoon

Italian seasoning, 2 teaspoons

paprika, 1¼ teaspoons

red pepper flakes, up to 2 teaspoons

rubbed dried sage, 1½ teaspoons

MISCELLANEOUS PANTRY ITEMS

black olives, sliced, 1 (2¼-ounce) can

coconut milk, full-fat, 4 (13½-ounce) cans + ¾ cup

diced tomatoes, 1 (28-ounce) can

fish sauce, 2 teaspoons

Thai red curry paste, 1 (4-ounce) jar + 3 tablespoons

tomato paste, 2 (6-ounce) cans

unflavored protein powder, 4 scoops

OPTIONAL DESSERT INGREDIENTS

For Roasted Fruit Pops *(choice of 5 flavors):*

extra-virgin olive oil, 1 tablespoon

lemon, 1

and one of the following:

• fresh blueberries, 4 ounces (1 cup)

• fresh cherries, ¾ pound (1 cup stemmed and pitted)

• fresh raspberries, 1 pint (2 cups)

• fresh strawberries, 1 pint (2 cups)

• grapefruits, 2

For Fudgesicles

coconut milk, full-fat, 1½ (13½-ounce) cans (2½ cups)

Medjool dates, 4

unflavored gelatin, 3 tablespoons

unsweetened cocoa powder, 1 ounce (¼ cup)

For all puddings:

coconut milk, full-fat, 1 (13½-ounce) can

Medjool dates, 2

unflavored gelatin, 2 teaspoons

and

for Vanilla Bean Pudding:
vanilla bean pods, 2

for Chocolate Pudding:
unsweetened cocoa powder, 2 tablespoons +extra for garnish

vanilla extract, 1 teaspoon

for Toasted Coconut Pudding:
unsweetened shredded coconut, 1½ ounces (½ cup) + extra for garnish

vanilla extract, 1 teaspoon

FRESH PRODUCE

avocado, 1

butternut squash, 1 large
(4 to 5 pounds)

carrots, 4

cauliflower, 6 heads

cherry tomatoes, large
handful (about ¼ pint)

cucumber, 1

garlic, 2 bulbs

golden beets, 2

green cabbage, 1 head

green onions, 3

hot red chili pepper, 1

kale, 5 bunches

mixed lettuce, 8 ounces
(4 cups)

parsnips, 3

potatoes, small fingerling,
new, or boiling, 1 pound

purple onion, ½

radishes, 1 bunch

red beets, 2

spinach, 8 ounces (4 cups)

sweet potatoes, 4 pounds
+ 2 large

white onion, ½

yellow onions, 5

yellow potatoes, 3½ pounds
(about 5 medium)

yellow summer squash or
zucchini, 3

Herbs:

basil, 1 large bunch

chives, 1 bunch

cilantro, 2 bunches

flat-leaf parsley, 1 small
bunch

mint, 1 bunch

Fruit:

bananas, 2

lemons, 14

limes, 6

in-scope fruit, 14 servings
(see page 76 for guidance)

MEAT & BROTH

bacon, 1½ pounds +
1⅔ pounds thick-cut

beef sirloin (or the best cut
of beef you have on hand),
1 pound

bone-in, skin-on chicken
thighs, 4 pounds

boneless pork chops,
3 pounds

boneless, skinless chicken
breasts, 5 pounds

bulk breakfast sausage,
3 pounds

chicken, 1 (4- to 5-pound),
or 1 precooked rotisserie
chicken

ground bison, 2 pounds

chicken broth, 8 cups
(64 ounces) *(If making
homemade, you will need
3 pounds chicken feet,
wings, or necks, 2 onions,
2 carrots, 2 cloves garlic,
2 tablespoons apple cider
vinegar, and 2 bay leaves.)*

EGGS & BUTTER

eggs, large, 3 dozen + 9

salted butter, 2¾ sticks
(1⅓ cups / 11 ounces) *(check
recipes for alternatives if
dairy-sensitive)*

FATS & OILS

extra-virgin olive oil,
8½ ounces (1 cup +
1 tablespoon)

SPICES & DRIED HERBS

chili powder, 2 tablespoons

dried oregano leaves,
1 teaspoon

dried thyme leaves,
2 tablespoons

garlic powder, 4 teaspoons

ginger powder, 4 teaspoons

ground cumin, 2 tablespoons

red pepper flakes,
1 teaspoon

MISCELLANEOUS PANTRY ITEMS

almonds, raw, 2 tablespoons

balsamic vinegar, 7½ ounces
(¼ cup + 3 tablespoons)

coconut milk, full-fat,
1 (13½-ounce) can +
4 ounces (½ cup)

fish sauce, 2 ounces (¼ cup)

mustard of choice, 2¼
ounces (¼ cup)

nutritional yeast, 1 ounce
(½ cup)

pine nuts, 1½ ounces
(about ⅓ cup)

prepared yellow mustard
or whole-grain mustard,
4½ ounces (about ½ cup)

sun-dried tomatoes packed
in olive oil, 3 tablespoons

OPTIONAL DESSERT INGREDIENTS

For Carrot Orange Juice
Gummies:

carrots, 3

oranges, 2

unflavored gelatin, ¼ cup

For Roasted Fruit Pops
(choice of 5 flavors):

extra-virgin olive oil,
1 tablespoon

lemon, 1

and one of the following:

- fresh blueberries,
  4 ounces (1 cup)

- fresh cherries, ¾ pound (1
  cup stemmed and pitted)

- fresh raspberries, 1 pint
  (2 cups)

- fresh strawberries, 1 pint
  (2 cups)

- grapefruits, 2

For Strawberry Raspberry
Jam Gummies:

fresh raspberries, 1 pint (2
cups)

fresh strawberries, 1 pint (2
cups)

unflavored gelatin, ¼ cup

For all puddings:

coconut milk, full-fat,
1 (13½-ounce) can

Medjool dates, 2

unflavored gelatin,
2 teaspoons

*and
for Vanilla Bean Pudding:*
vanilla bean pods, 2

for Chocolate Pudding:
unsweetened cocoa
powder, 2 tablespoons +
extra for garnish

vanilla extract, 1 teaspoon

for Toasted Coconut Pudding:
unsweetened shredded
coconut, 1½ ounces (½ cup)
+ extra for garnish

vanilla extract, 1 teaspoon

grocery shopping list

FRESH PRODUCE

avocados, 2

carrots, 1¼ pounds + 2 bunches slender (about 1 pound)

cauliflower, 3½ heads

celery, 7½ stalks

cherry tomatoes, 1 cup

garlic, 2 bulbs

ginger, 1 (2-inch) piece

green beans, 1 pound

green onions, 1 bunch

jalapeño peppers, 2

kale leaves, 4 ounces

napa cabbage, 1 large head

poblano or hatch green chili peppers, 10

potatoes, russet or other white, 2 pounds (about 6)

purple onion, ¼

romaine lettuce, 1 large head

shiitake mushrooms, 8 ounces

spaghetti squash, 1 medium (about 5 pounds)

spinach, 8 ounces

sweet potatoes, 4 pounds

tomatoes, 7

white onion, ½

yellow onions, 8

yellow potatoes, 5 pounds (1½ pounds preferably Baby Dutch)

Herbs:

chives, 1 small bunch

cilantro, 2 bunches

thyme, 6 sprigs

Fruit:

bananas, 2

cranberries, fresh or frozen, 7 ounces (2 cups)

lemons, 5

limes, 7

plantains, 2 ripe + 2 large green

in-scope fruit, 10 servings *(see page 76 for guidance)*

MEAT

bacon, 1 pound + 4 slices thick-cut

boneless sirloin or rib-eye steaks, 4 (4- to 6-ounce)

boneless turkey breast, 1 (4-pound)

boneless, skinless chicken breasts, 1 pound

bulk breakfast sausage or ground pork, 1 pound

chicken, 1 whole (about 3 pounds)

chorizo (bulk or link), 2 pounds

ground beef, 3 pounds

ground pork, 2 pounds

EGGS & BUTTER

eggs, large, 2 dozen + 5

salted butter, 3½ sticks (1¾ cups/14 ounces) *(check recipes for alternatives if dairy-sensitive)*

FATS & OILS

extra-virgin olive oil, 3 ounces (6 tablespoons)

sesame oil (untoasted), 1 tablespoon + 1 teaspoon

FROZEN FOODS

frozen blueberries, 12 ounces (2 cups)

SPICES & DRIED HERBS

chili powder, 5 teaspoons

dried dill weed, 1 teaspoon

dried Mexican oregano, 5 teaspoons

garlic powder, 3¼ teaspoons

ground cumin, 2 tablespoons

Italian seasoning, 1 tablespoon

paprika, ¼ teaspoon

red pepper flakes, up to 2 teaspoons

MISCELLANEOUS PANTRY ITEMS

almond butter, unsweetened, 4½ ounces (½ cup)

apple cider vinegar, 2 tablespoons + 1 teaspoon

balsamic vinegar, 4 ounces (½ cup)

barbecue sauce, ⅓ cup *[If using homemade, see note on page 99.]*

coconut aminos, 8½ ounces (1 cup + 1 tablespoon)

coconut milk, full-fat, 2 (13½-ounce) cans + 6 ounces (¾ cup)

diced green chilies, 1 (7-ounce) can

diced tomatoes, 1 (28-ounce) can

dill pickles or dill relish, 2¼ ounces (¼ cup)

fish sauce, 4 teaspoons

mayonnaise, Paleo-friendly, 16 ounces (2 cups) *[If making homemade, you will need 1 large egg, 1 lemon, and 12 ounces (1½ cups) avocado oil.]*

prepared yellow mustard, 1½ tablespoons

sunflower seeds, hulled raw, 4⅔ ounces (1 cup)

unflavored protein powder, 4 scoops

OPTIONAL DESSERT INGREDIENTS

For Roasted Fruit Pops for days 23 & 24 *(choice of 5 flavors)*:

extra-virgin olive oil, 1 tablespoon

lemon, 1

and one of the following:

- fresh blueberries, 4 ounces (1 cup)
- fresh cherries, ¾ pound (1 cup stemmed and pitted)
- fresh raspberries, 1 pint (2 cups)
- fresh strawberries, 1 pint (2 cups)
- grapefruits, 2

For Blueberry Cherry Jam Gummies:

fresh blueberries, ¾ pint (1½ cups)

fresh cherries, ¾ pound (1 cup stemmed and pitted)

limes, 2

unflavored gelatin, ¼ cup

For Roasted Fruit Pops for days 27 & 28 *(choice of 5 flavors)*:

extra-virgin olive oil, 1 tablespoon

lemon, 1

and one of the following:

- fresh blueberries, 4 ounces (1 cup)
- fresh cherries, ¾ pound (1 cup stemmed and pitted)
- fresh raspberries, 1 pint (2 cups)
- fresh strawberries, 1 pint (2 cups)
- grapefruits, 2

the diy food & fitness template

DAILY TEMPLATE	
BREAKFAST	PROTEIN + CRUNCHY VEGETABLE + STARCHY VEGETABLE + FAT + FRUIT
LUNCH	PROTEIN + CRUNCHY VEGETABLE + *optional* STARCHY VEGETABLE or FRUIT + FAT
DINNER	PROTEIN + CRUNCHY VEGETABLE + STARCHY VEGETABLE + FAT
DESSERT *(if desired)*	FAT + FRUIT
PRE-WORKOUT SNACK *(only if needed)*	See page 58 for options
POST-WORKOUT SNACK *(only if needed)*	See page 59 for options
WARM-UP	Warm-up of choice (page 382)
WORKOUT	30+ MINUTE WORKOUT — CARDIO + STRENGTH + MIXED BODY MOVEMENTS
MOBILITY	Mobility of choice (page 383) or yoga
TOTAL STEPS	Goal = 10,000
TOTAL WATER	Results from Water Equation on page 37
TOTAL SLEEP	Results from Sleep Analysis on page 32

journaling 101

why and how

Journaling your sleep, food, fitness activities, energy, mood, and lessons learned on a daily basis is a critical component of the Fed & Fit Project. Even more important than the contents of your meals or the specifics of last night's sleep, documenting your experiences in a strategic manner will give you a strong foothold that you can use to launch into your Perfect You Plan.

You can journal in one of three ways:

1.

Use the Journal Template provided here as a go-by while you record your entries in your own personal notebook.

2.

Join the Project Online, which includes an electronic journal template that you can use anytime!

3.

Download the Fed & Fit app and use the mobile journal there to record your notes.

when

• Upon waking: Document last night's sleep duration, sleep quality, measures you took to improve your sleep, and things that disturbed your sleep.

• Fitness activity: (move to where it fits your schedule) Detail your activity, the total length of the workout, and your feelings during and one hour after the workout (fatigued, shaky, energized, positive & happy, etc.).

• Just after breakfast: List the content of the meal and describe how you feel just after eating.

• Two hours after breakfast: Describe how you feel two hours after breakfast (hungry, still full, anxious, bloated, energized, etc.).

• Just after lunch: List the content of the meal and describe how you feel just after eating.

• Two hours after lunch: Describe how you feel two hours after lunch (hungry, still full, anxious, bloated, energized, etc.).

• Just after dinner: List the content of the meal and describe how you feel just after eating.

• Two hours after dinner: Describe how you feel two hours after dinner (hungry, still full, anxious, bloated, energized, etc.). Document you water intake for the day. Summarize the day's energy levels and mindset/outlook. List three or four specific lessons learned from the day regarding your sleep, water, nutritional needs, and/or fitness activities and how they relate to your overall energy level and/or mindset.

reading between the lines

I know that at first glance, this may seem like a considerable effort, but it will become easier a few days into the Project.

I highly recommend that you journal throughout the day. The details of how you felt when you woke up or what your breakfast included will become fuzzier as the hours go by, making your journal less reliable and significant as a resource.

As for journaling food, there's no need to get into highly specific weight measurements of each food you consume. Ballpark volume-based measurements will be highly telling: for example, ½ cup seasoned shredded chicken, 1 cup cilantro lime cauliflower rice, and 2 tablespoons crushed almonds.

REMEMBER: There are no such things as mistakes, missteps, cheats, or bandwagons in the Project; there are only opportunities to learn lessons. If you ever feel like you've gotten off track, use it as an opportunity to journal a new realization! If you happen to indulge in a few corn tortillas in the middle of your 28-day plan, no sweat! Just observe how you feel after eating the tortillas and make a note of it. While the tortillas may extend the time it takes to heal your gut, eating them might give you valuable insight into how you tolerate certain out-of-scope foods.

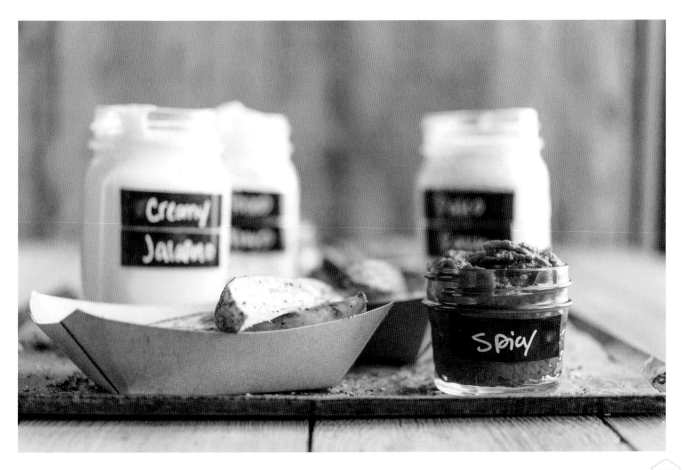

FED & fit journal

Date: _____ Day #: _____

SLEEP

Hours I slept last night: ....

Quality of my sleep: ....

Measures I took to improve sleep:
....
....

Things that disturbed my sleep:
....
....

WATER *(cross off 1 water drop for every 8 ounces you drank)* 🜄 🜄 🜄 🜄 🜄 🜄 🜄 🜄 🜄 🜄 🜄

Were you over, under, or right on your minimum water intake? ☐ Over ☐ Under ☐ At minimum

MINIMUM WATER INTAKE (in ounces) = WEIGHT/2

NUTRITION *(fill out throughout the day)*

	What I ate and how much	How I felt just after eating	How I felt 2 hours after eating
Meal	....	....	....
	....	....	....
	....	....	....
Meal	....	....	....
	....	....	....
	....	....	....
Meal	....	....	....
	....	....	....
	....	....	....
Meal	....	....	....
	....	....	....

FITNESS *(fill out throughout the day)*

Activity details	Length of workout	How I felt during workout	How I felt 1 hour after workout
....	....	....	....
....	....	....	....
....	....	....	....
....	....	....	....

ENERGY & MINDSET *(fill out at day's end)*

Describe your energy level today. ....
....
....

Describe your overall outlook and mindset today. ....
....
....

LESSONS LEARNED *(fill out at day's end)*

List 3 things you learned today regarding your sleep, water, nutritional needs, or fitness activities and how they correspond to your overall energy level and/or mindset.
....
....
....
....
....

FED & *fit* journal

Date: _____ Day #: _____

SLEEP *(fill out at beginning of day)*

Hours I slept last night: ....

Quality of my sleep: ....

Measures I took to improve sleep: | Things that disturbed my sleep:
....
....

WATER *(cross off 1 water drop for every 8 ounces you drank)*

MINIMUM WATER INTAKE (in ounces) = WEIGHT/2

Were you over, under, or right on your minimum water intake? ☐ Over ☐ Under ☐ At minimum

NUTRITION *(fill out throughout the day)*

	What I ate and how much	How I felt just after eating	How I felt 2 hours after eating
Meal	....	....	....
	....	....	....
	....	....	....
Meal	....	....	....
	....	....	....
	....	....	....
Meal	....	....	....
	....	....	....
	....	....	....
Meal	....	....	....
	....	....	....
	....	....	....

FITNESS *(fill out throughout the day)*

Activity details	Length of workout	How I felt during workout	How I felt 1 hour after workout
....	....	....	....
....	....	....	....
....	....	....	....
....	....	....	....

ENERGY & MINDSET *(fill out at day's end)*

Describe your energy level today. ....
....

Describe your overall outlook and mindset today. ....
....
....

LESSONS LEARNED *(fill out at day's end)*

List 3 things you learned today regarding your sleep, water, nutritional needs, or fitness activities and how they correspond to your overall energy and/or mindset. ....
....
....
....

the Perfect You Plan

what is it?

The Perfect You Plan is the ultimate destination of any Projecter. It's the plan that is custom-fit to your body, needs, tastes, preferences, and goals. It includes the number of hours of sleep you actually need at night to feel your best. It includes the experiential knowledge that tells you when you don't get enough sleep; you crave foods that your body doesn't necessarily need (like sweets). It includes the list of healing foods you love and the foods you don't love. It includes the healing foods that you know make you feel your best (maybe half a sweet potato after a workout) and a list of foods that don't make you feel your best (maybe you realized that you don't digest nuts very well). It includes best practices that help you get your workout in, the workouts you're more likely to stick with, and the workouts you should avoid. It includes your favorite kind of water, favorite herbal teas, favorite "in a pinch" snacks, and favorite places to stop for a healthy bite while out. It includes a newfound or re-found intuition about what your body needs (rest, water, food, fitness) and when it needs it.

The Perfect You Plan isn't a diet circumvented by the occasional "cheat meal." *There are no cheat meals* when you're just living your life. There are foods that heal and foods that sabotage. It's up to you to determine how often you indulge and what you're willing to compromise. There's no one single way for this plan to work, which is why it's called the Perfect (For) You Plan. Make it your own! Make a plan that supports your healthy living goals *and* allows you to live a life you love.

how to build it

As you work through the Project, be sure to journal the following when they come up as "lessons learned" for that day. At the end of the Project, I encourage you to rewrite all your lessons learned on a separate sheet of paper. These are the revelations, the important things to remember. These are the gems that you've just spent 28 days mining. Treasure these lessons learned and use *them* to build your Perfect You Plan.

Be on the lookout for these lessons learned:

Mindset:

- *Goals that you modified.*
- *Realizations about your abilities.*
- *Tricks that kept you positive.*

Sleep & Hydration:

- *The number of hours of sleep that left you energized the next day (a number more finely tuned than the DSN found on page 32).*
- *The bedtime that supports the most sleep.*
- *The wake time that supports a productive day and doesn't sacrifice sleep.*
- *Best sleep practices (darker room, colder temperatures, no blue lights, etc.).*
- *The amount of water you drink to feel energized the next day (a number more finely tuned than the DWN found on page 37).*
- *Favorite ways to hydrate (sparkling water, herbal tea with lemon, tap water, etc.)*

Food:

• *Healing or "in-scope" foods that you absolutely love.*

• *Healing or "in-scope" foods that make your body feel great.*

• *How you kicked your dependency on snacks.*

• *What breakfast felt the least overwhelming to prepare.*

• *Your favorite recipes from Fed & Fit.*

Fitness:

• *What motivated you to work out even when you didn't want to.*

• *Workouts that you found fun!*

• *Workouts that made your body feel great.*

• *Workouts that you did not enjoy.*

• *Whether you prefer to work out at home or at a gym, by yourself or with other people.*

• *The workouts that accomplish all Savvy Seven (page 64).*

• *Your favorite workouts (and why).*

Plus any other revelation you had during the 28 days that relates to you and your healthy lifestyle. These may be realizations about your family, work, scheduling, finances, and body image. Lessons learned are precious pieces of custom-fit feedback on your life; catch and keep as many as you can for as long as you can.

The pursuit of the Perfect You Plan may be something you stay in for a while. This is normal. Six years later, I still tweak my plan with new realizations about how to live my healthiest as my life continues to evolve. Stay the course and keep your chin up. All is good, and you're in the driver's seat! If you feel like you've gotten off track, use it as an opportunity to gauge whether you need another reset or just to revisit your previous lessons learned.

get ready to test foods!

This is the fun part. This is where, after the 28-Day Food & Fitness Plan is complete, you reintroduce foods that you're curious about. I recommend working with a single food group at a time. For example, if you're most curious about how dairy impacts you, then test dairy first. Enjoy some grass-fed heavy cream and take note of how you feel afterward. If your symptoms are minimal, then you know that kind of dairy can be part of your PYP!

HERE ARE SOME IDEAS OF FOODS TO TEST:

Organic corn (fresh corn, popcorn, or corn tortillas)	Natural sweeteners such as coconut sugar, honey, maple syrup, and molasses
Dairy from grass-fed cows	Beans
Goat or sheep dairy products	Other gluten-free grains, such as quinoa and rice

the five phases of a projecter

Before I send you off into the world of meal plans, fitness templates, and more recipes than you can shake a stick at, I'd like to briefly overview the mental and physical phases that you're likely to encounter while working through the Project. I review these because I want you to know that you're *not* alone! Even if you don't identify with the phases listed below, I promise you're not the only one. Keep working in the material to the best of your ability and trust the process. The clouds will lift and you will reap the benefits!

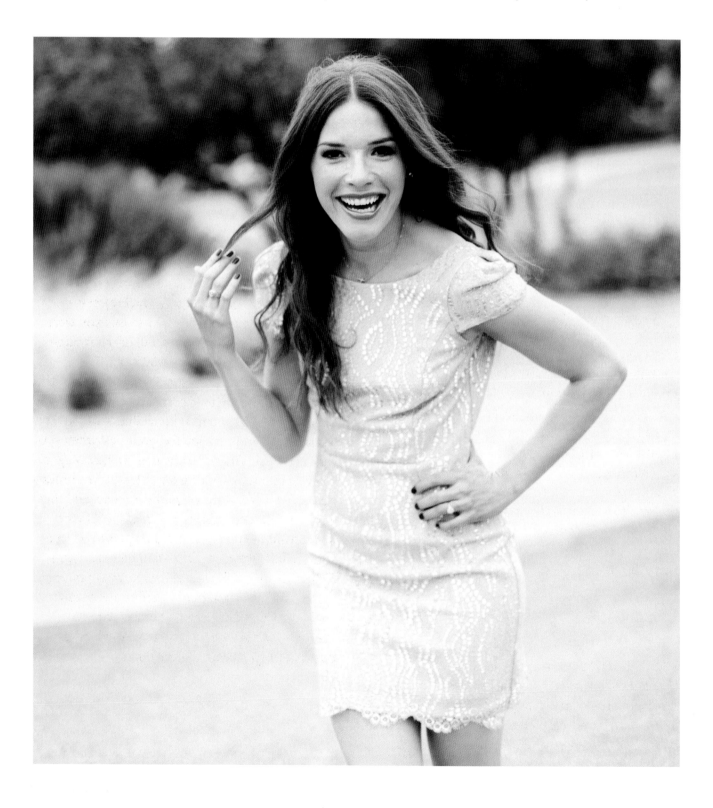

Phase 1: *from the moment you think "I want to do this" to the day before you begin the Project*

LET'S DO THIS!

High-five! You've totally got this. You've got a vision, you've got goals, and you're ready to commit! Maybe you've already cleaned out your pantry and refrigerator of all those sabotaging foods. Maybe you've started to grocery shop and meal plan! Maybe you've already sat your family down to tell them about the 28-day adventure you are about to embark on.

Phase 2: *from day 3 to about day 14 (or maybe even day 21 for some)*

Why am I doing this? This is a lot of work, and I'm uncomfortable.

This feeling is completely normal. If this is your first time pursuing a grain-free, refined sugar–free, Paleo lifestyle, you're going to work through some major adjustments while your body detoxes and you learn to live without bread (and all of the other sabotaging foods from your past). The good news is that you can rely on sleep, delicious food, and adequate amounts of water. Know that change is supposed to be uncomfortable. Comfort equals no change, so try to embrace the suck. Embrace the work that goes into making your meals, embrace the challenge of finding time to make it to the gym, embrace the water bottle you're always lugging around, and embrace the journal! Committing yourself to the plan *will* pay off. The clouds will part. These uncomfortable *new* habits that you're forming will, with a little time and consistency, become comfortable habits. As soon as your body starts to feel lighter, the challenge of this new lifestyle will disappear, too.

Phase 3: *from day 15 to day 21*

Okay, I'm finding a groove. I think I like this.

See? I told you! I knew you'd like it. Cooking isn't that difficult! In fact, you kind of enjoy it. You've discovered that you actually really love braised kale. Though they still make you a little nervous because they always seem difficult on paper, you look forward to your workouts because you love the way they make you feel! You're experiencing more energy and sleep more soundly at night, and people keep telling you how refreshed you look. The foggy detox cloud has lifted, and you love the way you feel.

Phase 4: *from day 22 to day 28*

I LOVE THIS!

The graduate high! You're in love with the way you feel. Cooking feels like second nature now, you've got a meal prep game plan on lockdown, you no longer have to talk yourself into working out (you just do it!), and you feel like you've found the fountain of youth and energy. This last week is going to fly by.

Phase 5: *from day 29 on*

I get it. I really, really get it.

This is the vision I have for you: days, weeks, or maybe months after you complete the Project, you realize that the 28 days on the Project were about helping you feel your best so that you were truly prepared to choose the foods, sleep routines, hydration habits, and fitness plans that fit you best. Maybe you've discovered that you tolerate the occasional dairy, organic corn, and glass of red wine well. Maybe you now know that breakfast is a must for you and that you feel your best when you eat a couple servings of leafy greens a day. Maybe you've found that working out at least three times a week is your recipe for a healthy mindset and that "off-track" indulgences are a part of life. There's no more punishment, no more wagons to be on or off of. You're living your life—a life that supports lasting physical and mental health. You're in your groove, and the mystery of a perfect diet doesn't hold any power over you anymore. You're the one with the power, and you get to decide what's included in your Perfect You Plan.

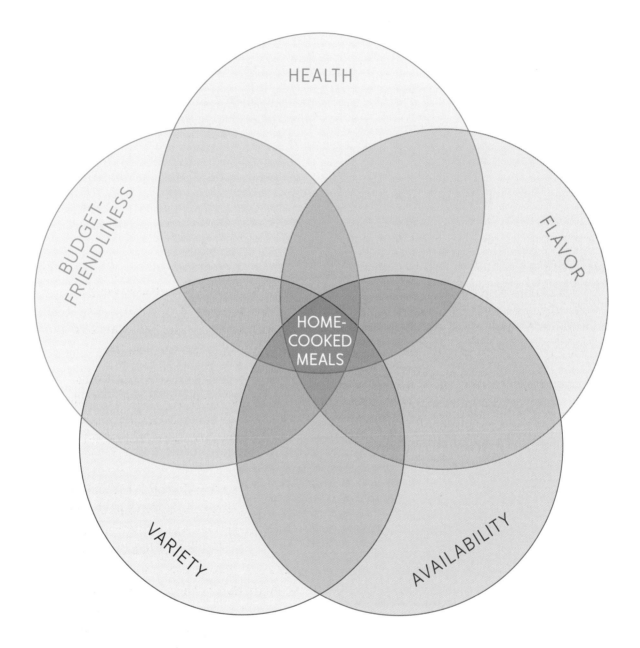

HEALTH

BUDGET-
FRIENDLINESS

FLAVOR

HOME-
COOKED
MEALS

VARIETY

AVAILABILITY

THE RECIPES

Let's get cooking!

When we look at a Venn diagram that links the food-related circles of health, budget-friendliness, flavor, variety, and availability (meaning: how far do you need to go to get it?), notice that they all meet in the middle at home-cooked meals. While home is where the heart is, it's also where affordable, delicious, and accessible health is.

Eating at home, at least most of the time, is the best way to ensure your success on a healthy lifestyle journey—whether you're at the very beginning or smack in the middle. I say this fully aware that not everyone likes to cook! I do love to cook, but I don't like to spend every spare minute in the kitchen. I prefer to make my time at the sink and stove as efficient as possible: minimum effort for maximum output.

So what kind of output are we looking for? We're looking for healthy foods that are as budget-friendly as possible (note that if you're eating in, you're probably spending less than if you ate out), are bursting with delicious flavor, and offer a good deal of variety. Flavor, variety, ease, and getting the most bang for your buck (in both dollars and time) were at the forefront of my mind when I developed the recipes in this book! These recipes are my very best work, you guys. They're the foods that have powered my consistent healthy lifestyle for years. They've helped me maintain dinner-table variety for my small family, successfully entertain large groups of picky eaters, and offer up a healthy addition (that's raved over) to a potluck family reunion. These recipes contain just about every healthy trick that I've got up my sleeve, and I'm beyond thrilled to put them in your hands.

stocking your kitchen

Before we jump into the recipes themselves, let's set the kitchen stage. In a Fed & Fit (or Paleo-friendly) kitchen, there are several ingredients you'll want to keep on hand and several ingredients that you won't need anymore. I like to break up the kitchen into three sections: pantry, refrigerator, and freezer. Let's discuss each of those sections individually.

stocking your pantry

Stocking your pantry for the 28-Day Fed & Fit Project is actually pretty simple. Because flours—even gluten-free and Paleo-friendly nut flours—are considered out of scope, you don't need to worry about buying those (sometimes expensive) baking ingredients. Here's what I recommend that you keep in the pantry:

Perishables:

Citrus fruits: grapefruit, lemons, limes, oranges, tangerines, etc.

Tomatoes and tomatillos

Plantains

Sweet potatoes

White potatoes: russet, red-skinned, Yukon Gold, etc.

Squash: acorn, butternut, spaghetti, etc.

Onions

Garlic

Dates

Raw nuts *(will keep longer if stored in the refrigerator or freezer)*: almonds, cashews, pecans, etc.

Raw seeds *(will keep longer if stored in the refrigerator or freezer)*: chia, pumpkin, sesame, sunflower, etc.

Unsweetened shredded coconut

Fats, sauces, and other ingredients:

Coconut oil

Extra-virgin olive oil *(from a reliable source; Kasandrinos is my preferred brand)*

Ghee

Apple cider vinegar

Balsamic vinegar

Frank's RedHot Sauce

Curry paste *(Thai Kitchen is my preferred brand)*

Coconut aminos *(Coconut Secret is my preferred brand)*

Canned full-fat coconut milk *(Native Forest is my preferred brand)*

Unsweetened cocoa powder

Unsweetened nut and seed butters: almond, cashew, sunflower, etc.

Organic spices: black pepper, chili powder, cumin, garlic powder, Italian seasoning, etc. *(Primal Palate is my preferred brand)*

Fine sea salt

Store-bought beef or chicken broth *(Pacific Foods is my preferred brand, if not making homemade)*

Caffeine-free herbal teas *(Traditional Medicinals is my preferred brand)*

Convenience foods:

RxBar Protein Bars: *These yummy bars are Project compliant!*

Beet chips: *Make sure that the ingredients include only beets, palm oil or another healthy fat, and salt.*

Chicharrones or pork skins: *Make sure that the ingredients include only pork skins and salt.*

Plantain chips: *Make sure that the ingredients include only plantains, palm oil or another healthy fat, and salt.*

Grass-fed, pasture-raised gelatin: *A number of the treat recipes in this book call for gelatin, which is an excellent dietary addition for bone, skin, hair, and joint health. I recommend using gelatin from grass-fed, pastured sources for maximum health benefits. Vital Proteins is my preferred brand.*

Grass-fed, pasture-raised collagen peptides: *Collagen peptides are one of the healthiest sources of powdered protein available. In addition to providing dietary protein, peptides promote healthy skin, strong nails, and hair growth. Collagen peptides, unlike gelatin, dissolve in cool water and do not gel. Most healthy options need to be ordered online, and I recommend that you seek peptides from grass-fed cows. Vital Proteins is my preferred brand.*

Grass-fed, pasture-raised whey protein powder: *If you prefer a whey-based protein powder, I recommend buying one with as few ingredients as possible, ideally sourced from grass-fed cows. Vital Proteins is my preferred brand; it includes just one ingredient: grass-fed whey. Try to avoid highly processed protein powders with long lists of ingredients.*

Here's what I recommend that you either donate to a food pantry, pass on to a neighbor, or store somewhere else in the house for your family (so that you don't have to see them when you're in the kitchen and going through withdrawal):

All baked goods *(including breads, muffins, cookies, and crackers)*

Candy

Chips

Dried fruit *(with the exception of dates, which may be used as a sweetener)*

Non-Project-compliant protein powders or bars

Cereals

Granola

Oatmeal

Pasta

Rice *(at least for the duration of the 28-Day Project)*

Non-Paleo canned soups

Conventional salad dressings

Sauces that contain sugars, food colorings, and other additives

Soda *(regular or diet)*

Sports drinks and mixes

note

If you have a collection of grain-free flours and natural sweeteners, it's okay to keep those on hand. They're expensive, and I don't expect you to toss them! Just remember that they're not considered in scope for the duration of the 28-Day Project.

JUST TO CONFIRM, BAKED GOODS ARE OUT?

That's right! There are zero bready baked goods (with the single quasi-exception of the protein pancakes on page 146) during the 28-Day Fed & Fit Project. This is because baked goods often promote overeating and a lack of nutrient awareness. While grain-free, Paleo-friendly baked goods are absolutely worth considering as an addition to your Perfect You Plan, I recommend going without for these four cleansing, rebalancing weeks.

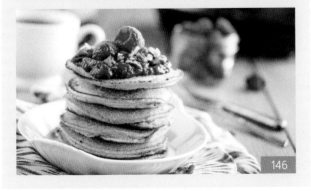

stocking your fridge

Produce and proteins:

Fresh berries: blueberries, raspberries, strawberries, etc.

Grapes

Leafy greens: collards, kale, lettuce, spinach, etc.

Crunchy vegetables: bell peppers, carrots, celery, cucumbers, parsnips, etc.

Pasture-raised beef, pork, poultry, and eggs

Responsibly sourced seafood *(see page 50 for advice on finding the best seafood choices)*

Game meat

Fats and sauces:

Butter from grass-fed cows (I use salted)

Lard, tallow, or duck fat from pastured or grass-fed animals

BBQ sauce *(homemade (page 336) or store-bought; Tessemae's is my preferred brand)*

Mayo *(homemade (page 349) or store-bought; Primal Kitchen is my preferred brand)*

Mustard *(whether grainy, yellow, or spicy, make sure that it's labeled gluten-free and abides by the label reading tips listed on page 116)*

Paleo-friendly salad dressings *(homemade (such as the ranch dressing on page 338) or store-bought; Tessemae's is my preferred brand)*

Pico de gallo *(homemade (page 342) or store-bought; be sure to buy only freshly made pico that's free of additives)*

Salsa *(homemade (pages 344 and 345) or store-bought; be sure to buy only freshly made salsa that's free of additives)*

Drinks:

Unflavored sparkling water or mineral water

Unsweetened coconut water *(enjoy in moderation)*

Cold-brew coffee *(see page 328 for my cold-brew coffee concentrate recipe)*

stocking your freezer

Fruits and vegetables:

Vegetables

Berries that were frozen when in season

Bananas, chopped and then bagged in ½-banana serving sizes for smoothies (recipes on page 150)

Homemade fruit pops for treats (page 318)

Proteins:

Beef: roasts, steaks, ground beef, etc. *(It's best to find a pasture-raised, grass-fed cow-share.)*

Pork: chops, roasts, steaks, ground pork, etc.

Fish

Other cuts of meat

If possible, I highly recommend investing in a separate deep freezer and then purchasing large amounts of healthy proteins and produce when they're on sale. A deep freezer will also give you extra room for freezing leftovers for future meals—a great time-saver.

label reading 101

Stocking your kitchen with high-quality ingredients that will heal your body and help you feel your best requires you to do a little sleuthing:

- Regardless of what's written on the front of a package, flip it over and read the full list of ingredients.

- For the duration of the Project, avoid any food that includes any of the artificial ingredients listed on page 47.

- Try to buy products that contain only ingredients you know and can personally source. For example, although carrageenan (often used as a stabilizer) is extracted from red seaweed, I'd have a hard time buying a batch of it myself, so I avoid it.

- Though these terms don't tell the whole story, look for labels that read organic, gluten-free, soy-free, GMO-free, and sugar- or sweetener-free.

- When buying protein powder, sparkling water, and other Project-compliant foods (like chicharrones), always opt for the "original" or "plain" flavor.

using the recipes in this book

While you're more than welcome to jump right into the recipes, I think it's important to cover a few bases first. In this section, I explain how I've set up my recipes and review the considerations I've made for those who are following specific nutrition programs. I also pass along some tricks for cooking in bulk and storing and reheating leftovers.

prep & cook times

The prep and cook times listed at the top of each recipe are totaled times. Please note that the time required to make cross-referenced subrecipes, such as mayonnaise or broth, is not included in the totaled times, so you will need to factor in the additional time to make those subrecipes. Inactive kitchen time, such as marinating, chilling, or resting, is noted separately.

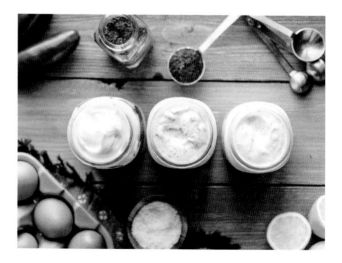

program compliance & recipe modifications

Before I jump into the efforts I've made to meet individual program compliance needs, I want to note that every recipe in this book is:

- Grain-free
- Dairy-free (with the exception of butter used as a cooking fat)
- Legume-free (with the exception of green beans)
- Free of refined sugars
- Free of added sweeteners (including all natural sugars, like honey, maple syrup, and stevia)
- Free of fruits that are especially high in fructose
- Flour-free (including nut flours, coconut flour, arrowroot starch, tapioca starch, and cassava flour)
- Free of baking additives (including baking powder, baking soda, guar gum, xanthan gum, and yeast)

In addition to the above, I've offered specific considerations for individual food intolerances and programs. This book includes recipes that comply with the following programs as noted by their individual icons:

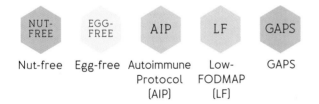

Nut-free   Egg-free   Autoimmune   Low-   GAPS
                       Protocol   FODMAP
                       (AIP)   (LF)

So, for example, if a recipe is marked with the GAPS icon, it is safe for those who are following a GAPS protocol.

I've also included modifications where possible. If a recipe is not AIP friendly when prepared as written but can be made AIP friendly by omitting the black pepper, for example, you'll see the word "Option" above the AIP icon. Look for the recommended modifications within the ingredient list or below it.

cooking fat substitutions

Most of the recipes in this book call for grass-fed salted butter as the preferred cooking fat. This is my personal preference and the way I've tested the recipes. That being said, you absolutely may substitute an equal amount of one of the following fats if you like:

- Coconut oil
- Extra-virgin olive oil (EVOO)
- Grass-fed ghee
- Cage-free duck fat
- Pasture-raised lard
- Palm shortening
- Grass-fed tallow

a couple notes about serving sizes

For almost every recipe, I've given the number of servings as a range: you'll find a smaller number (which represents larger portions) and a larger number (smaller portions). This is because I want the recipes to be as flexible as possible for the number and types of eaters in your household—not everyone eats the same amount of food, after all, and the appropriate portion sizes for different people are, of course, different! Typically, but not exclusively, the smaller number is meant to serve as a guide for men and the larger number as a guide for women. Above all, remember to listen to your body. If you're still hungry, eat more, and if you're absolutely stuffed, eat less. Satiety is a great thing to journal so that you can start to develop a better idea of how much food you personally require.

Note, too, that the recipes I've included produce a range of servings. A few serve just one person, and others feed a crowd. The majority fall somewhere in the middle, serving four to six people. Even if you're cooking for one or two, I encourage you not to shy away from the larger-yield dishes! While they are great to make when you are entertaining guests, they're also wonderful for preparing meals ahead of time. Whether you keep the leftovers in the fridge to enjoy later in the week or you freeze them for those no-time-to-cook days, these larger dishes are meant to help you get the most food for your cooking effort.

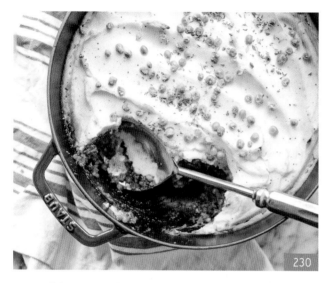
230

cooking in bulk

The biggest, baddest healthy-lifestyle trick I've got up my sleeve is that I intentionally make meals that are too big to eat within a few days so that I have leftovers to freeze for later meals. Though I cook often, there are still days when I'm low on groceries and don't have time to run out and shop so that I can make food. It's on these days that I'm the most tempted to eat an unhealthy meal out, and it's on these days that I'm the most thankful for my freezer-meal stash. After a quick reheat, I've got a healthy, delicious, Project-friendly meal that is sure to nourish my body.

Here's an example of how this works. Let's say I make Roasted Garlic Cottage Pie (page 230) for dinner one night, which makes 6 to 8 servings. My husband and I will likely enjoy two of those servings the night I make the pie, leaving us an extra 4 to 6 servings to store. I'll spoon two of those servings into containers for lunch the next day, and then I'll transfer the remainder into individual portion–size freezer-safe containers. I label each freezer container with the name of the recipe and the date I made it. Then they go into the special part of my freezer designated for healthy frozen meals.

These healthy frozen meals are a lifesaver. Despite our best intentions to cook fresh food every day, sometimes it's just not practical. Building up a supply of frozen meals is a great safety net for when you just don't have the time or the desire to cook.

leftovers 101

Storing leftovers

Which containers you choose to store your food in is a total judgment call, but I'll give you some "best," "good," and "these work" options as a starting point. Some are more practical than others, which is why, at the end of the day, it's up to you to decide.

Best: Glass or stainless-steel containers are great for leftovers and for storing food in the refrigerator. They can also be frozen, but then your best containers may be unavailable for a long time.

Good: Aluminum containers are great for freezing whole casseroles, roasts, and slow-cooker meals.

These Work: Plastic containers and bags, though not the ideal option for health, are super convenient. If I'm being totally transparent, I have to admit that almost every single individually portioned meal in my deep freezer is stored in a plastic bag (if it's a non-watery dish) or plastic container (if it's a soup or stew).

Although I've done my best to include with each recipe that might generate leftovers the approximate storage time for both fridge and freezer, the following table is helpful as a general guide.

HOW LONG ARE FOODS GOOD FOR?		
Food	Refrigerator	Freezer
Prepared proteins	3–5 days	5 months
Prepared vegetables	3–5 days	5 months
Full meals	3–5 days	5 months
Cooked eggs	1 week	5 months
Raw eggs	3 weeks	Not advised
Fresh fish	3 days	5 months
Fresh beef, pork, or game meat	4 days	5 months
Raw vegetables	10 days	5 months
Fresh berries	4 days	5 months
Fresh citrus	2 weeks	5 months

Reheating leftovers

Though I've included specific information about how to reheat leftovers for many of the recipes in this book, the following is a brief overview of your reheating options.

From the refrigerator:

• Oven: *While the oven is the slowest method of reheating, it does the best job of heating foods thoroughly and evenly. I recommend this method for all full casseroles, roasts, or slow-cooker meals. Though temperatures can vary, 350°F is a good temperature for reheating most foods. Simply place the food on a baking sheet or in a casserole dish when the oven reaches temperature. If you're reheating the food in its refrigerated container (like a casserole dish), it's best to let the dish sit out at room temperature while the oven preheats. Keep an eye on it, but smaller foods (like fries or tostones) will be ready after 10 to 15 minutes, while larger dishes (like full casseroles) may take 30 to 35 minutes to heat through. You can check the temperature either with a food thermometer or by cutting into the dish to test if it's warmed through.*

• Stovetop: *This is my preferred method for smaller-batch food that I want to crisp back up. I recommend starting with a small amount of cooking fat in a large frying pan. Once melted, add the food and cook until heated through. For soups and stews, you can simply add them to an appropriately sized pot, cover, place over medium heat, and enjoy once it comes to a simmer.*

• Microwave*: *If using a microwave, cover the food with a paper towel and microwave for 2 to 5 minutes (depending on the size of the dish) until it's warmed through.*

• A note about toaster ovens: *Though not found in every kitchen, a toaster oven can be a happy middle ground between an oven and a microwave. It typically heats foods quickly like a microwave, but thoroughly like an oven.*

* I understand that some people prefer not to use a microwave, and I support you whatever your stance. I've included oven, stovetop, and microwave instructions to cover all the bases, whatever your personal preferences.

From the freezer:

The only thing that's truly different about reheating food from the freezer versus the refrigerator is that the food needs to be defrosted first. Defrosting times vary for different kinds and sizes of foods. Follow this rough guide for defrosting practices, then choose one of the reheating methods listed at left.

• *For a large dish (casserole, whole roast, etc.) or raw protein, I recommend placing it in the refrigerator for a slow defrost at a safe temperature two full days in advance.*

• *For a cooked single-serving meal, you can either place it in the refrigerator to defrost one day in advance or defrost it as you cook it. To do the latter, simply add time to your reheating method: 5 to 7 minutes for the oven, 3 to 4 minutes for the stovetop, or 1 to 2 minutes for the microwave.*

Note that if you choose to defrost in the microwave, you can use the defrost feature. If you're planning to reheat your food in the microwave, using the defrost setting will result in a more even defrost.

a note for new cooks

I want to get this out there: there was a time when I didn't know the first thing about how to cook. I wasn't born with this knowledge or skill, and it didn't come to me overnight. Everyone has to start somewhere, so don't think that you're not capable! Keep your chin up, have fun, know that not every dish is going to turn out exactly the way you hoped, and remember that at the end of the day, at least you're cooking with healthy ingredients. Take care with your food and have patience while you cook. One of my biggest lessons learned in the kitchen is that rushed meals don't always work out, but the meals that I take my time on (making sure to brown the meat, not crowd the pan, etc.) are always favorites.

Pat yourself on the back each and every time you try something new, and remember that, just like learning a new sport (shout-out to the soccer story on page 23), cooking will get easier the more you do it.

You got this!

Download the Fed & Fit iPhone and Android app! You can scan the adjacent QR codes directly in the app, which will then populate a consolidated grocery shopping list for the scanned recipes.

CHAPTER 1:
SIMPLE MEAL COMPONENTS

No more than 5 ingredients and 5 steps

Proteins

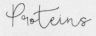 Perfect Baked Chicken Breast
122

Crispy Baked Chicken Thighs
122

Simple Shredded Chicken
123

Basic Pork Tenderloin
123

Basic Pork Chops
124

Simple Sautéed Shrimp
124

Pan-Seared Steak
125

Easy Tuna Steak
125

Pan-Seared Salmon
126

Roasted Turkey Breast
126

Simple Seasoned Ground Beef
127

Veggies

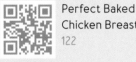 Crispy Brussels Sprouts
127

Grilled Summer Squash
128

Simple Roasted Cauliflower
128

Roasted Broccoli
129

Braised Greens
129

Basic Cauliflower Rice
130

Crispy Okra
130

Roasted Cherry Tomatoes
131

Starches

Roasted Acorn Squash
131

Caramelized Carrots
132

Perfect Parsnips
132

Baked Potatoes—Sweet Potatoes
133

Baked Potatoes—Russets
133

Roasted Potatoes—Yukon Golds
133

Roasted Potatoes—Fingerlings
133

Boiled Potatoes—New Potatoes
134

Simple Hash Browns
134

Easy Parsnip Mash
135

Roasted Butternut Squash
135

Simple Spaghetti Squash
136

Easy Baked Beets
136

Boiled Yuca
137

Green Peas
137

Proteins

Perfect Baked Chicken Breast

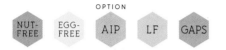

| *prep time: 5 minutes* | *cook time: 18 minutes* | *yield: 2 to 3 servings* |

1 pound boneless, skinless chicken breasts, rinsed and patted dry

2 teaspoons extra-virgin olive oil

½ teaspoon fine sea salt

¼ teaspoon ground black pepper (omit for AIP)

1. Preheat the oven to 450°F. Line a rimmed baking sheet with parchment paper.

2. Coat the chicken breasts with the olive oil and sprinkle with the salt and pepper. Place them on the prepared baking sheet and bake for 15 to 18 minutes, until the juices run clear and the chicken is starting to brown.

3. Let rest for 5 minutes before cutting.

APPROXIMATE NUTRITION BREAKDOWN	
(based on 1 of 3 servings)	
CALORIES: 208	FAT: 7 g
PROTEIN: 34 g	CARBS: 0 g

Crispy Baked Chicken Thighs

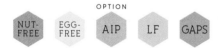

| *prep time: 5 minutes* | *cook time: 45 minutes* | *yield: 2 to 3 servings* |

2 pounds bone-in, skin-on chicken thighs, rinsed and patted dry

½ teaspoon fine sea salt

¼ teaspoon ground black pepper (omit for AIP)

1. Preheat oven to 400°F. Line a rimmed baking sheet with parchment paper.

2. Sprinkle the tops of the chicken thighs with the salt and pepper. Place them on the prepared baking sheet and bake for 45 minutes, or until the juices run clear and the tops are browned but not burned.

3. Let rest for 5 minutes before cutting.

APPROXIMATE NUTRITION BREAKDOWN	
(based on 1 of 3 servings)	
CALORIES: 633	FAT: 46 g
PROTEIN: 52 g	CARBS: 0 g

Simple Shredded Chicken

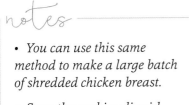

prep time: 5 minutes | cook time: 4 to 10 hours | yield: 3 to 4 servings (about 4 cups)

1 whole chicken (4 to 5 pounds), rinsed and patted dry

Fine sea salt and ground black pepper (optional) (omit pepper for AIP)

notes

• *You can use this same method to make a large batch of shredded chicken breast.*

• *Save the cooking liquid and use it as an extremely basic broth.*

APPROXIMATE NUTRITION BREAKDOWN *(based on 1 of 4 servings)*			
CALORIES:	220	FAT:	2 g
PROTEIN:	52 g	CARBS:	0 g

Slow cooker method: Place the chicken in the slow cooker and cover with water. Place the lid on the slow cooker and cook on low for 8 to 10 hours or on high for 4 to 6 hours, until the chicken falls apart easily. When the chicken is cool enough to handle, transfer it to a large bowl and work to separate the meat from the bones and skin; discard the skin and bones or save the bones to make broth. Shred the meat and moisten it with some of the liquid from the slow cooker. Season with salt and pepper or use as desired.

Pressure cooker method: Place the chicken in the pressure cooker and cover with water. Seal and, following the pressure cooker manufacturer's instructions for cooking a whole chicken, cook until the chicken is done. Slowly release the pressure and let sit for 30 minutes once the pressure dissipates. Transfer the cooked chicken to a large bowl and work to separate the meat from the bones and skin; discard the skin and bones or save the bones to make broth. Shred the meat and moisten it with some of the liquid from the pressure cooker. Season with salt and pepper or use as desired.

Basic Pork Tenderloin

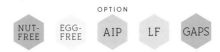

prep time: 5 minutes | cook time: 30 minutes | yield: 3 to 4 servings

1 tablespoon salted butter (use EVOO for AIP)

1 (1¼-pound) pork tenderloin, trimmed

½ teaspoon fine sea salt

¼ teaspoon ground black pepper (omit for AIP)

APPROXIMATE NUTRITION BREAKDOWN *(based on 1 of 4 servings)*			
CALORIES:	226	FAT:	8 g
PROTEIN:	36 g	CARBS:	0 g

1. Preheat the oven to 375°F.

2. In a large cast-iron or other oven-safe frying pan, melt the butter over high heat. While the butter melts, sprinkle all sides of the pork with the salt and pepper.

3. Once the butter has melted, sear the tenderloin on all sides for about 2 minutes per side, until it develops a nice char. Transfer the pan to the oven and bake for 25 minutes, or until the internal temperature reads 160°F.

4. Let rest for 10 minutes, then slice and serve.

Basic Pork Chops

NUT-FREE | EGG-FREE | OPTION AIP | LF | GAPS

prep time: 5 minutes | *cook time: 10 minutes* | *yield: 2 to 3 servings*

2 tablespoons salted butter (use EVOO for AIP)

2 (1-inch-thick) boneless pork chops (about 1 pound)

1 teaspoon fine sea salt

½ teaspoon ground black pepper (omit for AIP)

1. Melt the butter in a large cast-iron, enameled, or stainless-steel frying pan over medium-high heat. Sprinkle the pork chops with the salt and pepper.

2. Sear the chops for 4 minutes per side, or until the inside is just lightly pink and the outside has a nice brown sear. Let rest for 5 minutes before serving.

APPROXIMATE NUTRITION BREAKDOWN
(based on 1 of 3 servings)

CALORIES: 254	FAT: 13 g
PROTEIN: 33 g	CARBS: 0 g

Simple Sautéed Shrimp

NUT-FREE | EGG-FREE | OPTION AIP | OPTION LF | GAPS

prep time: 20 minutes | *cook time: 8 minutes* | *yield: 2 to 3 servings*

1 tablespoon salted butter (use EVOO for AIP)

1 pound large shrimp, peeled and deveined

½ teaspoon garlic powder (omit for low-FODMAP)

½ teaspoon fine sea salt

2 tablespoons fresh lemon juice (about 1 small lemon)

1. Melt the butter in a large frying pan over high heat. Sprinkle the shrimp with the garlic powder and salt. Add the shrimp to the pan and reduce the heat to medium. Cook for 3 minutes per side, or until pink.

2. Once cooked, add the lemon juice and stir to combine.

APPROXIMATE NUTRITION BREAKDOWN
(based on 1 of 3 servings)

CALORIES: 197	FAT: 6 g
PROTEIN: 31 g	CARBS: 0 g

Pan-Seared Steak

| NUT-FREE | EGG-FREE | OPTION AIP | LF | GAPS |

prep time: 5 minutes | *cook time: 5 to 10 minutes* | *yield: 1 serving*

1 tablespoon salted butter (use EVOO for AIP)

1 (4- to 6-ounce) boneless sirloin or rib-eye steak, about 1 inch thick

½ teaspoon fine sea salt

¼ teaspoon ground black pepper (omit for AIP)

1. Melt the butter in a large cast-iron, enameled, or stainless-steel frying pan over medium-high heat. Sprinkle the steak with the salt and pepper.

2. Sear the steak on each side for 2 minutes for rare, 3 minutes for medium-rare, and 4 minutes for well-done. Let rest for 5 minutes, then enjoy warm.

APPROXIMATE NUTRITION BREAKDOWN	
(based on 1 serving)	
CALORIES: 436	FAT: 18 g
PROTEIN: 33 g	CARBS: 0 g

Easy Tuna Steak

| OPTION NUT-FREE | EGG-FREE | OPTION AIP | LF | GAPS |

prep time: 5 minutes | *cook time: 5 minutes* | *yield: 1 to 2 servings*

1 tablespoon salted butter (use EVOO for AIP)

1 (8-ounce) tuna steak, about 1 inch thick

1 tablespoon black sesame seeds (omit for AIP and nut-free)

½ teaspoon fine sea salt

¼ teaspoon ground black pepper (omit for AIP)

1. Melt the butter in a frying pan over medium-high heat. Dust both sides of the tuna with the sesame seeds, salt, and pepper.

2. Once the butter has melted, sear the tuna for 2 minutes per side, or until a light brown crust develops on the outside and the inside is still pink. (This cook time results in medium-done tuna; if you like your tuna slightly more or less done, adjust the time accordingly.)

3. Let the tuna rest for 5 to 10 minutes before serving. Enjoy warm or chilled and sliced over a salad.

APPROXIMATE NUTRITION BREAKDOWN	
(based on 1 of 2 servings)	
CALORIES: 197	FAT: 9 g
PROTEIN: 29 g	CARBS: 1 g

Pan-Seared Salmon

NUT-FREE   EGG-FREE   OPTION AIP   LF   GAPS

prep time: 5 minutes | *cook time: 6 minutes* | *yield: 2 to 3 servings*

1 tablespoon salted butter (use EVOO for AIP)

1 (1-pound) salmon fillet, cut into 2 or 3 portions

½ teaspoon fine sea salt

¼ teaspoon ground black pepper (omit for AIP)

1. Melt the butter in a large cast-iron, enameled, or stainless-steel frying pan over high heat. Sprinkle the salmon with the salt and pepper.

2. Sear the salmon for 3 minutes per side, or until the fish flakes at the thickest part. Let rest for 5 minutes before serving.

APPROXIMATE NUTRITION BREAKDOWN (based on 1 of 3 servings)	
CALORIES: 248	FAT: 12 g
PROTEIN: 32 g	CARBS: 0 g

Roasted Turkey Breast

NUT-FREE   EGG-FREE   OPTION AIP   OPTION LF   GAPS

prep time: 5 minutes | *cook time: 1 hour 30 minutes* | *yield: 8 to 12 servings*

1 (5- to 7-pound) bone-in turkey breast, thawed

1 tablespoon extra-virgin olive oil

1 teaspoon fine sea salt

1 teaspoon garlic powder (omit for low-FODMAP)

½ teaspoon ground black pepper (omit for AIP)

1. Preheat the oven to 325°F. Massage the turkey breast with the olive oil, salt, garlic powder, and pepper, then place it breast side down on a rack in a roasting pan. Cover loosely with aluminum foil and bake for 1 hour.

2. Remove from the oven and carefully flip the turkey over so that it is breast side up. Increase the oven temperature to 400°F and return the turkey, uncovered, to the oven for an additional 30 minutes, or until a meat thermometer reads 165°F when inserted in the thickest part of the breast.

3. Let rest covered loosely with foil for 15 minutes before carving.

APPROXIMATE NUTRITION BREAKDOWN (based on 1 of 12 servings)	
CALORIES: 384	FAT: 17 g
PROTEIN: 49 g	CARBS: 0 g

Simple Seasoned Ground Beef

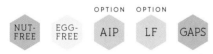

NUT-FREE EGG-FREE OPTION AIP OPTION LF GAPS

prep time: 5 minutes | *cook time: 15 minutes* | *yield: 2 to 3 servings*

1 tablespoon salted butter (use EVOO for AIP)

1 pound ground beef

1 teaspoon chili powder (omit for AIP)

1 teaspoon garlic powder (omit for low-FODMAP)

½ teaspoon fine sea salt

1. Melt the butter in a large frying pan over high heat. Add the beef and, using a rubber spatula or spoon, break it up into clumps. Cook, stirring occasionally, until the meat is no longer pink, about 10 minutes.

2. Season the beef with the chili powder, garlic powder, and salt. Stir to combine and continue to cook until most of the moisture has evaporated, about 5 minutes.

APPROXIMATE NUTRITION BREAKDOWN *(based on 1 of 3 servings)*	
CALORIES: 364	FAT: 26 g
PROTEIN: 28 g	CARBS: 0 g

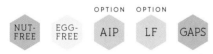

Crispy Brussels Sprouts

NUT-FREE EGG-FREE OPTION AIP OPTION LF GAPS

prep time: 15 minutes | *cook time: 45 minutes* | *yield: 4 servings*

12 ounces Brussels sprouts*, cut in half

2 tablespoons fresh lemon juice (about 1 small lemon)

1 tablespoon extra-virgin olive oil

½ teaspoon fine sea salt

¼ teaspoon ground black pepper (omit for AIP)

1. Preheat the oven to 375°F. Line a rimmed baking sheet with parchment paper.

2. Toss the Brussels sprouts in the lemon juice, olive oil, salt, and pepper. Spread them out on the prepared baking sheet.

3. Bake for 45 minutes, or until the tops are crispy but not burned.

*Consume Brussels sprouts on a low-FODMAP protocol only if well tolerated.

APPROXIMATE NUTRITION BREAKDOWN *(per serving)*	
CALORIES: 68	FAT: 4 g
PROTEIN: 3 g	CARBS: 8 g

Grilled Summer Squash

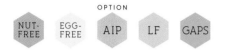

prep time: 10 minutes | *cook time: 10 minutes* | *yield: 2 to 4 servings*

4 zucchini or yellow squash, cut in half lengthwise

2 teaspoons extra-virgin olive oil

½ teaspoon fine sea salt

¼ teaspoon ground black pepper (omit for AIP)

1. Preheat a grill or grill pan over high heat. Rub the cut sides of the zucchini with the olive oil. Sprinkle with the salt and pepper.

2. Grill the zucchini for 5 minutes per side, or until grill marks are visible.

APPROXIMATE NUTRITION BREAKDOWN *(based on 1 of 4 servings)*	
CALORIES: 54	FAT: 3 g
PROTEIN: 2 g	CARBS: 6 g

Simple Roasted Cauliflower

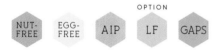

prep time: 10 minutes | *cook time: 40 minutes* | *yield: 3 servings*

1 large head cauliflower*

1 tablespoon extra-virgin olive oil

½ teaspoon garlic powder (omit for low-FODMAP)

½ teaspoon fine sea salt

1. Preheat the oven to 375°F. Line a rimmed baking sheet with parchment paper.

2. Cut the cauliflower florets away from the head and separate or cut into bite-sized pieces. Toss the cauliflower in the olive oil, garlic powder, and salt. Spread it out on the prepared baking sheet.

3. Bake for 40 minutes, or until the tops are golden brown.

Consume cauliflower on a low-FODMAP protocol only if well tolerated.

APPROXIMATE NUTRITION BREAKDOWN *(per serving)*	
CALORIES: 88	FAT: 5 g
PROTEIN: 4 g	CARBS: 10 g

Roasted Broccoli

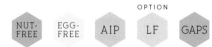

prep time: 10 minutes | *cook time: 25 minutes* | *yield: 4 servings*

2 medium to large heads broccoli*

1 tablespoon extra-virgin olive oil

½ teaspoon garlic powder (omit for low-FODMAP)

½ teaspoon fine sea salt

APPROXIMATE NUTRITION BREAKDOWN *(per serving)*	
CALORIES: 134	FAT: 4 g
PROTEIN: 9 g	CARBS: 20 g

1. Preheat the oven to 400ºF. Line a rimmed baking sheet with parchment paper.

2. Cut the broccoli florets away from the head, leaving the long stem attached. Peel and slice the stem and add to the florets.

3. Toss the broccoli in the olive oil, garlic powder, and salt. Spread it out on the prepared baking sheet.

4. Bake for 15 minutes, flip each piece over, and bake for an additional 10 minutes, or until the tops are golden brown.

*Consume broccoli on a low-FODMAP protocol only if well tolerated.

Braised Greens

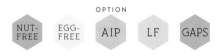

prep time: 10 minutes | *cook time: 10 minutes* | *yield: 4 servings*

1 tablespoon salted butter (use EVOO for AIP)

1 small bunch collard greens, kale, or other braising green of choice (about 1 pound), destemmed and roughly chopped

1 tablespoon fresh lemon juice (about ½ small lemon)

½ teaspoon fine sea salt

APPROXIMATE NUTRITION BREAKDOWN *(per serving)*	
CALORIES: 62	FAT: 3 g
PROTEIN: 3 g	CARBS: 6 g

1. Melt the butter over medium heat in a large frying pan that has a matching lid. Add the greens, toss to coat in the butter, and cover to steam until wilted, about 5 minutes.

2. Add the lemon juice and salt and stir to combine with the wilted greens. Serve warm.

Basic Cauliflower Rice

OPTION

NUT-FREE · EGG-FREE · AIP · LF · GAPS

prep time: 5 minutes | *cook time: 10 to 15 minutes, depending on method* | *yield: 4 servings*

1 large head cauliflower*

1 tablespoon salted butter (use EVOO for AIP)

APPROXIMATE NUTRITION BREAKDOWN	
(per serving)	
CALORIES: 78	FAT: 3g
PROTEIN: 4g	CARBS: 11g

1. To "rice" cauliflower, you can either grate it by hand using the largest holes on a box grater or affix the grating attachment to a food processor and let it do the work for you. One large head of cauliflower should give you 3 cups of "rice."

2. Steam the cauliflower rice using one of these two methods:

   Microwave option: Place the riced cauliflower in a microwave-safe bowl with ¼ cup water. Cover and microwave on high for 10 minutes, or until cooked through. Let cool slightly, then drain. Add the butter and toss to combine.

   Stovetop option: Melt the butter in a large frying pan or sauté pan with a tight-fitting lid over medium heat, then add the riced cauliflower. Stir to incorporate, cover, and let steam over medium-low heat for 12 to 15 minutes, until the cauliflower is cooked through.

*Consume cauliflower on a low-FODMAP protocol only if well tolerated.

Crispy Okra

OPTION

NUT-FREE · EGG-FREE · AIP

prep time: 10 minutes | *cook time: 40 minutes* | *yield: 4 servings*

1 pound fresh okra, cut into ½-inch-thick discs

2 teaspoons extra-virgin olive oil

1 teaspoon fine sea salt

¼ teaspoon ground black pepper (omit for AIP)

1. Preheat the oven to 375°F. Line a rimmed baking sheet with parchment paper.

2. Toss the okra with the olive oil, salt, and pepper. Spread it out on the prepared baking sheet.

3. Bake for 40 minutes, or until it just begins to darken in color.

APPROXIMATE NUTRITION BREAKDOWN	
(per serving)	
CALORIES: 58	FAT: 2g
PROTEIN: 2g	CARBS: 9g

Roasted Cherry Tomatoes

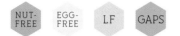

prep time: 5 minutes | *cook time: 40 minutes* | *yield: 2 servings*

1 pint cherry tomatoes

1 teaspoon extra-virgin olive oil

½ teaspoon fine sea salt

¼ teaspoon ground black pepper

1. Preheat the oven to 375°F. Line a rimmed baking sheet with parchment paper.

2. Toss the tomatoes with the olive oil, salt, and pepper. Spread them out on the prepared baking sheet.

3. Bake for 40 minutes, or until they just begin to burst and darken in color.

APPROXIMATE NUTRITION BREAKDOWN *(per serving)*			
CALORIES:	60	FAT:	2 g
PROTEIN:	2 g	CARBS:	8 g

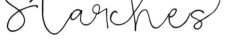

Roasted Acorn Squash

OPTION

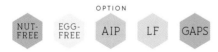

prep time: 10 minutes | *cook time: 40 minutes* | *yield: 4 servings*

1 acorn squash, cut into quarters and seeded

2 teaspoons extra-virgin olive oil

½ teaspoon fine sea salt

¼ teaspoon ground black pepper (omit for AIP)

1. Preheat the oven to 375°F.

2. Rub the cut sides of the squash with the olive oil and sprinkle with the salt and pepper. Place the squash wedges cut side up in a baking dish.

3. Bake for 40 minutes, or until fork-tender.

APPROXIMATE NUTRITION BREAKDOWN *(per serving)*			
CALORIES:	63	FAT:	2 g
PROTEIN:	1 g	CARBS:	11 g

Caramelized Carrots

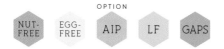

OPTION

NUT-FREE · EGG-FREE · AIP · LF · GAPS

prep time: 10 minutes | *cook time: 45 minutes* | *yield: 4 servings*

2 bunches slender carrots (about 1 pound), peeled

1 tablespoon fresh lemon juice (about ½ small lemon)

2 teaspoons extra-virgin olive oil

½ teaspoon fine sea salt

¼ teaspoon ground black pepper (omit for AIP)

1. Preheat the oven to 375°F. Line a rimmed baking sheet with parchment paper.

2. Toss the carrots with the lemon juice, olive oil, salt, and pepper. Spread them out on the prepared baking sheet.

3. Bake for 45 minutes, or until the tops start to brown.

APPROXIMATE NUTRITION BREAKDOWN *(per serving)*			
CALORIES:	68	FAT:	3 g
PROTEIN:	1 g	CARBS:	11 g

Perfect Parsnips

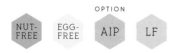

OPTION

NUT-FREE · EGG-FREE · AIP · LF

prep time: 10 minutes | *cook time: 35 minutes* | *yield: 4 servings*

2 pounds parsnips, peeled and cut crosswise into ½-inch discs

2 teaspoons extra-virgin olive oil

½ teaspoon fine sea salt

¼ teaspoon ground black pepper (omit for AIP)

1. Preheat the oven to 375°F. Line a rimmed baking sheet with parchment paper.

2. Toss the parsnips with the olive oil, salt, and pepper. Spread them out in an even layer on the prepared baking sheet.

3. Bake for 35 minutes, or until the tops start to brown.

APPROXIMATE NUTRITION BREAKDOWN *(per serving)*			
CALORIES:	190	FAT:	3 g
PROTEIN:	3 g	CARBS:	41 g

Baked Potatoes—Sweets or Russets

OPTION

NUT-FREE · EGG-FREE · AIP · LF

prep time: varies | *cook time: 35 to 45 minutes* | *yield: 1, 4, or 12 servings*

Sweet* or russet potato(es):
1 medium (for 1 serving), 1 pound (for 4 servings), or 3 pounds (for 12 servings)

1. Preheat the oven to 425°F. Wash and pat dry the potato(es). Poke each potato four or five times with a fork.

2. Bake the potato(es) until soft to the touch: about 35 minutes for 1 medium potato, 40 minutes for 1 pound, or 45 minutes for 3 pounds.

Use sweet potatoes for AIP. If following a low-FODMAP protocol, consume sweet potatoes only if well tolerated.

APPROXIMATE NUTRITION BREAKDOWN	
(per serving)	
CALORIES: 110	FAT: 0 g
PROTEIN: 2 g	CARBS: 25 g

Roasted Potatoes—Yukon Golds or Fingerlings

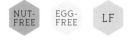

NUT-FREE · EGG-FREE · LF

prep time: varies | *cook time: 30 to 45 minutes* | *yield: 1, 4, or 12 servings*

Yukon Gold or fingerling potato(es):
1 medium Yukon Gold or a handful of fingerlings (for 1 serving), 1 pound (for 4 servings), or 3 pounds (for 12 servings)

½ teaspoon to 2 tablespoons extra-virgin olive oil

1. Preheat the oven to 375°F.

2. Wash and pat dry the potato(es).

3. If using Yukon Golds, cut each potato lengthwise into four long wedges. If using fingerlings, cut each potato in half lengthwise. Toss the potato wedges or halves in olive oil, using ½ teaspoon of oil for a single serving, 2 teaspoons for 1 pound, or 2 tablespoons for 3 pounds. Spread out the potatoes on a rimmed baking sheet.

4. Bake until crispy: 30 minutes for 1 medium potato, 35 minutes for 1 pound, or 45 minutes for 3 pounds.

APPROXIMATE NUTRITION BREAKDOWN	
(per serving)	
CALORIES: 140	FAT: 0 g
PROTEIN: 3 g	CARBS: 26 g

Boiled Potatoes—New Potatoes

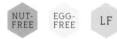

prep time: varies | *cook time: 15 minutes* | *yield: 1, 4, or 12 servings*

Round red-skinned or white-skinned potatoes: 2 to 3 potatoes, depending on size (for 1 serving), 1 pound (for 4 servings), or 3 pounds (for 12 servings)

1. So that all of the potatoes cook at the same rate, cut any large potatoes so that they're roughly the same size as the smallest whole potatoes.

2. Place the potatoes in a pot, cover with water, and bring to a boil. Reduce the heat to medium and simmer until fork-tender, about 15 minutes, depending on size.

APPROXIMATE NUTRITION BREAKDOWN *(per serving)*	
CALORIES: 360	FAT: 0 g
PROTEIN: 10 g	CARBS: 81 g

Simple Hash Browns

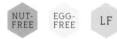

prep time: 15 minutes | *cook time: 20 minutes* | *yield: 4 servings*

3 medium-sized russet potatoes (about 1 pound), shredded

2 tablespoons salted butter

1 teaspoon fine sea salt, divided

¼ teaspoon ground black pepper, divided

1. Place the shredded potatoes in a large bowl and cover with lukewarm water. Let the potatoes sit in the water for about 5 minutes or until the water is cloudy (this indicates excess starch has been removed). Place the potatoes in a nut bag, dish towel, or piece of cheesecloth and squeeze out as much water as possible.

2. Heat a large cast-iron skillet over high heat. Once hot, add the butter and, when the butter is melted, spread the shredded and drained potatoes out in the pan in an even layer. Season the top with half of the salt and pepper. Reduce the heat to medium-high and let the potatoes cook for 10 to 12 minutes, or until the bottoms look browned and crispy.

3. Working in several sections, use a metal spatula to flip pieces of the hash browns. Season with the rest of the salt and pepper and cook on the second side for 5 to 6 minutes, or until browned and crispy. Enjoy warm. To reheat leftovers, simply cook in a hot dry cast-iron frying pan until warmed through.

APPROXIMATE NUTRITION BREAKDOWN *(per serving)*	
CALORIES: 159	FAT: 6 g
PROTEIN: 3 g	CARBS: 22.5 g

Easy Parsnip Mash

NUT-FREE EGG-FREE OPTION AIP

prep time: 15 minutes | *cook time: 45 minutes* | *yield: 6 servings*

6 large parsnips, peeled and cut into 1-inch pieces

2 tablespoons extra-virgin olive oil

1 (13½-ounce) can full-fat coconut milk

¼ cup fresh lemon juice (about 2 small lemons)

1 teaspoon fine sea salt

½ teaspoon ground black pepper (omit for AIP)

1. Preheat the oven to 350°F and line a rimmed baking sheet with parchment paper. Toss the cut parsnips in the olive oil and spread them out in one even layer on the baking sheet. Bake for 45 minutes, or until they're easily pierced with a fork.

2. When the parsnips are finished roasting, place them in a food processor or blender. Pour in the coconut milk, lemon juice, salt, and pepper. Blend until smooth.

3. If the mixture doesn't have enough liquid to blend, add up to ¼ cup water. Enjoy warm.

APPROXIMATE NUTRITION BREAKDOWN *(per serving)*	
CALORIES: 209	FAT: 34.3 g
PROTEIN: 1.6 g	CARBS: 12.8 g

Roasted Butternut Squash

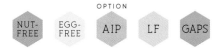

NUT-FREE EGG-FREE OPTION AIP LF GAPS

prep time: 15 minutes | *cook time: 40 minutes* | *yield: 5 servings*

1 medium butternut squash (about 2½ pounds)

1 tablespoon extra-virgin olive oil

1 teaspoon fine sea salt

¼ teaspoon ground black pepper (omit for AIP)

1. Preheat the oven to 375°F. Line a rimmed baking sheet with parchment paper.

2. Peel the squash, cut it in half lengthwise, and remove the seeds, then cut it into ½-inch cubes. Toss the squash with the olive oil, salt, and pepper. Spread out the squash on the lined baking sheet.

3. Bake for 40 minutes, or until the tops start to turn brown. Serve warm.

APPROXIMATE NUTRITION BREAKDOWN *(per serving)*	
CALORIES: 106	FAT: 3 g
PROTEIN: 2 g	CARBS: 21 g

Simple Spaghetti Squash

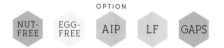

prep time: 10 minutes | *cook time: 30 minutes* | *yield: 6 servings*

1 large spaghetti squash (about 7 pounds)

2 tablespoons salted butter (use EVOO for AIP)

½ teaspoon fine sea salt

¼ teaspoon ground black pepper (omit for AIP)

1. Preheat the oven to 375°F.

2. Cut the squash in half lengthwise and scrape out the seeds with a large spoon. Place the squash cut side down on a rimmed baking sheet.

3. Bake for 30 minutes, or until the flesh is easily pierced with a fork.

4. Scrape the squash "threads" into a large bowl and toss with the butter, salt, and pepper. Serve warm.

APPROXIMATE NUTRITION BREAKDOWN			
(per serving)			
CALORIES:	54	FAT:	4 g
PROTEIN:	0 g	CARBS:	5 g

Easy Baked Beets

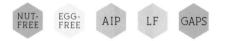

prep time: 10 minutes | *cook time: 45 minutes to 1 hour* | *yield: 4 servings*

3 to 4 large beets*, trimmed

2 teaspoons extra-virgin olive oil

1 teaspoon dried thyme leaves

½ teaspoon fine sea salt

1. Preheat the oven to 400°F.

2. Wrap each beet in a piece of aluminum foil. Bake for 45 minutes to 1 hour, until the beets give when squeezed.

3. Let the beets cool to room temperature, then rub the skins off. Cut the beets into wedges and toss with the olive oil, thyme, and salt. Serve at room temperature or chilled.

*Consume beets on a low-FODMAP protocol only if well tolerated.

APPROXIMATE NUTRITION BREAKDOWN			
(per serving)			
CALORIES:	56	FAT:	2 g
PROTEIN:	1 g	CARBS:	8 g

Boiled Yuca

NUT-FREE   **EGG-FREE**   **AIP**   **LF**

prep time: 10 minutes | *cook time: 25 minutes* | *yield: 4 servings*

1 pound fresh yuca, peeled and cut crosswise into 1-inch rounds

2 tablespoons fresh lime juice (about 1 lime)

½ teaspoon fine sea salt

1. Place the yuca in a large saucepan and cover with water. Bring to a boil over high heat, then reduce the heat to medium and let simmer for 15 minutes, or until the yuca is fork-tender.

2. Drain the yuca, then toss with the lime juice and salt. Serve warm.

APPROXIMATE NUTRITION BREAKDOWN *(per serving)*	
CALORIES: 182	FAT: 1 g
PROTEIN: 5 g	CARBS: 41 g

Green Peas

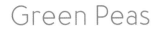

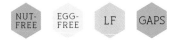

NUT-FREE   **EGG-FREE**   **LF**   **GAPS**

prep time: 10 minutes | *cook time: 10 minutes* | *yield: 4 servings*

1 tablespoon salted butter

10 ounces frozen green peas*

2 tablespoons fresh lemon juice (about 1 small lemon)

1 teaspoon dried dill weed

½ teaspoon fine sea salt

1. Melt the butter in a medium-sized saucepan over medium heat. Add the peas and stir to combine. Cover and let steam for 5 minutes.

2. Add the lemon juice, dill, and salt and stir to combine. Serve warm.

Consume peas on a low-FODMAP protocol only if well tolerated.

APPROXIMATE NUTRITION BREAKDOWN *(per serving)*	
CALORIES: 82	FAT: 3 g
PROTEIN: 4 g	CARBS: 10 g

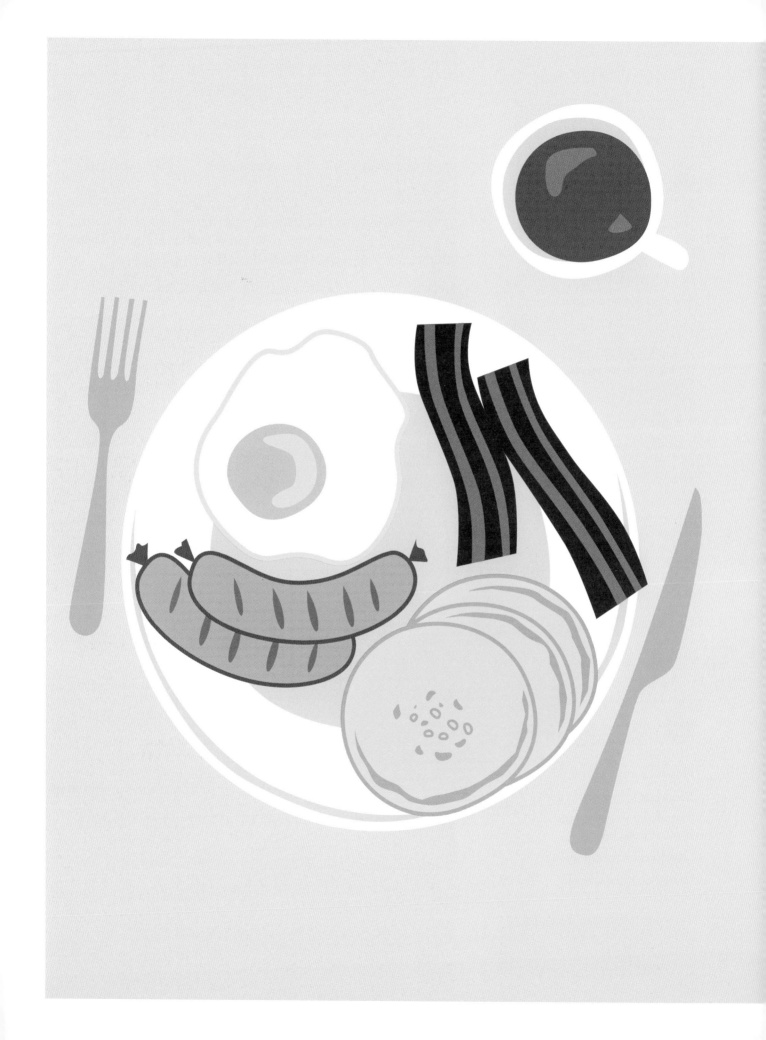

CHAPTER 2:
BREAKFAST LIKE YOU MEAN IT

Bubble & Squeak

This is comfort food at its finest, and it's what I crave after an especially late night. Bubble & Squeak is traditionally made with whatever leftover potatoes and vegetables you find in your refrigerator—so feel free to get creative with what you have on hand! Just in case you're out of leftovers, I've written this recipe so that you can make it from scratch.

NUT-FREE

prep time: 10 minutes | *cook time: 40 minutes* | *yield: 2 to 3 servings*

½ pound small fingerling potatoes, new potatoes, or boiling potatoes, scrubbed

½ head green cabbage, shredded (about 4 cups)

1 tablespoon extra-virgin olive oil

2 tablespoons salted butter, ghee, or coconut oil

1 teaspoon fine sea salt

½ teaspoon ground black pepper

½ teaspoon dried oregano leaves

6 large eggs

½ teaspoon red pepper flakes, or to taste (optional)

1. Place the potatoes in a large pot and cover with water. Cover with a lid and bring to a boil over medium heat. Once boiling, reduce the heat to a simmer and cook for 15 minutes, or until the potatoes are easily pierced with a fork. Drain and set aside to cool for 10 minutes.

2. Preheat the oven to 400°F. Line a rimmed baking sheet with parchment paper.

3. Toss the shredded cabbage in the olive oil, then spread it evenly on the lined baking sheet. Bake for 20 minutes, or until the cabbage is starting to brown around the edges.

4. While the cabbage is baking and when the potatoes have cooled, smash the potatoes. Place one potato at a time on a baking sheet and, using either a mallet or the bottom of a glass, flatten each potato until it is about ½ inch thick.

5. Melt the butter in a large frying pan over high heat. Add the smashed potatoes and cook for 4 to 5 minutes per side, until slightly crispy. Add the cabbage, salt, pepper, and oregano and stir to combine.

6. Create 6 wells in the pan and crack an egg into each well. Reduce the heat to low and cook until the whites of the eggs are no longer translucent, 7 to 10 minutes. Sprinkle the red pepper flakes, if using, and any additional salt desired over the top, and serve warm.

tips

• *Add any random bits of unused peppers, carrots, or other crunchy vegetables you find in your fridge to the cabbage roasting pan for extra flavor!*

• *If you have leftover boiled fingerling potatoes on hand, skip Step 1 and jump ahead to Steps 4 and 5 for smashing and pan-frying instructions.*

• *If you don't plan to eat the entire batch the day of, I recommend setting aside the extra servings of potato mixture. To reheat the leftovers, return the mixture to the frying pan and repeat Step 6 so that the cooked eggs are fresh and have the best texture.*

APPROXIMATE NUTRITION BREAKDOWN *(based on 1 of 3 servings)*	
CALORIES: 341	FAT: 22 g
PROTEIN: 15 g	CARBS: 20 g

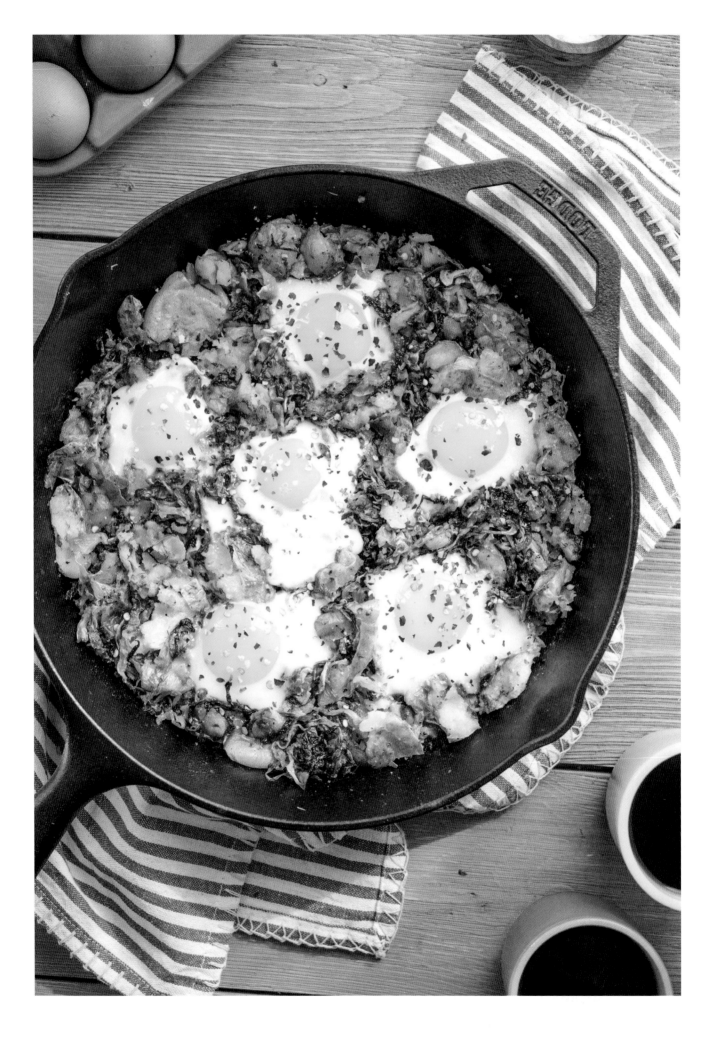

Chorizo & Egg Breakfast Scramble

I find myself making a couple recipes over and over again when we have company. This scramble is in my regular rotation for anyone who stays at our house! It's always a crowd-pleaser and takes so little time in the kitchen. I recommend serving it alongside Oven-Baked Tostones (page 291), which make a great tortilla substitute.

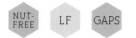

NUT-FREE   LF   GAPS

prep time: 5 minutes | *cook time: 20 minutes* | *yield: 4 to 6 servings*

1 tablespoon salted butter, ghee, or coconut oil

1 pound chorizo (bulk or link style)

12 large eggs, beaten

2 tablespoons fresh lime juice (about 1 lime)

¼ teaspoon fine sea salt

⅛ teaspoon ground black pepper

¼ cup chopped fresh cilantro, divided

4 to 6 lime wedges, for garnish (optional)

1. Melt the butter in a frying pan or heavy-bottomed pot over high heat. If using link-style chorizo, squeeze the sausage out of its casings. When the butter is completely melted, reduce the heat to medium-high and add the chorizo, breaking it up using a spoon or heat-resistant rubber spatula. Cook until crispy, 10 to 15 minutes.

2. When the chorizo is crispy, pour the eggs into the pan and lower the heat to medium. Using your rubber spatula or spoon, slowly stir the eggs until they're combined with the chorizo and cooked through, 5 to 6 minutes.

3. Add the lime juice, salt, pepper, and most of the cilantro to the pan, reserving some cilantro for garnish. Stir to combine.

4. Serve warm, garnished with the remaining cilantro and lime wedges, if using.

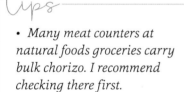

- *Many meat counters at natural foods groceries carry bulk chorizo. I recommend checking there first.*

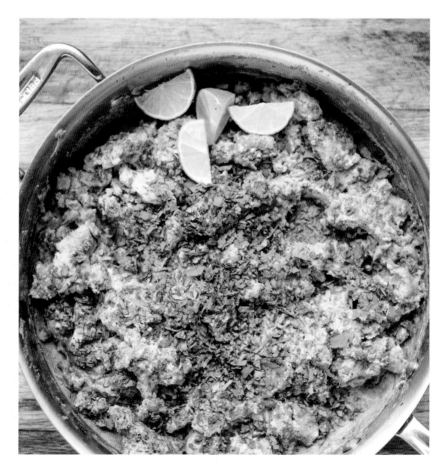

APPROXIMATE NUTRITION BREAKDOWN	
(based on 1 of 6 servings)	
CALORIES: 400	FAT: 31 g
PROTEIN: 25 g	CARBS: 6 g

Cinnamon Sage Sausage Patties

I think I've emailed this recipe to my nutrition clients more often than any other. Which means that it needs to be documented somewhere! This is a great breakfast protein option for folks who are following an Autoimmune Protocol or just want to avoid eggs. They're delicious, easy to make in bulk, and keep well either refrigerated or frozen.

NUT-FREE   EGG-FREE   OPTION AIP   LF   GAPS

prep time: 5 minutes | *cook time: 10 minutes (per batch)* | *yield: 6 to 7 servings (about 2 patties per serving)*

2 pounds ground pork

2 tablespoons rubbed dried sage

1 tablespoon ground cinnamon

1½ to 2 teaspoons fine sea salt (see Tips)

½ teaspoon ground black pepper (omit for AIP)

1 tablespoon bacon fat, salted butter, ghee, or coconut oil

1. In a large bowl, thoroughly mix together the pork, sage, cinnamon, salt, and pepper. Form the mixture into ¼-cup balls, then flatten those balls into ½-inch-thick patties.

2. Melt the bacon fat in a large cast-iron or other frying pan over high heat. Lower the heat to medium-high and cook half of the patties for 4 to 5 minutes per side, until they're cooked to your liking. Repeat with the second half of the patties.

Tips

- *I like crispier, more well-done breakfast sausage, so I cook mine for 5 minutes on each side.*

- *If you prefer saltier breakfast meat, I recommend that you add 2 teaspoons of salt. If not, 1½ teaspoons is sufficient.*

- *Store the sausage patties in the refrigerator for up to 4 days or in the freezer for up to 4 months.*

- *To reheat, defrost the patties if frozen and place them in a greased frying pan over medium heat. Cook for about 5 minutes on each side, until they're warmed through. You can also place them on a rimmed baking sheet and warm them in a preheated 350°F oven for about 20 minutes (if frozen) or 10 minutes (if just chilled). Or you can microwave each patty for 4 minutes (if frozen) or 2 minutes (if just chilled).*

APPROXIMATE NUTRITION BREAKDOWN *(based on 1 of 7 servings)*	
CALORIES: 353	FAT: 27 g
PROTEIN: 23 g	CARBS: 1 g

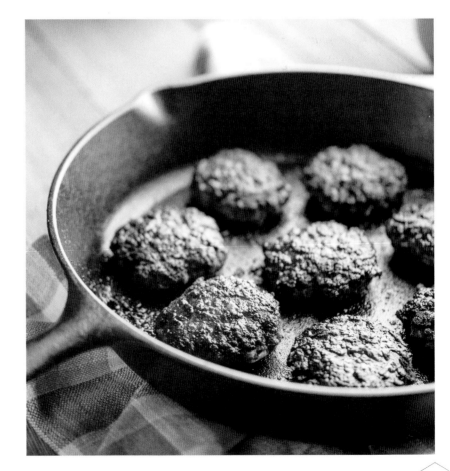

Jicama Breakfast Cakes

If you love hash browns, like I do, but don't always want or need that many carbohydrates, these jicama cakes will blow you away. With less than half the carbs of a potato, jicama makes a seriously delicious and comforting savory addition to your breakfast table.

NUT-FREE

prep time: 10 minutes, plus at least 30 minutes to disgorge the jicama | *cook time: 20 minutes* | *yield: 3 to 4 servings (2 to 3 cakes per serving)*

2 large jicamas (about 1¾ pounds), shredded

2 teaspoons fine sea salt

2 large eggs, beaten

¼ teaspoon garlic powder

¼ teaspoon ground black pepper

3 tablespoons bacon fat

tips

- *I recommend using a nut milk bag to squeeze the excess water out of the jicama.*

1. Place the shredded jicama in a colander and toss with the salt. Place the colander in a bowl or sink and let the jicama sit for 30 minutes (or overnight), then squeeze out as much liquid as possible—the jicama will have lost about 1 pound of its weight after you squeeze the water out. Blot dry on a paper towel, then transfer to a mixing bowl.

2. Mix the eggs, garlic powder, and pepper with the jicama in the bowl.

3. In a large frying pan over high heat, melt the bacon fat. Working in batches, add the jicama batter to the pan in ¼-cup increments. Flatten the cake with the back of a spatula and cook for 3 to 5 minutes on each side, or until slightly brown and crispy. Transfer to a paper towel–lined dish to drain. Repeat with the rest of the batter.

4. Sprinkle the finished cakes with salt and serve warm.

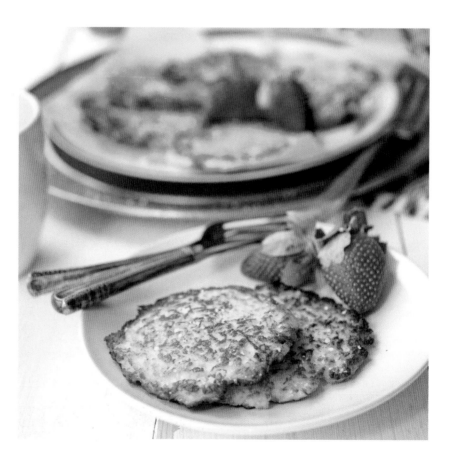

APPROXIMATE NUTRITION BREAKDOWN *(based on 1 of 4 servings)*			
CALORIES:	200	FAT:	12 g
PROTEIN:	5 g	CARBS:	18 g

Pan-Fried Plantains

Although these plantains are a delicious starch option for any time of the day, I usually make them for breakfast. They offer a punch of healthy carbohydrate, potassium, and vitamin B6. Serve them alongside some eggs, sliced tomatoes, sautéed kale, and sliced avocado for a beautiful and balanced breakfast or next to a delicious burger (pages 242 to 245) for a balanced dinner.

NUT-FREE · EGG-FREE · AIP (OPTION) · LF

prep time: 2 to 5 minutes | *cook time: 10 minutes* | *yield: 2 dozen discs (6 discs per serving)*

1 tablespoon salted butter (use coconut oil or ghee for AIP)

2 ripe plantains, peeled and sliced crosswise into ¼-inch-thick discs

½ teaspoon fine sea salt

tips

- *Plantains are easier to peel if you score them first with three long marks.*

1. Melt the butter in a large frying pan over high heat. When the butter is bubbling, reduce the heat to medium and add the plantains. If the plantains don't all fit in the pan at once without crowding, work in batches. Cook the plantains on one side for 4 minutes, then flip and cook the other side for an additional 4 minutes, until golden brown.

2. Transfer the cooked plantains to a paper towel–lined plate and immediately sprinkle the tops with the salt. Enjoy warm.

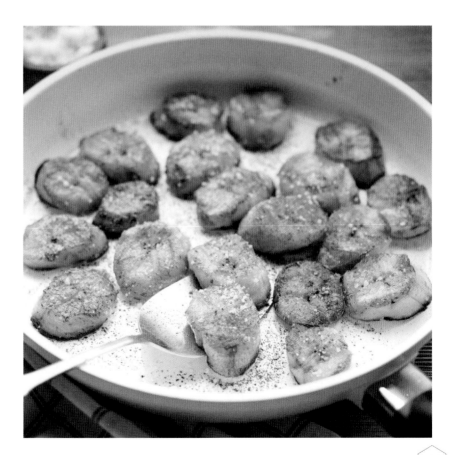

APPROXIMATE NUTRITION BREAKDOWN *(per serving)*			
CALORIES:	108	FAT:	2 g
PROTEIN:	1 g	CARBS:	23 g

Plantain Protein Pancakes

WITH SALTED RASPBERRY JAM

These pancakes have come in handy more times than I can remember. I especially love grabbing a couple out of the freezer to enjoy post-workout! They defrost nicely and allow me to continue my day without having to run home for a small meal. The protein from the egg and powder and the carbohydrates from the plantains make them an ideal recovery snack.

OPTION   OPTION

NUT-FREE   **LF**

prep time: 5 minutes	cook time: 20 minutes	yield: 3 to 5 servings (2 to 3 pancakes per serving)

SALTED RASPBERRY JAM

1 cup fresh raspberries

1 teaspoon fresh lemon juice

¼ teaspoon fine sea salt

PANCAKES

2 ripe plantains, peeled and cut into chunks

2 scoops unflavored protein powder

3 large eggs

1 teaspoon vanilla extract

¼ teaspoon fine sea salt

1 tablespoon salted butter, ghee, or coconut oil, or more as needed

¼ teaspoon ground cinnamon, for garnish (optional)

¼ cup coarsely chopped raw pecans, for garnish (optional) (omit for nut-free)*

*If sensitive to pecans and on a low-FODMAP plan, omit them entirely.

1. For the salted raspberry jam, place all of the ingredients in a small sauce pot, stir, and simmer over medium heat, covered, for 5 minutes. Remove the lid and simmer for an additional 10 minutes, until thickened, stirring regularly to make sure that it doesn't burn.

2. In a large bowl, blend the plantains, protein powder, eggs, vanilla, and salt until smooth.

3. Melt the butter in a large frying pan over medium-high heat. When the butter has melted, pour two ¼-cup portions of the batter into the frying pan. Cook the pancakes for 1½ to 2 minutes on one side, flip, and cook for an additional 1½ to 2 minutes on the other side, until golden brown. Repeat with the remaining batter, adding more fat to the pan as needed.

4. Enjoy the pancakes warm with a drizzle of jam, a sprinkle of cinnamon, and pecans (if using).

PANCAKES

APPROXIMATE NUTRITION BREAKDOWN (based on 1 of 5 servings)	
CALORIES: 243	FAT: 9 g
PROTEIN: 15 g	CARBS: 26 g

JAM

APPROXIMATE NUTRITION BREAKDOWN (based on 1 of 5 servings)	
CALORIES: 13	FAT: 0 g
PROTEIN: 0 g	CARBS: 3 g

tips

• Make the Salted Raspberry Jam in advance to save yourself time the day of. The jam will keep refrigerated for up to 4 days.

• To freeze the pancakes, layer them between pieces of parchment paper and place in a freezer-safe container for up to 4 months.

• To reheat, either place the frozen pancake in a lightly greased frying pan over medium-low heat or microwave for 2 minutes, or until warm.

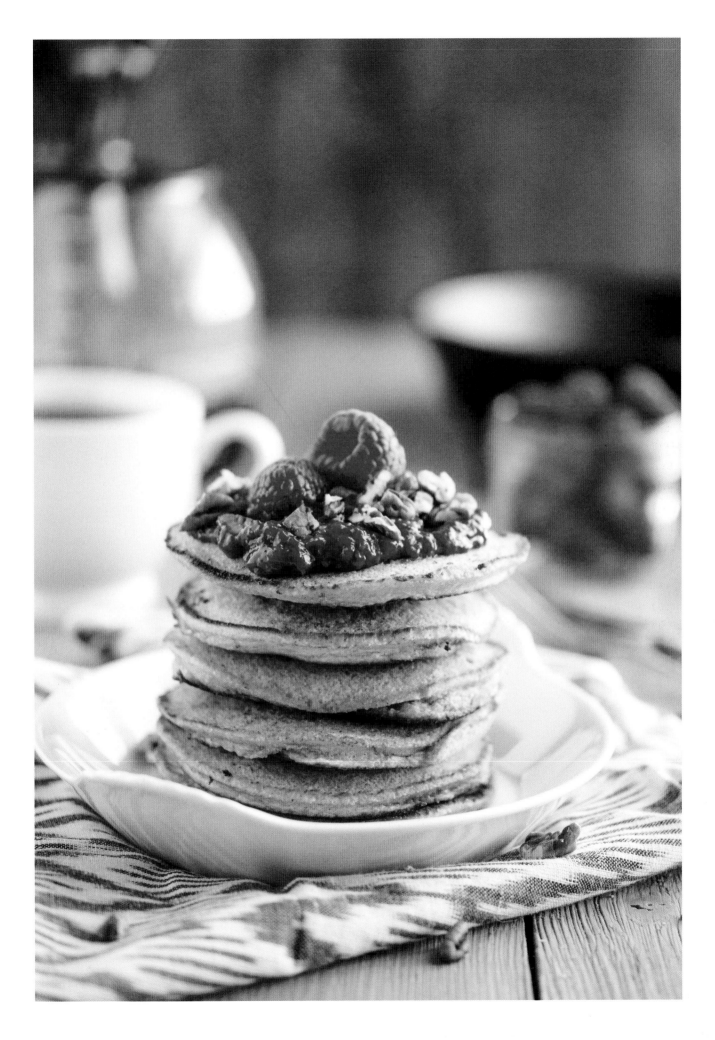

Sausage & Tomato Frittata

I've lost count of the number of times I've made this frittata. It's one of those meals that calls for ingredients I always seem to have on hand, requires little early-morning brain power, always pleases a crowd, and makes for the very best refrigerated leftovers. It reheats well for a quick breakfast.

NUT-FREE | **LF** | **GAPS**

prep time: 5 minutes | *cook time: 45 minutes* | *yield: 4 to 6 servings*

1 pound bulk breakfast sausage or ground pork*

1 dozen large eggs, lightly beaten

3 or 4 medium tomatoes, sliced into ¼-inch rounds

1½ teaspoons fennel seeds

½ teaspoon fine sea salt

¼ teaspoon ground black pepper

If using breakfast sausage and following a GAPS protocol, read the label to make sure that the ingredients are GAPS compliant.

1. Preheat the oven to 350°F.

2. In a large ovenproof sauté pan over medium heat, brown the sausage until crispy, 10 to 15 minutes. Drain off the excess grease, then pour the eggs over the sausage and stir together over medium heat until the eggs just start to set, about 4 minutes.

3. Lay the tomato slices evenly over the top of the eggs. Sprinkle the tomatoes with the fennel seeds, salt, and pepper.

4. Transfer the frittata to the oven and bake for 25 minutes, or until the middle doesn't jiggle when the pan is shaken. Let cool for 5 minutes, then serve warm.

tips

• *Leftovers will keep refrigerated for up to 4 days. To reheat, either place the frittata in a preheated 350°F oven for 20 minutes, microwave for about 2 minutes, or heat it up on the stovetop in a frying pan over medium heat for about 10 minutes.*

APPROXIMATE NUTRITION BREAKDOWN *(based on 1 of 6 servings)*	
CALORIES: 377	FAT: 27 g
PROTEIN: 24 g	CARBS: 4 g

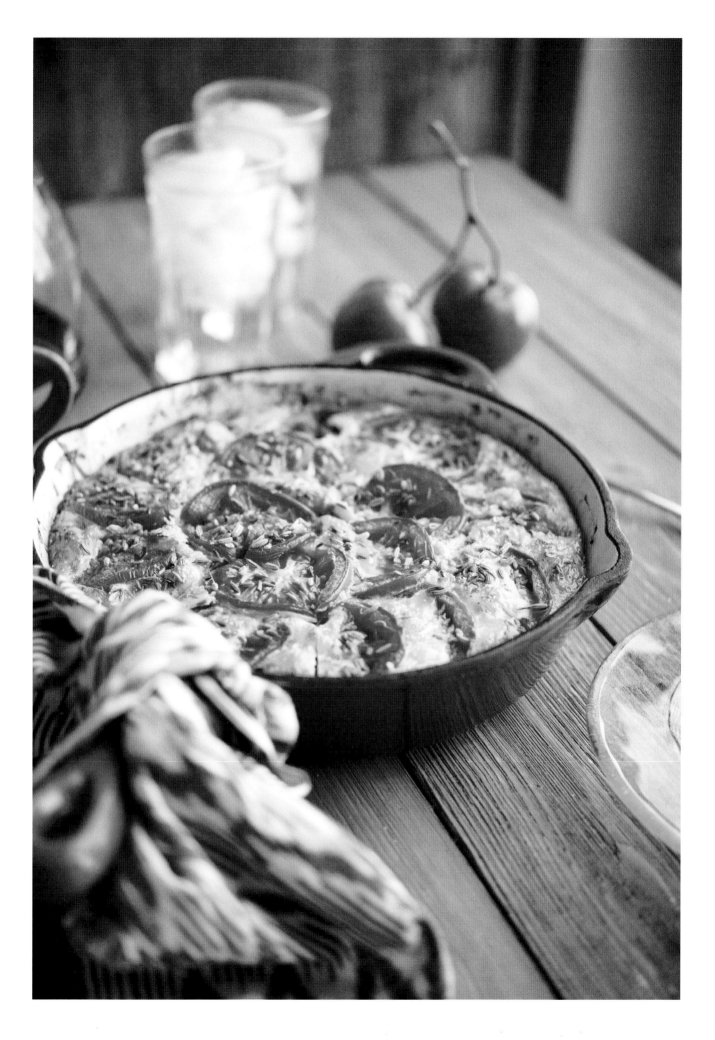

Smoothies:

ANTI-INFLAMMATORY, GREEN DETOX, ONE-STOP-SHOP, AND PURPLE PROTEIN

Though it's no secret that I usually opt for meals that require a chair, fork, knife, and company, I love a healthy smoothie when I'm on the go. With four varieties to choose from, I encourage you to experiment and keep things fresh! The Anti-Inflammatory and Green Detox Smoothies are ideal for the morning after an indulgent night or weekend, while the One-Stop-Shop and Purple Protein Smoothies are wonderful for especially busy mornings.

NUT-FREE · EGG-FREE · AIP · GAPS

prep time: 10 minutes | *yield: 1 serving each*

ANTI-INFLAMMATORY SMOOTHIE

½ orange, peeled and seeded

1 cup frozen strawberries

2 teaspoons turmeric powder

1 teaspoon ginger powder

2 tablespoons full-fat coconut milk

½ banana, cut into chunks and frozen (about ½ cup)

½ cup cold water

GREEN DETOX SMOOTHIE

½ banana, cut into chunks and frozen (about ½ cup)

1 packed cup kale leaves

1 packed cup fresh spinach

¼ avocado

¼ packed cup fresh cilantro or parsley leaves and stems

1 teaspoon ginger powder

2 tablespoons fresh lemon juice (about 1 small lemon)

½ cup cold water

PURPLE PROTEIN SMOOTHIE

¾ cup frozen blueberries

1 scoop unflavored protein powder*

2 tablespoons full-fat coconut milk

½ cup cold water

If following a GAPS protocol, read the protein powder label to make sure that the ingredients are compliant.

ONE-STOP-SHOP SMOOTHIE

½ banana, cut into chunks and frozen (about ½ cup)

1 scoop unflavored protein powder*

½ packed cup kale leaves

1 packed cup fresh spinach

2 tablespoons full-fat coconut milk

½ cup frozen blueberries

½ cup cold water

If following a GAPS protocol, read the protein powder label to make sure that the ingredients are compliant.

1. Place all of the ingredients in a blender. Blend for 2 minutes, or until entirely smooth.

2. Enjoy right away, refrigerate for up to 2 days, or freeze for up to 5 months.

tips

- *If you prefer your smoothies on the colder side, you can add ¼ cup ice cubes.*

- *If your smoothie is too thick, add more cold water 1 tablespoon at a time.*

ANTI-INFLAMMATORY

APPROXIMATE NUTRITION BREAKDOWN *(per serving)*	
CALORIES: 226	FAT: 7 g
PROTEIN: 1 g	CARBS: 40 g

ONE-STOP-SHOP

APPROXIMATE NUTRITION BREAKDOWN *(per serving)*	
CALORIES: 270	FAT: 6 g
PROTEIN: 20 g	CARBS: 33 g

GREEN DETOX

APPROXIMATE NUTRITION BREAKDOWN *(per serving)*	
CALORIES: 160	FAT: 6 g
PROTEIN: 5 g	CARBS: 25 g

PURPLE PROTEIN

APPROXIMATE NUTRITION BREAKDOWN *(per serving)*	
CALORIES: 217	FAT: 7 g
PROTEIN: 19 g	CARBS: 21 g

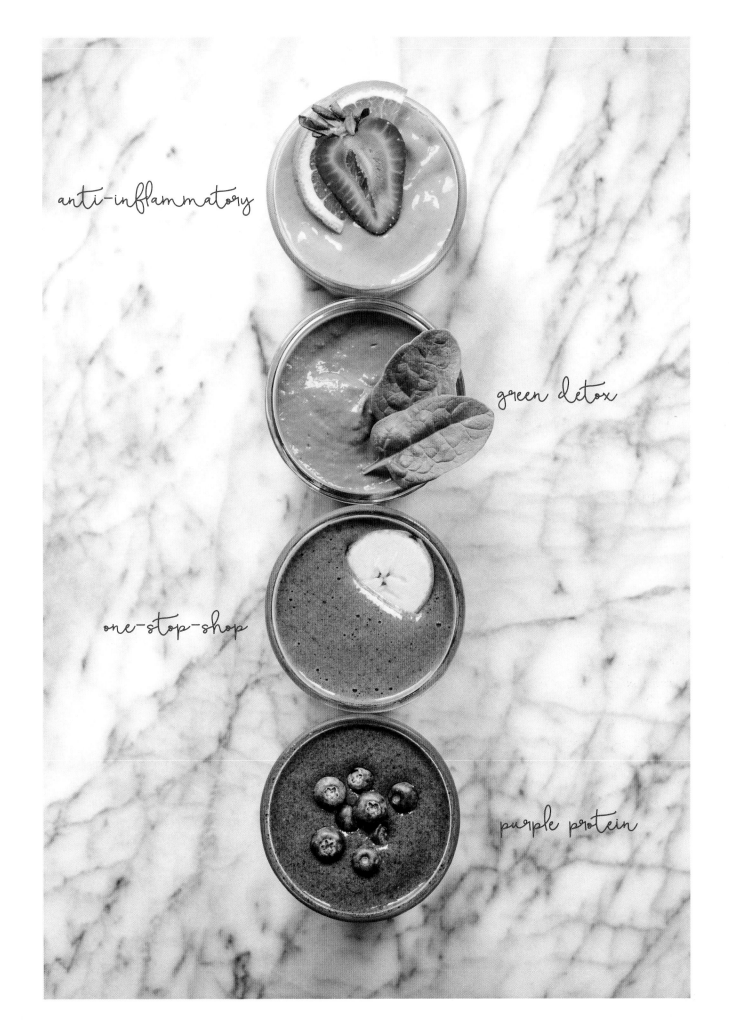

anti-inflammatory

green detox

one-stop-shop

purple protein

Spaghetti Squash & Dill Egg Cups

Are you catching on to a theme here? I'm a big fan of large-batch breakfasts that provide leftovers for the week. For some reason, my weekday mornings seem to grow shorter the longer I spend making breakfast. However, if I just need to reheat something I made over the weekend, my morning meals become efficient, productive, nutritious fuel for the whole day!

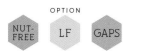

OPTION

NUT-FREE · LF · GAPS

prep time: 5 minutes | *cook time: 1 hour 15 minutes* | *yield: 12 egg cups (2 to 3 per serving)*

1 medium spaghetti squash (about 5 pounds)

1 tablespoon extra-virgin olive oil

1 teaspoon fine sea salt

½ teaspoon garlic powder (omit for low-FODMAP)

¼ teaspoon ground black pepper

12 large eggs

1 teaspoon dried dill weed

1. Preheat the oven to 375°F.

2. Using a sharp knife and working carefully, pierce the spaghetti squash 4 to 5 times through the flesh and into the center. Place the squash on a rimmed baking sheet and bake for 1 hour, or until it gives when gently poked with a large spoon or your hand in an oven mitt. Let cool for at least 30 minutes, until it's cool enough to handle.

3. Cut the squash in half lengthwise and scrape out and dispose of the seeds using a large spoon. Scrape the spaghetti squash flesh into a large mixing bowl.

4. Add the olive oil, salt, garlic powder, and pepper to the squash and stir to combine.

5. Preheat the oven to 350°F and grease the wells of a 12-well muffin pan or line the wells with parchment paper or silicone cupcake liners. Place about ¼ cup of the squash mixture in each greased muffin cup. Using your fingers, press some of the squash mixture along the bottom and all the way up the sides of each well, then crack an egg into each well. Bake for 15 minutes, or until the egg whites are cooked through.

6. Let cool for 5 minutes, then use a knife to pry out each egg cup. Sprinkle the tops with dill and enjoy!

tips

• *Pre-roast the spaghetti squash the day before to save yourself some time the day of!*

• *I recommend using a silicone muffin pan to prevent sticking. If you use a silicone pan, you don't need to grease or line the wells.*

• *The egg cups will keep for up to 5 days in the refrigerator.*

• *To reheat, either place the egg cups in a preheated 350°F oven for 10 minutes or microwave for 1 minute.*

APPROXIMATE NUTRITION BREAKDOWN *(based on 2 egg cups per serving)*			
CALORIES:	189	FAT:	12 g
PROTEIN:	13 g	CARBS:	9 g

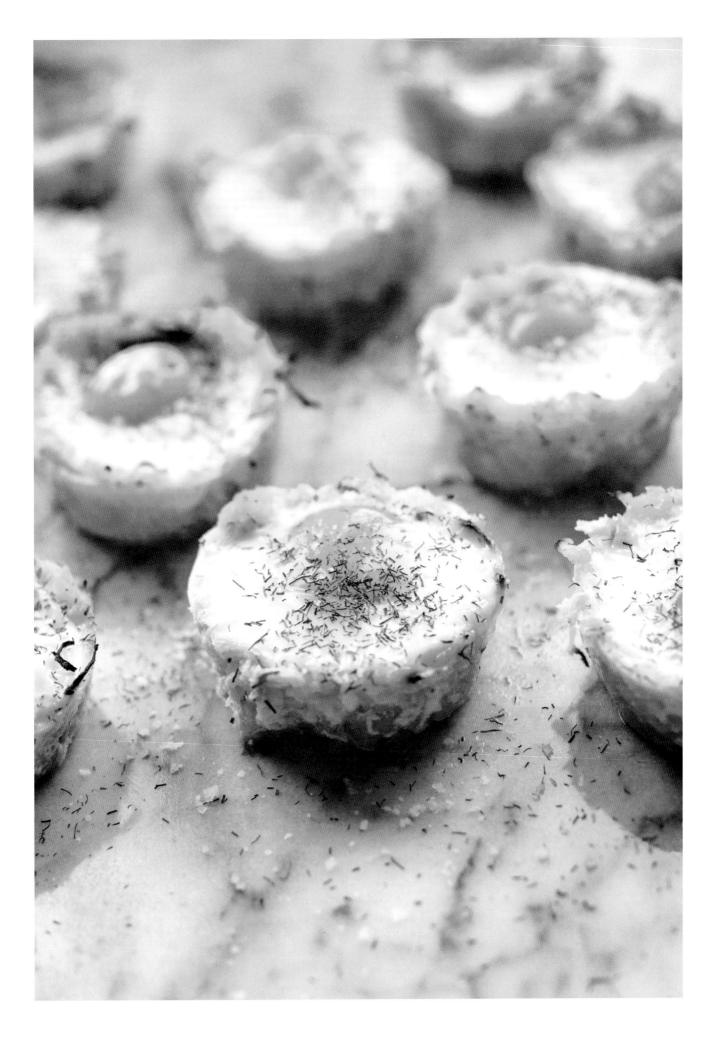

Sweet Potato Breakfast Hash Casserole

This recipe marries ~~two~~ THREE of my favorite things: sweet potato hash (a longtime Fed & Fit fan favorite), casseroles, and a hot breakfast. This dish is ideal if you've got a houseful of visitors or you need a post-workout morning carbohydrate. Serve it alongside some fresh berries and avocado slices for a complete meal!

NUT-FREE

prep time: 10 minutes	cook time: 1 hour 35 minutes to 1 hour 45 minutes	yield: 4 to 6 servings

1 pound bulk breakfast sausage

½ medium white onion, chopped

2 pounds sweet potatoes (about 4), peeled and shredded

1 tablespoon salted butter, ghee, or coconut oil

½ pound kale, destemmed and finely chopped

Juice of 1 lime (about 2 tablespoons)

1 teaspoon fine sea salt

½ teaspoon ground black pepper

12 large eggs

1 tablespoon chopped fresh cilantro, for garnish

tips

• *Leftovers will keep refrigerated for up to 5 days.*

• *To reheat, either place a serving in a preheated 350°F oven for 10 minutes or microwave for 1 minute.*

1. In a large frying pan over high heat, cook the sausage for 10 to 15 minutes, breaking it up into small crumbles with a spatula, until brown and crispy. Using a slotted spoon, transfer the sausage to a large mixing bowl, leaving the grease behind.

2. Add the onion to the sausage grease and cook over medium heat until translucent, about 10 minutes. Add the sweet potatoes, stir, cover, and cook for 10 to 15 minutes, stirring often. When the sweet potatoes are cooked and softened, add the kale, stir, and cook for an additional 5 minutes, or until wilted.

3. Preheat the oven to 350°F.

4. Transfer the sweet potato mixture to the bowl with the sausage. Add the lime juice, salt, and pepper and stir to combine. Transfer this mixture to a 9 by 13-inch baking dish.

5. Create 12 wells in the sweet potato hash. Crack an egg into each well. Bake the casserole for 30 minutes for slightly runny eggs or 35 to 40 minutes for more well-done eggs.

6. Let cool for 5 minutes, then top with fresh cilantro and serve.

APPROXIMATE NUTRITION BREAKDOWN (based on 1 of 6 servings)	
CALORIES: 471	FAT: 29 g
PROTEIN: 26 g	CARBS: 24 g

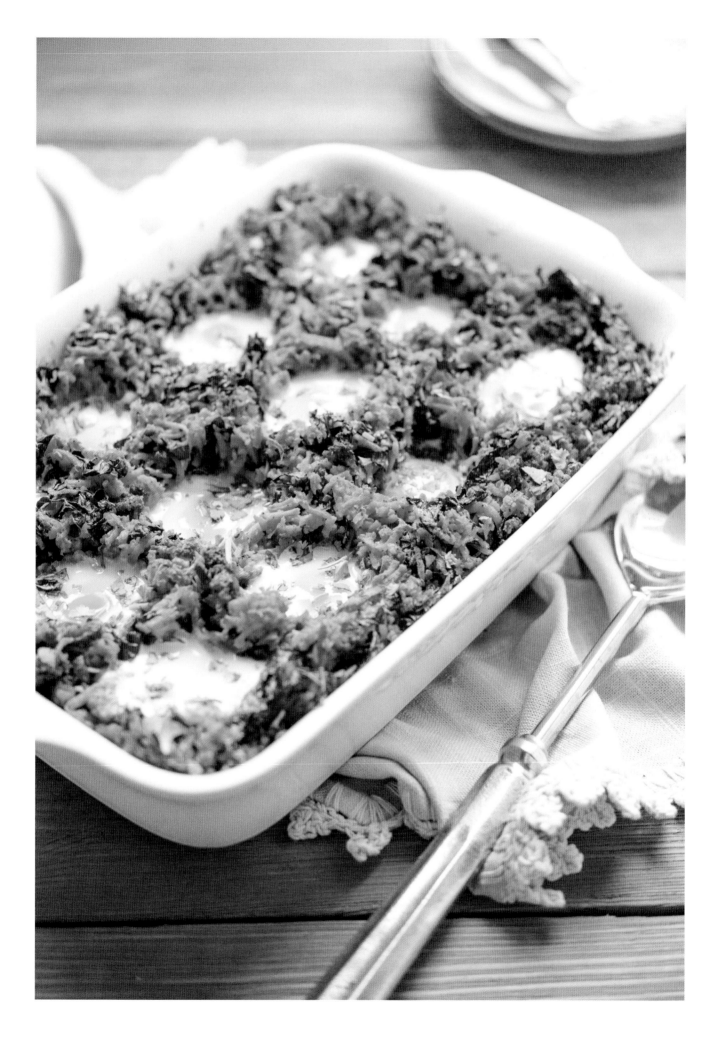

Tuscan Chicken Frittata

I could literally devote an entire chapter, and maybe even an entire cookbook (one day?), to the incredible, edible frittata. There are so many possibilities! Frittatas are a great way to seamlessly incorporate vegetables, extra proteins, and fun flavors on a plate. The pesto, sun-dried tomatoes, and pine nuts in this frittata add excitement to the breakfast hour. This recipe is portioned for a crowd, but you could easily cut it in half and prepare it in a 6-inch oven-safe skillet if you prefer.

OPTION

LF   GAPS

prep time: 15 minutes (not including the pesto) | cook time: 1 hour | yield: 8 to 10 servings

2 pounds boneless, skinless chicken breasts, rinsed and patted dry

½ teaspoon fine sea salt

¼ teaspoon ground black pepper

¾ pound thick-cut bacon (about 8 strips), sliced crosswise (about ⅛ inch thick)

1 bunch kale, destemmed and finely chopped

18 large eggs, lightly beaten

¼ cup Roasted Garlic Pesto 2.0 (page 348)

⅓ cup sun-dried tomatoes packed in olive oil, thinly sliced

2 tablespoons pine nuts, toasted

1. Preheat the oven to 450°F. Line a rimmed baking sheet with parchment paper.

2. Sprinkle the tops of the chicken breasts with the salt and pepper and place them on the lined baking sheet. Bake for 15 to 18 minutes, until the juices run clear. Remove from the oven and set aside to rest for 5 minutes.

3. In a 12-inch oven-safe frying pan or sauté pan, cook the bacon over medium heat until crispy, 10 to 12 minutes. Add the kale and cook until wilted, about 5 minutes.

4. When the chicken breasts are cool enough to handle, slice them thinly crosswise and add them to the pan with the bacon and kale. Pour the eggs over the mixture and stir together over medium heat for 4 to 5 minutes, until the eggs barely start to stiffen.

5. Preheat the oven to 350°F.

6. Drizzle the pesto over the top of the frittata, then sprinkle with the sun-dried tomatoes and toasted pine nuts.

7. Bake the frittata for 25 minutes, or until the middle doesn't jiggle when the pan is shaken.

8. Let cool for 5 minutes, then serve warm.

tips

- To make this meal low-FODMAP friendly, omit the roasted garlic pesto or make the pesto without the garlic.

- Leftovers will keep in the refrigerator for up to 4 days.

- To reheat, either place the frittata in a preheated 350°F oven for 20 minutes, microwave it for about 2 minutes, or heat it up on the stovetop in a frying pan over medium heat for about 10 minutes.

APPROXIMATE NUTRITION BREAKDOWN *(based on 1 of 10 servings)*	
CALORIES: 369	FAT: 22 g
PROTEIN: 36 g	CARBS: 7 g

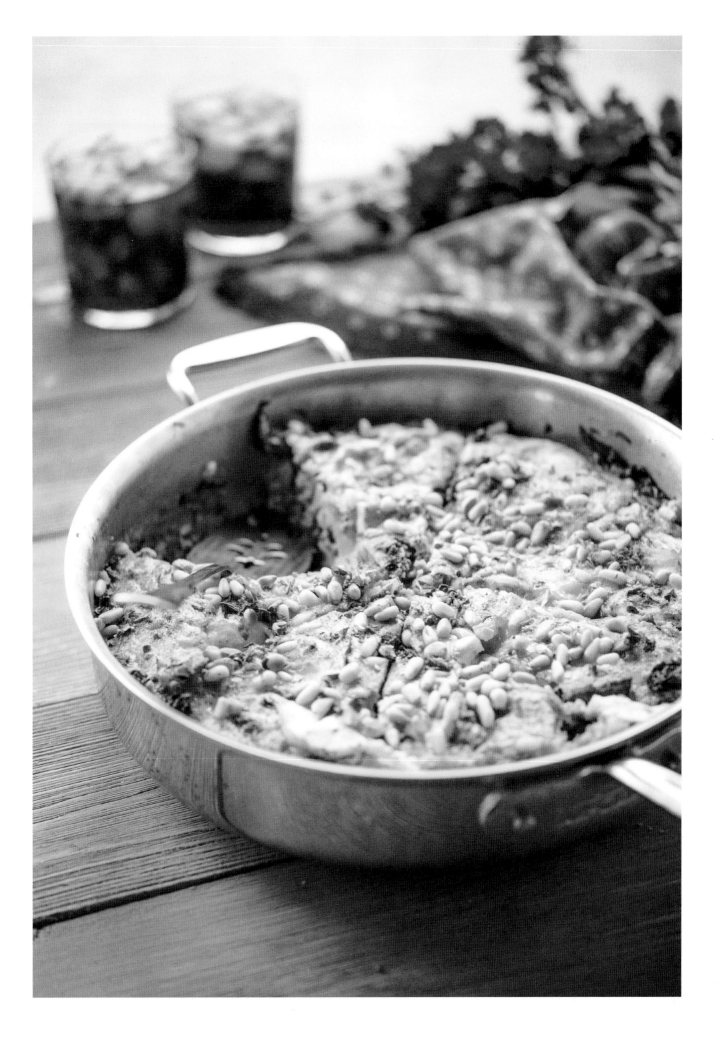

Paleo Diner Breakfast Plate

I've made a version of this breakfast just about every single week for the last six years. While I love frittatas, scrambles, and casseroles as much as the next gal, diner-style breakfasts have the key to my heart. I love to pile my plate with healthy proteins (eggs), a couple forms of fat (fresh avocado and a few slices of bacon), a serving of healthy starch (breakfast potatoes, anyone?), some cooked greens, and a serving of fresh fruit. I encourage you to customize this diner-style plate to your taste! If you need to go egg-free, I suggest you add some Cinnamon Sage Sausage Patties (page 143) instead!

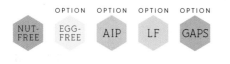

prep time: 20 minutes (not including the braised collards) | cook time: 45 minutes | yield: 4 servings

BREAKFAST POTATOES
(omit for AIP and GAPS)

1½ pounds round red-skinned or white-skinned potatoes (about 4 large potatoes), cut into ½-inch pieces

1 tablespoon extra-virgin olive oil

½ teaspoon dried ground oregano

½ teaspoon fine sea salt

¼ teaspoon ground black pepper

¼ teaspoon paprika

BREAKFAST PLATE

½ pound bacon

8 large eggs (omit for egg-free and AIP)

½ teaspoon fine sea salt

¼ teaspoon ground black pepper (omit for AIP)

1 avocado, sliced thin (see Tips) (omit for low-FODMAP)

1 batch Braised Greens made with kale or collards (page 129)

2 cups fresh berries or 8 wedges or sections of citrus

1. To make the breakfast potatoes, preheat the oven to 400°F and line a rimmed baking sheet with parchment paper. Toss the potatoes in the olive oil, then spread them out in an even layer on the baking sheet. Sprinkle the potatoes with the oregano, salt, pepper, and paprika. Bake for 45 minutes, or until slightly crispy and golden on all sides, but not burned.

2. While the potatoes are in the oven, cook the bacon in a frying pan over medium heat for 5 to 7 minutes, flipping often, until crispy. Place the bacon on a paper towel–lined plate to help absorb excess grease while you prepare the eggs. Remove all but 1 tablespoon of bacon grease from the pan.

3. When the potatoes are nearly done, prepare the eggs. For sunny-side eggs, working in batches, crack 2 to 4 eggs into the hot frying pan over medium heat. After the whites start to turn opaque, season with some of the salt and pepper and then turn the heat to low and cook for an additional 4 minutes, or until the whites are cooked through. Transfer the cooked eggs to serving plates and repeat with the rest of the eggs.

4. To plate, spoon one-quarter of the breakfast potatoes, bacon, eggs, avocado, collards, and berries onto each plate. Enjoy!

5. To reheat leftover potatoes, I recommend adding them from the refrigerator to a large cast-iron or frying pan over medium heat. Sauté until heated through.

tips

- *I recommend chilling the avocado overnight to make it easier to slice thin, delicate pieces.*

APPROXIMATE NUTRITION BREAKDOWN (based on 1 of 4 servings)			
CALORIES:	619	FAT:	36 g
PROTEIN:	26 g	CARBS:	54 g

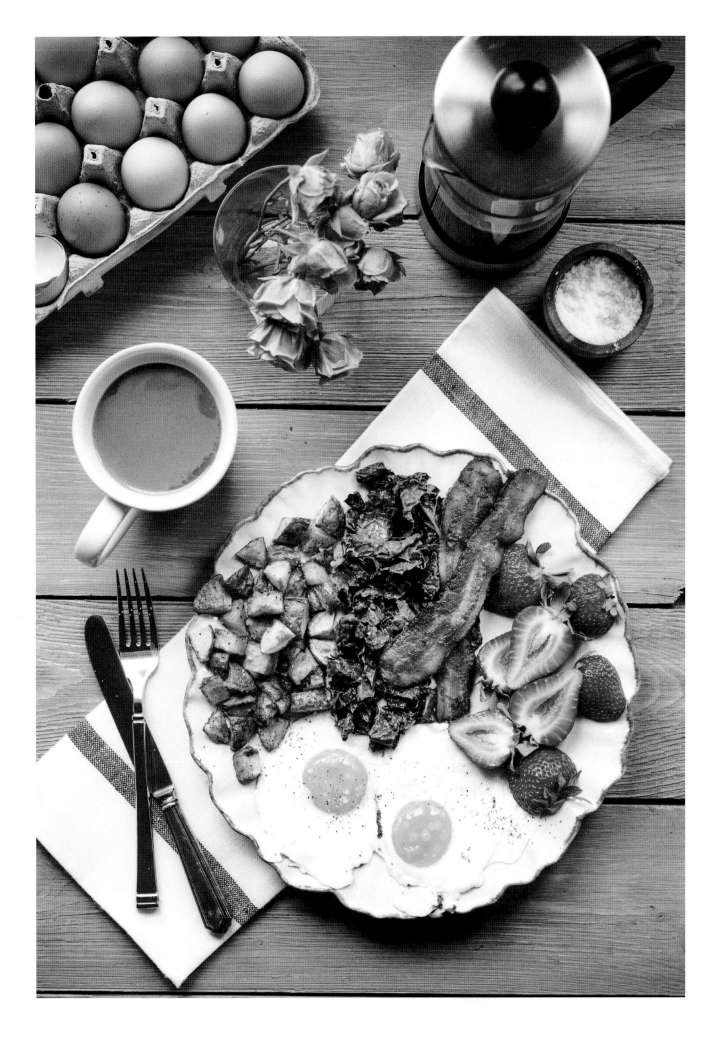

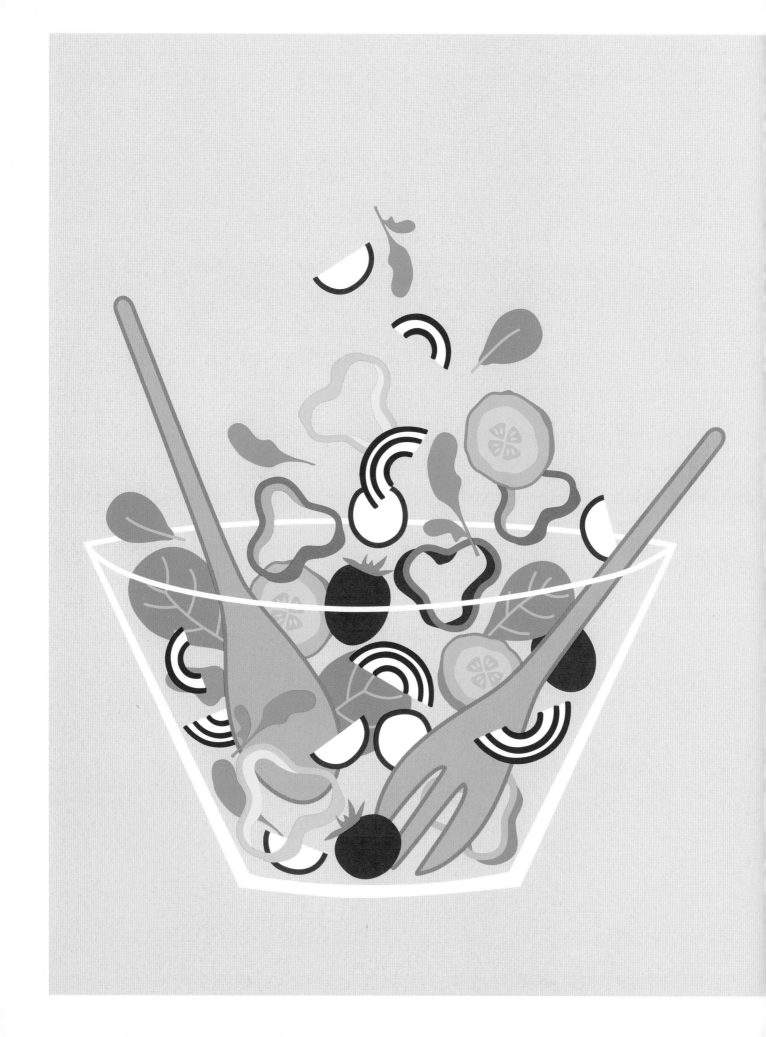

CHAPTER 3:
SOUPS & SALADS THAT MEAN BUSINESS

Download the Fed & Fit iPhone and Android app! You can scan the above QR codes directly in the app, which will then populate a consolidated grocery shopping list for the scanned recipes.

Chicken No-Tortilla Soup

Tortilla soup is a secret go-to of mine. Well, maybe it's not so secret anymore, but now it can be your secret! It's dang delicious, simple to whip up, reminds me of eating out, and leaves me feeling like a million bucks. I like to top it with avocado and fresh cilantro for a genuine restaurant finish, though it's delicious as is. Try chilling the avocado: it makes the avocado easier to cut and offers a contrasting temperature to the hot soup.

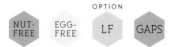

OPTION

NUT-FREE   EGG-FREE   LF   GAPS

prep time: 10 minutes | *cook time: 25 minutes* | *yield: 4 to 6 servings*

4 boneless, skinless chicken breast halves (about 2¼ pounds), rinsed and patted dry

1 teaspoon chipotle powder

1 teaspoon ground cumin

1 teaspoon fine sea salt

½ teaspoon ground black pepper

2 tablespoons salted butter

8 cups water (or chicken broth for extra flavor!)

1 (28-ounce) can diced tomatoes, with juice

⅓ cup fresh lime juice (about 3 limes)

1 bunch green onions, chopped (omit for low-FODMAP)

2 jalapeño peppers, thinly sliced

1 avocado, cubed, for garnish*

½ cup chopped fresh cilantro, for garnish

4 to 6 lime wedges, for garnish

Okay in moderation for low-FODMAP.

1. Sprinkle the chicken with the chipotle powder, cumin, salt, and pepper.

2. Melt the butter in a heavy-bottomed pot over high heat. When the butter has melted, add the chicken and sear for 4 minutes on one side, or until the chicken starts to develop a brown crust. Flip the chicken over, then pour in the water and simmer for 20 minutes. Remove the chicken, shred with two forks, and return to the cooking liquid in the pot.

3. To the pot, add the diced tomatoes with juice, lime juice, green onions, and jalapeños. Stir and cook until warmed through.

4. Spoon the soup into individual serving bowls. Garnish each bowl with avocado cubes, cilantro, and a lime wedge.

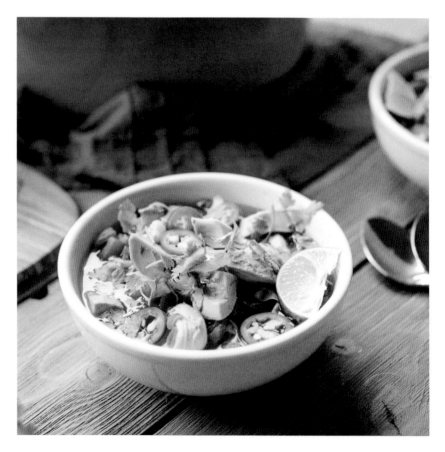

APPROXIMATE NUTRITION BREAKDOWN	
(based on 1 of 6 servings)	
CALORIES: 297	FAT: 10 g
PROTEIN: 44 g	CARBS: 9 g

Lemony Kale & Sausage Soup

I invented this soup recipe after an especially indulgent weekend a few years ago. I wanted something really healthy but also really comforting. It has a distinct lemon flavor and is an excellent vehicle for kale! I make it at least once a week and freeze the leftovers for convenient healthy soup meals when a craving strikes.

NUT-FREE   EGG-FREE   OPTION AIP   LF   GAPS

prep time: 15 minutes | *cook time: 25 minutes* | *yield: 4 to 6 servings*

2 pounds bulk breakfast sausage*

12 ounces kale, bottom stems removed and leaves coarsely chopped

8 cups chicken broth, store-bought or homemade (page 332)

½ teaspoon fine sea salt

¼ teaspoon ground black pepper (omit for AIP)

½ cup fresh lemon juice (about 4 small lemons)

If following an AIP or GAPS protocol, read the breakfast sausage label to make sure that the ingredients are compliant.

1. In a stockpot, cook the sausage over medium-high heat for 10 to 15 minutes, until crispy and brown, using a wooden spoon to break it up as it cooks.

2. Once the sausage is crispy, add the kale, stir, and cover to steam for 5 minutes. Once the kale is wilted and bright green, add the chicken broth, salt, and pepper and bring to a simmer.

3. To finish, add the lemon juice and spoon the soup into individual serving bowls.

Tips

- *This soup freezes really well! I recommend spooning individual portions into freezer-safe containers so that you can defrost each serving as you need it. To defrost, simply let it soften enough on the countertop so that it will slide out of the container and into a pot to be reheated on the stovetop. Or you can microwave it on high for 3 minutes and then 2 minutes.*

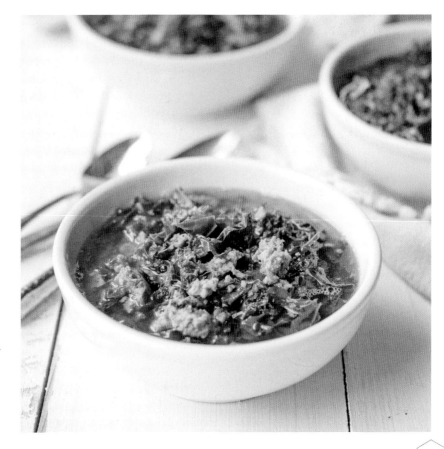

APPROXIMATE NUTRITION BREAKDOWN *(based on 1 of 6 servings)*	
CALORIES: 433	FAT: 30 g
PROTEIN: 32 g	CARBS: 8 g

A Really Good Chicken & Sausage Gumbo

Everyone wins with this gumbo. EVERYONE. You like sausage? You like chicken? Okra? Things that are delicious? Filling? Comforting? How about things that are ridiculously good for you? My husband swore that he'd propose to me all over again when I made this dish for him. Serve it with some Dirty Rice [page 264] for a complete meal!

NUT-FREE | EGG-FREE | OPTION AIP | OPTION LF | OPTION GAPS

prep time: 15 minutes | *cook time: 45 minutes* | *yield: 10 to 12 servings*

2 pounds andouille sausage, cut on the diagonal into ½-inch thick ovals [omit for low-FODMAP]*

2 pounds boneless, skinless chicken thighs, rinsed, patted dry, and cut into ½-inch pieces**

1 teaspoon fine sea salt

¼ teaspoon ground black pepper [omit for AIP]

1 yellow onion, chopped [omit for low-FODMAP]

4 cloves garlic, minced [omit for low-FODMAP]

2 tablespoons dried thyme leaves

1 tablespoon dried basil

1 tablespoon dried oregano leaves

¼ teaspoon cayenne pepper [omit for AIP]

¼ cup paprika [omit for AIP]

8 cups chicken or beef broth, store-bought or homemade [page 332]

4 cups diced fresh or frozen okra [about 14 ounces] [omit for GAPS]

¼ cup fresh lemon juice [about 2 small lemons]

3 tablespoons chopped fresh flat-leaf parsley, for garnish

*If following an AIP or GAPS protocol, read the andouille sausage label to make sure that the ingredients are compliant.

**Double the quantity of chicken for low-FODMAP.

1. In a Dutch oven or other heavy-bottomed pot over high heat, cook the sliced sausage for 10 to 15 minutes, until both sides are browned and slightly crispy. Using a slotted spoon, transfer the cooked sausage to a bowl, leaving the drippings in the pot.

2. Sprinkle the chicken pieces with the salt and pepper. Add the chicken to pot with the sausage drippings and cook over medium-high heat for 7 to 10 minutes, until each piece is browned and cooked through. Using a slotted spoon, transfer the chicken to the bowl with the sausage, again leaving the drippings in the pot.

3. To the drippings, add the onion and cook for about 5 minutes, until translucent. Add the garlic and cook for an additional 3 minutes, or until fragrant.

4. Add the thyme, basil, oregano, cayenne pepper, and paprika to the pot and stir to combine. Cook until fragrant, about 5 minutes, then add the broth and okra.

5. Bring the ingredients in the pot to a simmer, then add the cooked sausage and chicken. Simmer for an additional 10 minutes. Stir in the lemon juice, check for seasoning, and add more salt if needed.

6. Spoon into bowls and serve garnished with the parsley.

tips

• *Leftovers will keep refrigerated for up to 5 days.*

APPROXIMATE NUTRITION BREAKDOWN *(based on 1 of 12 servings)*	
CALORIES: 316	FAT: 18 g
PROTEIN: 31 g	CARBS: 6 g

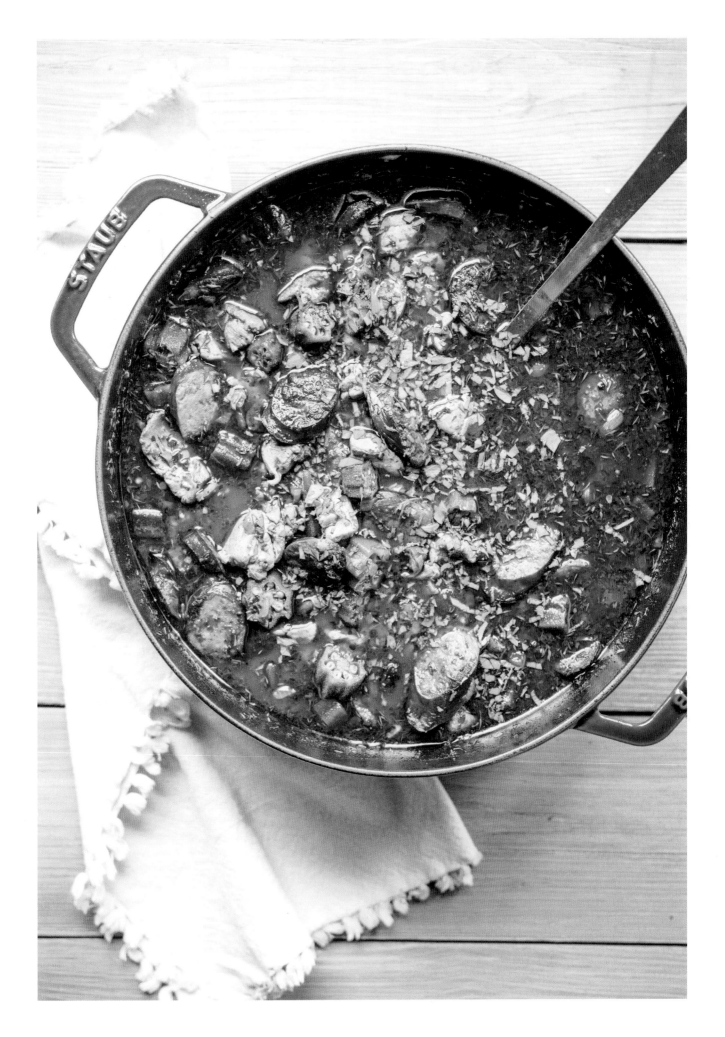

Weeknight Leafy Green & Beef Chili

I probably make this recipe more often in my own kitchen than any other that I've ever written. It's my husband's most requested meal, and I'm happy to oblige, as it's incredibly healthy and an awesome way to integrate cooked leafy greens! It's also very satisfying and filling.

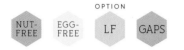

NUT-FREE · EGG-FREE · LF (OPTION) · GAPS

prep time: 15 minutes (not including the sour cream | *cook time: 30 minutes* | *yield: 4 to 6 servings*

2 tablespoons salted butter

1 medium white onion, chopped (omit for low-FODMAP)

4 cloves garlic, minced (omit for low-FODMAP)

2 pounds ground beef

1 pound kale, destemmed and chopped

2 (28-ounce) cans diced tomatoes with juice

2 (24-ounce) jars tomato puree or tomato sauce

¼ cup fresh lemon juice (about 2 small lemons)

¼ cup plus 1 tablespoon chili powder

¼ cup ground cumin

2 teaspoons fine sea salt

1 teaspoon ground black pepper

1 jalapeño pepper, finely sliced, for garnish

¼ cup chopped green onions, for garnish

½ cup Paleo Sour Cream (page 341), for garnish

1. In a large pot or Dutch oven over medium heat, melt the butter. Add the onion and cook for about 5 minutes, until translucent. Add the garlic and cook for an additional 3 minutes, until fragrant.

2. Add the ground beef and use a spoon or spatula to break it up and mix it with the onion and garlic. Cook for about 10 minutes, until completely browned and crumbled.

3. Once the beef is cooked, add the kale and stir to combine with the beef. Cover and let steam for 5 minutes, still over medium heat.

4. Once the kale is bright green and wilted, add the diced tomatoes with juice, tomato puree, lemon juice, chili powder, cumin, salt, and pepper. Stir to combine and bring to a simmer.

5. To serve, spoon into bowls and top with the jalapeños, green onions, and sour cream.

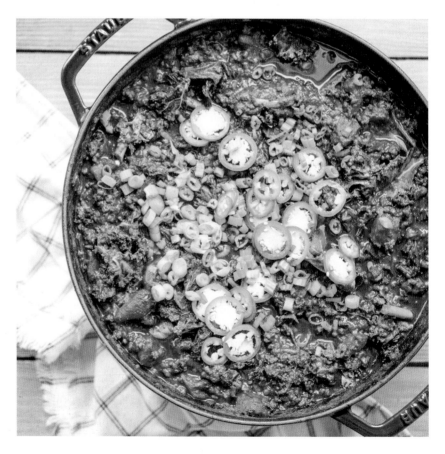

APPROXIMATE NUTRITION BREAKDOWN	
(based on 1 of 6 servings)	
CALORIES: 563	FAT: 29 g
PROTEIN: 40 g	CARBS: 42 g

The Great Beef Taco Salad

I'll admittedly go to a Tex-Mex restaurant just because I want a giant taco salad. Once you get past the puzzled look on the waiter's face when you say, "but no shell, please," you can settle in for an awesomely satisfying meal. There is one problem, though. If you're at a real-deal hole-in-the-wall Tex-Mex restaurant (my favorite kind of place), the ingredients used to make that tasty dish are pretty mysterious. This homemade version tastes, dare I say, even better and is even more satisfying—minus the mystery ingredients.

NUT-FREE EGG-FREE GAPS

prep time: 10 minutes (not including the sour cream | *cook time: 25 minutes* | *yield: 3 to 4 servings*

2 tablespoons salted butter

1 small yellow onion, chopped (about ½ cup)

3 cloves garlic, minced

1 pound ground beef

2 teaspoons chili powder

2 teaspoons ground cumin

2 teaspoons dried Mexican oregano leaves

½ teaspoon fine sea salt

Juice of 2 limes

4 cups chopped romaine lettuce (about 1 head)

1 cup pico de gallo, store-bought or homemade (page 342)

¼ cup chopped fresh cilantro

½ avocado, sliced

3 tablespoons Paleo Sour Cream (page 341)

Pickled sliced jalapeños (optional)

1 lime, cut into wedges

1. Melt the butter in a large frying pan or sauté pan over medium heat. Add the onion and cook for 5 minutes, or until translucent. Add the garlic and cook for an additional 3 minutes, or until fragrant. Add the ground beef and, using a spoon or spatula, break it up and mix it evenly with the onion and garlic. Cook until the beef is browned and cooked through, 10 to 15 minutes.

2. Add the chili powder, cumin, oregano, salt, and lime juice to the ground beef mixture. Stir to combine, then remove from the heat.

3. To serve the salad, divide the lettuce among three or four plates or bowls. Top with the ground beef, pico, cilantro, avocado slices, sour cream, and pickled jalapeños, if using. Serve with lime wedges.

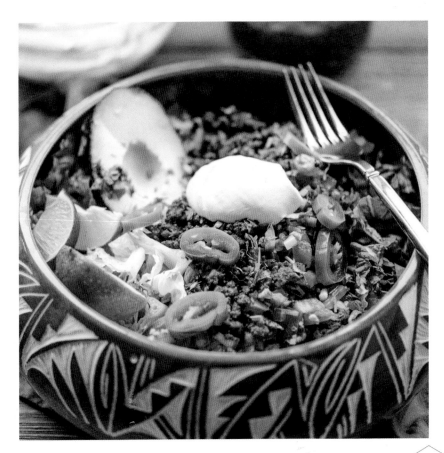

APPROXIMATE NUTRITION BREAKDOWN *(based on 1 of 4 servings)*		
CALORIES: 351	FAT:	21 g
PROTEIN: 23 g	CARBS:	13 g

BBQ Cobb Chicken Salad

WITH CREAMY JALAPEÑO RANCH

Here's a salad that makes a statement—a salad that you can serve at any time of the year, to any crowd of people, and get the same "WOW, that was GOOD" response from anyone lucky enough to enjoy your kitchen handiwork. This prized recipe is filling, bursting with great nutrition, and so flavorful that you'll want to put it on repeat.

NUT-FREE · GAPS

prep time: 15 minutes, plus at least 15 minutes to brine	cook time: 18 minutes	yield: 3 to 4 servings

BRINE

2 tablespoons fine sea salt

2 cups warm water

SALAD

1 pound boneless, skinless chicken breasts, rinsed

⅓ cup BBQ sauce, store-bought or homemade (page 336)

1 large head romaine lettuce, chopped (4 heaping cups)

2 hard-boiled eggs, quartered

4 slices thick-cut bacon, diced and fried until crispy

1 avocado, sliced or cubed

½ cup halved cherry tomatoes

½ teaspoon fine sea salt

⅛ teaspoon ground black pepper

1 tablespoon finely chopped purple onion, for garnish (optional)

½ cup Creamy Jalapeño Ranch (page 339)

2 tablespoons fresh cilantro leaves, finely chopped, for garnish (optional)

1. To make the brine: Dissolve the salt in the warm water and allow the water to cool. Place the chicken in the brine for at least 15 minutes, or up to overnight. If brining the chicken for longer than 30 minutes, place it in the refrigerator. After the chicken is finished brining, rinse and pat it dry. (If you have brined the chicken in the refrigerator, let it come to room temperature before baking.)

2. Preheat the oven to 450°F. Coat the chicken breasts with the BBQ sauce. Set them on a rimmed baking sheet and bake for 15 to 18 minutes, until the sauce on the chicken starts to turn brown.

3. While the chicken is baking, prepare the rest of the salad ingredients: Arrange the lettuce on one large platter or three or four individual plates. Top the lettuce with rows of egg, bacon, avocado, and tomato.

4. When the chicken is cooked, let it rest for 5 minutes before cutting.

5. Slice the chicken crosswise or cut it into 1-inch cubes and plate its row alongside the others.

6. Sprinkle the salt, pepper, and purple onion (if using) over the top. Drizzle the salad with the dressing and garnish with cilantro, if desired. Enjoy warm or cold.

tips

• *This amount of dressing will dress the salad lightly. If you prefer a more heavily dressed salad, double the amount of dressing.*

SALAD

APPROXIMATE NUTRITION BREAKDOWN (based on 1 of 4 servings)	
CALORIES: 332	FAT: 16 g
PROTEIN: 32 g	CARBS: 14 g

DRESSING

APPROXIMATE NUTRITION BREAKDOWN (based on 1 of 4 servings)	
CALORIES: 404	FAT: 44 g
PROTEIN: 0 g	CARBS: 0 g

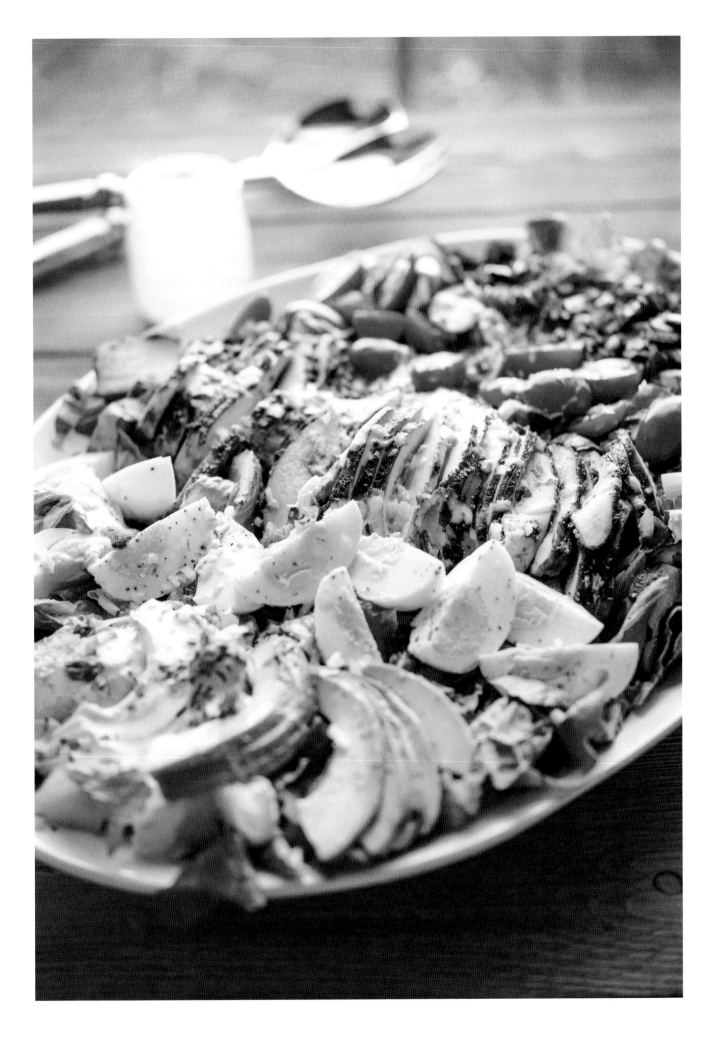

Chicken Caesar Salad

WITH POTATO CROUTONS

Let's get one thing straight—I don't avoid bread because I don't like it, I avoid it because it makes me feel sick. Sure, there are some foods (like cheesy French bread) that are hard to replicate sans grains, but croutons . . . croutons I took a stab at. This Caesar salad, which relies on a traditional dressing for authenticity, also uses a clever oven trick that turns ordinary potatoes into the perfect crouton replacement.

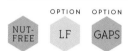

NUT-FREE   OPTION LF   OPTION GAPS

prep time: 15 minutes | *cook time: 1 hour* | *yield: 3 to 4 servings*

CROUTONS (omit for GAPS)

4 russet potatoes, peeled and cut into 1-inch cubes

1 tablespoon extra-virgin olive oil

1 teaspoon fine sea salt

1½ pounds boneless, skinless chicken breasts

½ teaspoon fine sea salt

¼ teaspoon ground black pepper

1 head romaine lettuce, leaves separated

1 pint grape tomatoes, halved

2 tablespoons finely chopped fresh flat-leaf parsley, for garnish

CAESAR DRESSING

2 large egg yolks

6 anchovy fillets packed in oil, drained

1 whole clove garlic (omit for low-FODMAP)

1 teaspoon Dijon mustard

2 tablespoons fresh lemon juice (about 1 small lemon)

½ teaspoon fine sea salt

¼ teaspoon ground black pepper

⅓ cup extra-virgin olive oil

1. Evenly space two oven racks in the middle of the oven and preheat the oven to 350°F. Line two rimmed baking sheets with parchment paper.

2. To make the croutons: Toss the potato cubes in the olive oil, then spread them out evenly one of the lined baking sheets. Sprinkle with 1 teaspoon salt, then bake for 30 minutes. Flip each cube over and bake for an additional 30 minutes, until each potato crouton is fork-tender and lightly browned.

3. While the potatoes are baking, prepare the chicken: Rinse and pat the chicken breasts dry, then sprinkle each side with the salt and pepper. Place the chicken on the other lined baking sheet. When the potatoes have 30 minutes left in the oven, place the chicken in the oven and roast for 30 minutes, until the juices run clear. Let the chicken rest for 5 minutes before slicing crosswise into ½-inch-thick pieces.

4. To prepare the dressing, blend the egg yolks, anchovies, garlic, mustard, lemon juice, salt, and pepper in a food processor or blender for about 30 seconds, until smooth. With the blender running, slowly pour in the olive oil—this should take about 1 minute.

5. To prepare the salad, lay the lettuce leaves on a large platter. Top with the sliced chicken, grape tomato halves, and potato croutons, drizzle with the dressing, and garnish with the chopped parsley.

SALAD WITH CROUTONS

APPROXIMATE NUTRITION BREAKDOWN *(based on 1 of 4 servings)*	
CALORIES: 426	FAT: 6 g
PROTEIN: 45 g	CARBS: 46 g

DRESSING

APPROXIMATE NUTRITION BREAKDOWN *(based on 1 of 4 servings)*	
CALORIES: 197	FAT: 21 g
PROTEIN: 3 g	CARBS: 1 g

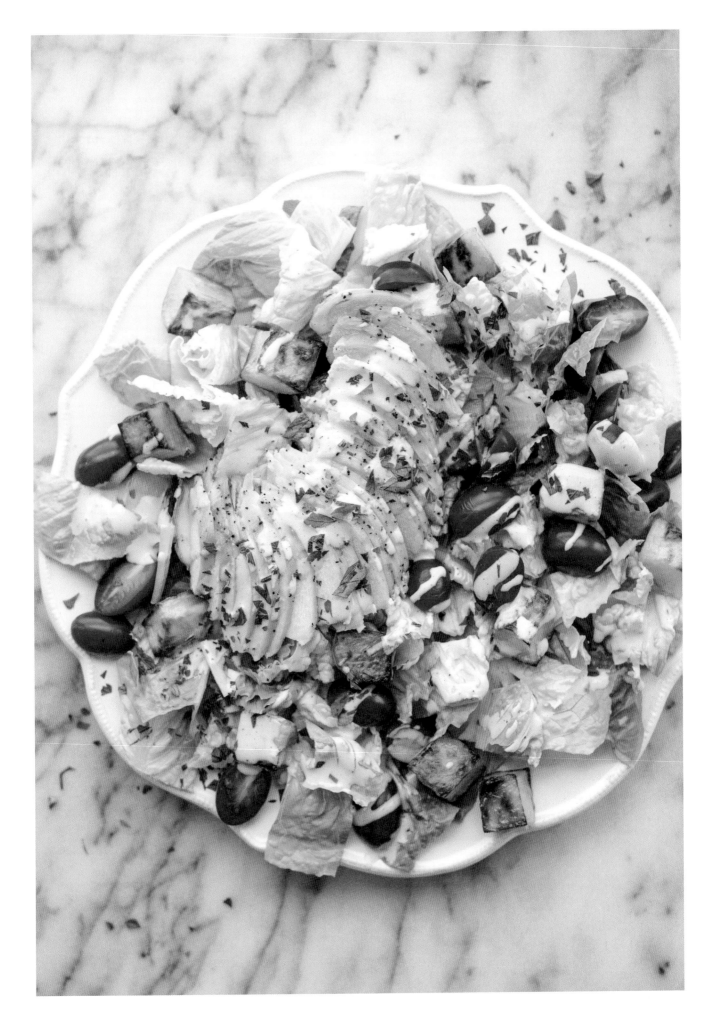

My Big Fat Greek Salad

I had an insatiable lunchtime craving for Greek salad topped with grilled chicken for an entire year of my life. There's something about the balance of zesty dressing, peppers, salty olives, crunchy vegetables, and savory chicken that kept me coming back for more. Because the vegetables in this salad keep really well once cut, this is an ideal candidate for pre-prepped lunchtime meals. Just add the dressing to each serving as you go.

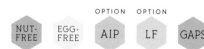

OPTION OPTION
NUT-FREE · EGG-FREE · AIP · LF · GAPS

prep time: 20 minutes, plus at least 15 minutes to marinate | *cook time: 8 minutes* | *yield: 4 to 6 servings*

SALAD

1½ pounds chicken breast strips

1 tablespoon salted butter (for stovetop option; use coconut oil for AIP)

1 head romaine lettuce, chopped (about 4 cups)

1 large cucumber, chopped into ½-inch pieces (about 2 cups)

1 cup halved grape tomatoes (omit for AIP)

½ cup pitted Kalamata olives

¼ purple onion, thinly sliced (about ¼ cup) (omit for low-FODMAP)

½ cup pepperoncini peppers (omit for AIP and if sensitive to food dyes)

2 tablespoons chopped fresh flat-leaf parsley, for garnish

GREEK MARINADE/DRESSING

¼ cup capers, finely chopped

¼ cup fresh lemon juice (about 2 small lemons)

¼ cup apple cider vinegar

½ cup extra-virgin olive oil

2 tablespoons dried oregano leaves

1 teaspoon fine sea salt

½ teaspoon ground black pepper (omit for AIP)

1. Rinse the chicken with cool water, pat dry, and place in a large glass bowl.

2. Combine all of the dressing ingredients in a bowl or large measuring cup and whisk to combine. When the dressing is well mixed, pour half of it over the chicken. Stir to coat the chicken evenly, then transfer to the refrigerator to marinate for at least 15 minutes or up to 4 hours.

3. Either grill the chicken or cook it on the stovetop:

   Grill option: Oil the grill grates and preheat the grill to high. When it reaches approximately 500°F, remove the chicken from the marinade and place it on the grill. Discard the marinade. Grill the chicken for 4 minutes on one side, or until char marks start to appear. Flip the chicken over and grill for an additional 3 minutes, or until there are char marks. Transfer to a plate to rest for 5 minutes.

   Stovetop option: Melt the butter in a large frying pan or sauté pan over high heat. When melted, remove the chicken breasts from the marinade, letting the excess marinade drip off, and place them in the pan. Discard the marinade. Cook the chicken for 5 minutes on one side, or until it starts to brown. Flip the chicken over and cook for an additional 3 minutes, or until the other side starts to brown. Transfer to a plate to rest for 5 minutes.

4. While the chicken is cooking and then resting, prepare the rest of the salad ingredients: Place the lettuce in a large bowl or on a large platter. Top with the cucumber, tomatoes, olives, onion, and pepperoncini.

5. When the chicken is done resting, slice it crosswise into bite-sized pieces. Add the chicken over the top of the salad and pour the remaining dressing on top. Finish with a sprinkle of fresh parsley and enjoy!

• If you think you're going to have leftovers, dress individual servings as needed, not the whole salad at once. The vegetables and chicken will keep in the refrigerator for up to 5 days if left undressed until serving.

• Using salad dressing as a marinade for the salad protein is one of my favorite flavor-boosting tricks. If you're short on time, you can absolutely forgo this step and make a simple chicken that's seasoned with salt and pepper.

SALAD

APPROXIMATE NUTRITION BREAKDOWN *(based on 1 of 6 servings)*	
CALORIES: 177	FAT: 4 g
PROTEIN: 28 g	CARBS: 9 g

DRESSING (excludes use as marinade)

APPROXIMATE NUTRITION BREAKDOWN *(based on 1 of 6 servings)*	
CALORIES: 83	FAT: 9 g
PROTEIN: 0 g	CARBS: 1 g

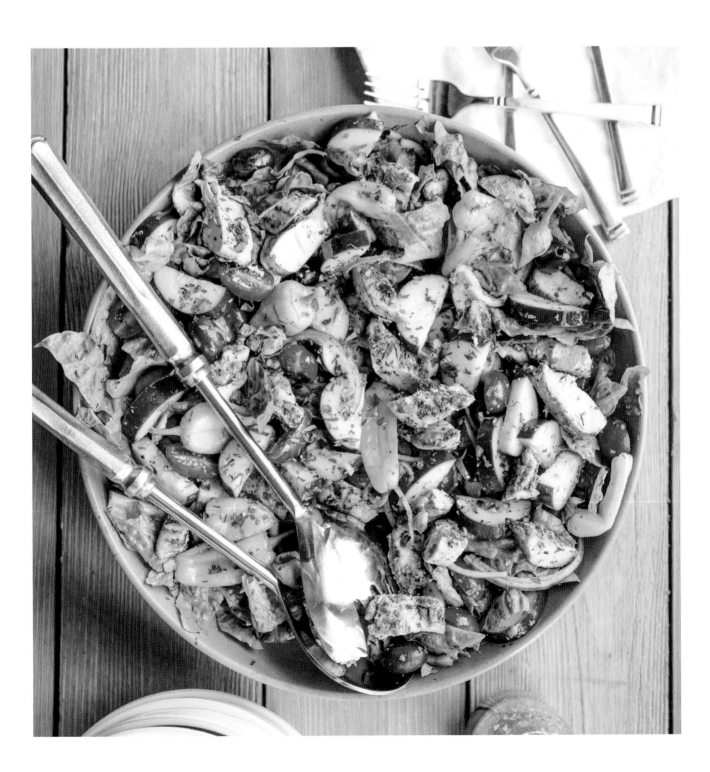

Spring Has Sprung Salad

WITH CRISPY CHICKEN &
LEMON DRESSING

Though the start of spring is still a little chilly and reminiscent of the cold, dark months just experienced, I always find myself craving bright, fresh flavors that remind me of new beginnings and sunshine. This spring salad calls for the dressing that I make more often than any other: lemon dressing. While it's absolutely delicious on this salad, don't be surprised if you start creating excuses to make it again and again.

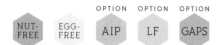

| NUT-FREE | EGG-FREE | OPTION AIP | OPTION LF | OPTION GAPS |

prep time: 15 minutes | *cook time: 45 minutes* | *yield: 3 to 4 servings*

SALAD

1 pound Yukon gold potatoes, quartered lengthwise (omit for GAPS and AIP)

2 tablespoons extra-virgin olive oil, divided

2 teaspoons fine sea salt, divided

½ teaspoon ground black pepper, divided (omit for AIP)

1 pound bone-in, skin-on chicken thighs, rinsed and patted dry

1 bunch thin asparagus spears (about 1 pound), tough bottoms removed (omit for low-FODMAP)

1 head butter lettuce

1 bunch radishes, sliced as thinly as possible (about 1½ cups)

2 tablespoons chopped fresh parsley, for garnish

LEMON DRESSING

1 tablespoon grated lemon zest (about 1 lemon)

¼ cup fresh lemon juice (about 2 small lemons)

¼ cup extra-virgin olive oil

1 teaspoon fine sea salt

½ teaspoon ground black pepper (omit for AIP)

1. Evenly space two oven racks in the middle of the oven and preheat the oven to 400°F. Line two rimmed baking sheets with parchment paper.

2. In a large mixing bowl, toss the potatoes with 1 tablespoon of the olive oil, 1 teaspoon of the salt, and ¼ teaspoon of the pepper. Spread them out evenly on one of the prepared baking sheets so that no two pieces are touching. Place the potatoes in the oven and roast until golden brown and crispy, about 45 minutes.

3. While the potatoes are roasting, prepare the chicken: Place the chicken thighs skin side up on the other prepared baking sheet. Rub the remaining 1 tablespoon of olive oil over the top of the chicken, then sprinkle the chicken with the remaining 1 teaspoon of salt and ¼ teaspoon of pepper. When the potatoes have 30 minutes left in the oven, place the chicken in the oven and cook until the tops are golden brown and crispy, 25 to 30 minutes.

4. To prepare the asparagus, bring a pot of water to a boil and prepare an ice bath. Boil the asparagus for 5 minutes, or until they turn bright green, then immediately place them in the ice bath. Let them sit in the ice bath for 5 minutes to lock in the bright green color and stop the cooking, then blot dry with paper towels.

5. While the chicken and potatoes are in the oven, prepare the rest of the salad. Coarsely chop the lettuce and lay it out in a large bowl or platter. Top the lettuce with the radishes and asparagus.

6. To prepare the dressing, whisk the ingredients together in a small bowl.

7. When the chicken and potatoes are cooked, remove them from the oven and let them rest for 5 minutes. After the chicken has cooled some, carefully pull the meat and skin away from the bones, roughly chop the meat and crispy skin together, and then add the chicken and potatoes to the salad. Drizzle the salad with the dressing, sprinkle with the chopped parsley, and serve warm.

SALAD		DRESSING	
APPROXIMATE NUTRITION BREAKDOWN *(based on 1 of 4 servings)*		**APPROXIMATE NUTRITION BREAKDOWN** *(based on 1 of 4 servings)*	
CALORIES: 418	FAT: 24 g	CALORIES: 183	FAT: 20 g
PROTEIN: 24 g	CARBS: 26 g	PROTEIN: 0 g	CARBS: 0 g

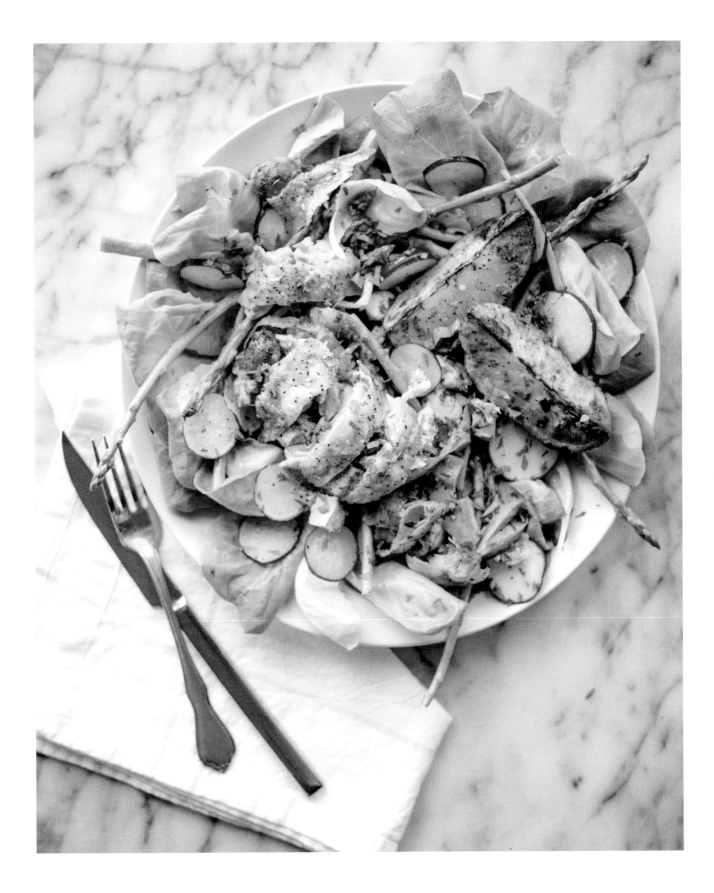

Summer Beach Babe Salmon Salad

WITH AVOCADO DILL DRESSING

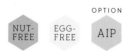

This is one of those salads that makes me want to pack a picnic lunch so I can kick back and enjoy it in the sunshine sitting on a lawn somewhere. It packs a lot of flavor and awesome raw vegetables. Don't be intimidated by the salmon—you may be surprised at how easily it comes together.

NUT-FREE   EGG-FREE   OPTION AIP

prep time: 25 minutes | *cook time: 6 minutes* | *yield: 2 to 3 servings*

SALAD

1 (8-ounce) salmon fillet, skin removed

½ teaspoon fine sea salt

¼ teaspoon ground black pepper (omit for AIP)

1 tablespoon salted butter (use coconut oil for AIP)

4 cups fresh baby spinach

3 small tomatillos, peeled, washed, and sliced as thinly as possible (about ½ cup) (omit for AIP)

4 ounces fresh okra, cut into ½-inch-thick discs (about 1 cup)

½ jicama, peeled and julienned (about ½ cup)

AVOCADO DILL DRESSING

½ avocado

2 tablespoons fresh lemon juice (about 1 small lemon)

2 tablespoons apple cider vinegar

2 tablespoons water

1 tablespoon chopped fresh dill leaves

½ teaspoon fine sea salt

¼ teaspoon ground black pepper (omit for AIP)

GARNISHES

1 tablespoon chopped fresh dill

2 tablespoons flax seeds (omit for AIP)

1. Rinse and pat the salmon dry. Using a sharp knife, carefully slice the salmon into 1-inch cubes. Sprinkle the fish with the salt and pepper.

2. Melt the butter in a large frying pan over high heat. When the butter has melted, add the salmon pieces and cook for 3 minutes, or until golden and starting to crisp. Flip each piece over and cook for an additional 3 minutes, or until golden and starting to crisp.

3. While the salmon is cooking, prepare the dressing. Place all of the dressing ingredients in a blender and blend on high speed for 1 minute, or until smooth. If your dressing is too thick, add more water 1 teaspoon at a time until it reaches the desired consistency.

4. When the salmon is cooked, transfer it to a plate to rest while you plate the salad.

5. Place the spinach in a large bowl or platter, then top with the sliced tomatillos, okra, and jicama. Place the salmon pieces on top of the salad and drizzle with the dressing. Finish with the fresh dill and flax seeds. Enjoy warm or cold!

tips

- *I like to prepare the salmon so that it's in bite-sized pieces, but feel free to pan-fry the salmon fillet as one whole piece!*

- *If you prefer your salmon a little more pink in the center, reduce the cooking time by at least 1 minute per side.*

SALAD			
APPROXIMATE NUTRITION BREAKDOWN *(based on 1 of 3 servings)*			
CALORIES:	242	FAT:	10 g
PROTEIN:	19 g	CARBS:	20 g

DRESSING			
APPROXIMATE NUTRITION BREAKDOWN *(based on 1 of 3 servings)*			
CALORIES:	46	FAT:	4 g
PROTEIN:	1 g	CARBS:	4 g

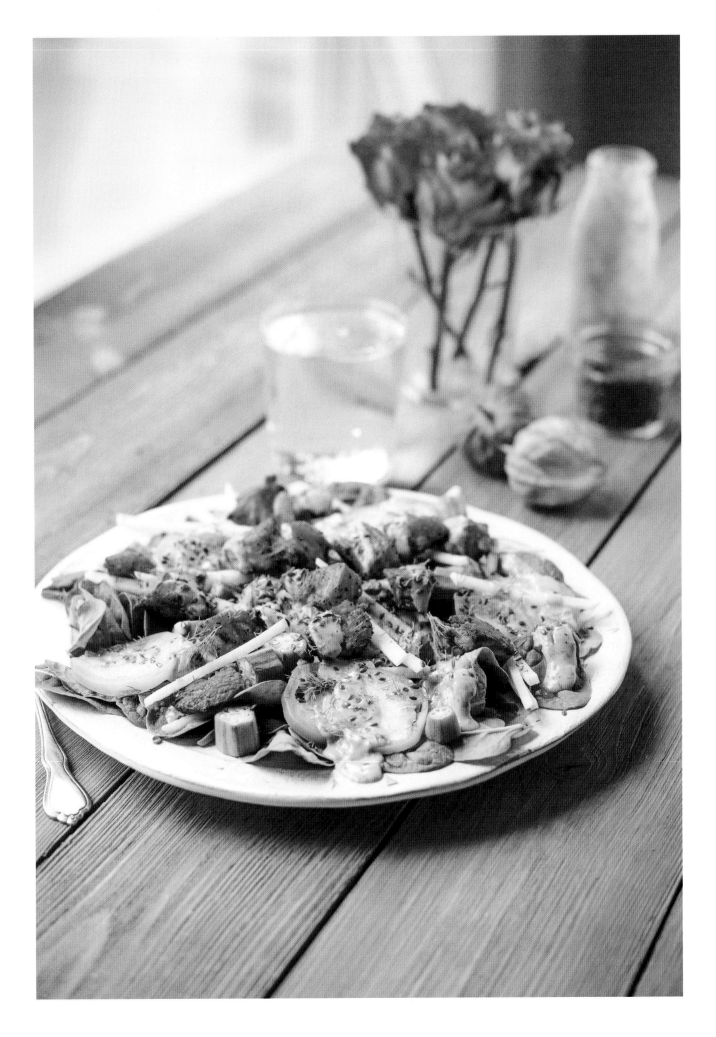

Massaged Kale & Turkey Harvest Salad

WITH SEA SALT & LIME DRESSING

I could eat this salad every day of my life. Something truly magical happens when you lovingly massage kale with fresh lime juice and sea salt. I've watched the magical combination make real kale lovers out of self-proclaimed kale haters. The wow factor is upped even higher by the awesome roasted turkey, acorn squash wedges, pecans, and bright pomegranate seeds. This salad would be perfect for a pre-Thanksgiving lunch or fall brunch!

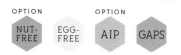

OPTION NUT-FREE · EGG-FREE · OPTION AIP · GAPS

prep time: 15 minutes | *cook time: 1 hour* | *yield: 3 to 4 servings*

SALAD

1 acorn squash (about 3 pounds), cut in half, seeded, and cut into 2-inch wedges

2 tablespoons extra-virgin olive oil, divided

1½ teaspoons fine sea salt, divided

1 boneless, skinless turkey breast half (about 1½ pounds)

1 tablespoon finely chopped fresh rosemary

½ teaspoon ground black pepper (omit for AIP)

2 bunches kale

1 cup fresh flat-leaf parsley, coarsely chopped, plus extra for garnish

½ cup raw pecans (omit for nut-free and AIP)

½ cup pomegranate seeds

SEA SALT & LIME DRESSING

¼ cup fresh lime juice (about 2 limes)

3 tablespoons extra-virgin olive oil

1 teaspoon fine sea salt

1. Place one oven rack near the top of the oven and one near the bottom. Preheat the oven to 375°F. Line two rimmed baking sheets with parchment paper.

2. Place the acorn squash wedges, cut side up, on one of the prepared baking sheets. Rub the cut sides with 1 tablespoon of the olive oil, then sprinkle with ½ teaspoon of the salt. Bake for 1 hour, until they're easily pierced with a fork and the tops are just starting to turn brown.

3. While the acorn squash is cooking, prepare the turkey breast, aiming to place it in the oven when the acorn squash has 30 minutes left on the timer. Rinse the turkey breast with cool water and pat dry. Place the breast on the other prepared baking sheet. Rub the top with the remaining tablespoon of olive oil, then sprinkle with the rosemary, remaining teaspoon of salt, and ½ teaspoon pepper. Bake for 30 minutes, or until the top is starting to turn golden brown and the internal temperature reads at least 165°F. Remove from the oven and let rest for at least 5 minutes before slicing.

4. While the turkey is in the oven, prepare the kale: Remove the stems, stack several leaves, and roll them up like a cigar. Then thinly slice them crosswise into ribbons. Place the kale in a large mixing bowl.

5. Prepare the dressing: Whisk together the lime juice, olive oil, and salt.

6. Pour three-quarters of the dressing over the kale, reserving the rest for final plating. With clean hands, massage the dressing into the kale so that each piece is well coated. Toss the kale with the parsley, then place in a serving bowl or on individual plates.

7. Slice the cooked and rested turkey into about ¼-inch pieces and place them on top of the kale. Sprinkle the pecans and pomegranate seeds on top of the salad and place the roasted acorn squash wedges alongside. Finish the salad with the remaining dressing and some fresh parsley and serve.

SALAD

APPROXIMATE NUTRITION BREAKDOWN *(based on 1 of 4 servings)*	
CALORIES: 657	FAT: 35 g
PROTEIN: 45 g	CARBS: 83 g

DRESSING

APPROXIMATE NUTRITION BREAKDOWN *(based on 1 of 4 servings)*	
CALORIES: 90	FAT: 11 g
PROTEIN: 0 g	CARBS: 1 g

tips

- *If you have trouble finding a turkey breast, you can substitute boneless, skinless chicken breasts. Just reduce the baking time from 25 minutes to 18 minutes.*

- *If you can't find acorn squash, a 2-pound butternut squash, peeled, seeded, and cut into cubes, or 2 large sweet potatoes, scrubbed and cut lengthwise into wedges, makes a great substitute!*

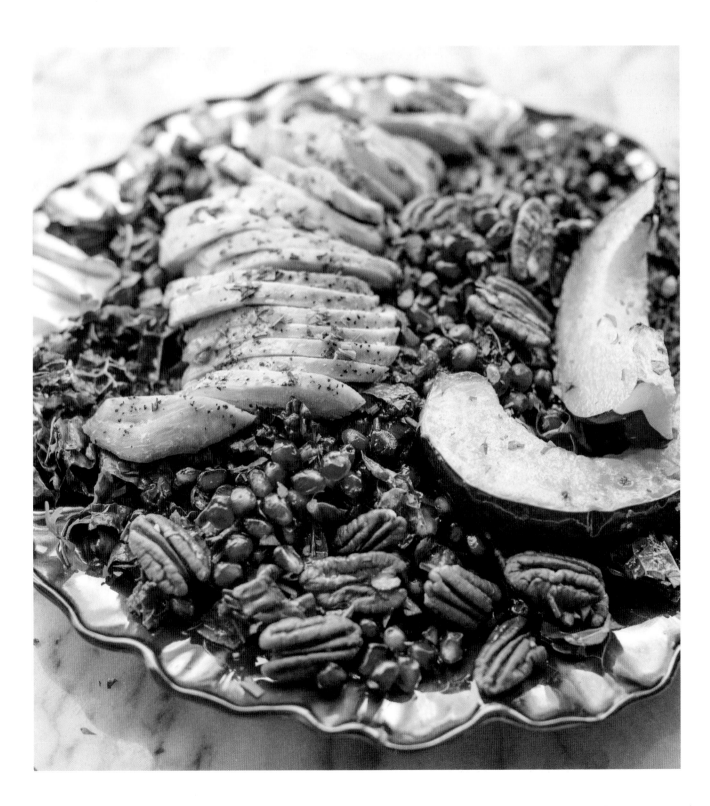

Winter Beef Salad

WITH ROASTED BEET VINAIGRETTE

Talk about salads that satisfy! This salad is like a warm, delicious, comforting hug. Full of flavorful roasted Brussels sprouts and sweet potatoes and pan-seared steak, it won't leave you hungry or wanting. If you'd prefer to meal-prep this salad, I recommend that you store the components separately and then combine them just before serving.

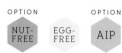

OPTION   OPTION
NUT-FREE   EGG-FREE   AIP

prep time: 20 minutes | cook time: 1 hour 45 minutes (see Tips) | yield: 2 to 3 servings

ROASTED BEET VINAIGRETTE

1 red beet

2 tablespoons extra-virgin olive oil, plus more for the beet

½ grapefruit, peeled and seeded

¼ cup apple cider vinegar

¼ cup water

¼ teaspoon fine sea salt

SALAD

½ pound Brussels sprouts, halved (about 1 cup)

1 pound sweet potatoes (about 2 medium), cut crosswise into ¼-inch discs

2 tablespoons extra-virgin olive oil

1½ teaspoons fine sea salt, divided

½ teaspoon ground black pepper, divided (omit for AIP)

8 ounces beef sirloin (or the best cut of beef you have on hand)

1 tablespoon salted butter (use coconut oil for AIP)

1 bunch Swiss chard, bottom stems removed and leaves coarsely chopped

1 bulb fennel, thinly sliced (reserve fronds)

¼ cup raw walnut pieces (omit for nut-free and AIP)

Chopped fennel fronds (reserved from fennel bulb, above)

1 tablespoon coarsely chopped fresh thyme, for garnish

1. To roast the beets for the vinaigrette, preheat the oven to 375°F. Scrub the beets clean, cut off the stems, and rub the outsides with a little olive oil. Wrap each beet in aluminum foil, place on a rimmed baking sheet, and bake for 45 minutes, until they can be easily pierced with a paring knife. Let cool completely, then peel off the skins and cut into quarters. While the beets are cooling, prepare the roasted vegetables.

2. Leave the oven temperature at 375°F. Line a rimmed baking sheet with parchment paper. Toss the halved Brussels sprouts and sliced sweet potatoes in the olive oil. Pour them out onto the prepared baking sheet and spread them out to make sure that no two pieces are touching. (Use an additional lined baking sheet if necessary.) Sprinkle the tops with 1 teaspoon of the salt and ¼ teaspoon of the pepper. Bake for 40 minutes, or until each piece is turning golden brown and starting to look crispy.

3. Prepare the vinaigrette: Place the roasted beets, grapefruit, vinegar, water, olive oil, and salt in a high-powered blender. Blend for at least 1 minute, until smooth. If your dressing is too thick, add 1 teaspoon of water at a time until you get the consistency you want.

4. To prepare the salad, toss the chopped Swiss chard with the fennel. Place this mixture on a serving platter, in a serving bowl, or on individual plates.

5. When the Brussels sprouts and potatoes have about 15 minutes left in the oven, prepare the steak: Season each side with the remaining ½ teaspoon of salt and ¼ teaspoon of pepper. Melt the butter in a frying pan over high heat. When the butter has melted, add the steak and cook for 4 minutes, or until it starts to turn brown, then flip it over to cook for an additional 4 minutes on the other side, or until it's starting to brown and develop a slight char. When finished, place on a plate to rest for 5 minutes before slicing into ¼-inch-thick pieces.

6. Top the chard and fennel with the roasted Brussels sprouts and sweet potatoes followed by the walnut pieces, chopped fennel fronds, and sliced steak. Finish with the vinaigrette and a sprinkle of fresh thyme.

SALAD

APPROXIMATE NUTRITION BREAKDOWN (based on 1 of 3 servings)	
CALORIES: 556	FAT: 29 g
PROTEIN: 26 g	CARBS: 53 g

VINAIGRETTE

APPROXIMATE NUTRITION BREAKDOWN (based on 1 of 3 servings)	
CALORIES: 114	FAT: 9 g
PROTEIN: 1 g	CARBS: 7 g

tips

- *Prepare the roasted beets in advance and save yourself time the day of! If you use pre-roasted beets for this recipe, the cook time will be reduced to 40 minutes. I like to roast about a dozen beets at a time and store them in individual serving-sized bags in the freezer. Unlike raw beets, roasted beets freeze and defrost well.*

- *You do not need to segment the grapefruit, discarding the membrane, for this vinaigrette. Most blenders will be able to sufficiently break up the membrane, saving you a step and adding even more nutrients to the salad.*

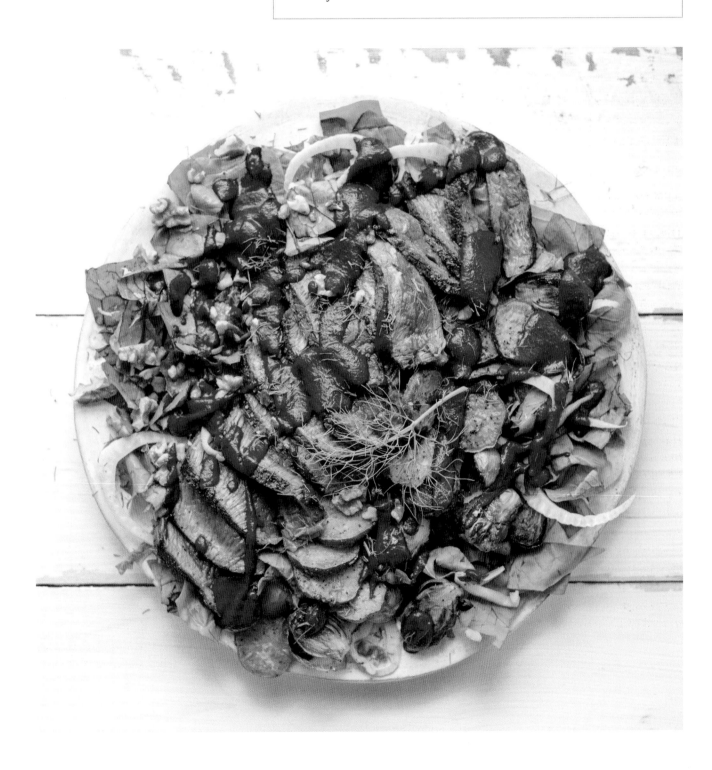

Thai Beef Salad

WITH ZESTY LIME DRESSING

This salad is one of my most favorite foods on this earth. It's always so fresh and packed with diverse flavors. If you're new to using fish sauce in your food, I encourage you not to be intimidated. Give it a go and see what you think! I could literally swim in this dressing, it's so good.

OPTION **NUT-FREE**   **EGG-FREE**   OPTION **AIP**   OPTION **LF**

| *prep time: 25 minutes* | *cook time: 8 minutes* | *yield: 2 to 3 servings* |

SALAD

1 tablespoon salted butter, ghee, or coconut oil

8 ounces beef sirloin (or the best cut of beef you have on hand)

½ teaspoon fine sea salt

¼ teaspoon ground black pepper

2 cups mixed lettuce

¼ cup cherry tomatoes, halved (omit for AIP)

⅛ purple onion, thinly sliced (omit for low-FODMAP)

½ cucumber, thinly sliced

¼ cup fresh coarsely chopped cilantro leaves and stems

¼ cup fresh mint leaves, coarsely chopped

ZESTY LIME DRESSING

½ hot red chili pepper, thinly sliced (omit for AIP)

¼ teaspoon fine sea salt

2 tablespoons fish sauce

¼ cup fresh lime juice (about 2 limes)

1 tablespoon extra-virgin olive oil

OPTIONAL GARNISHES

1 tablespoon raw almonds, coarsely chopped (omit for nut-free and AIP)

2 tablespoons coarsely chopped fresh cilantro

2 tablespoons coarsely chopped fresh mint

1. Place the butter in a small sauté or frying pan over high heat. While the butter is melting, season both sides of the steak with the salt and pepper. When the butter has finished bubbling, it's ready for the steak. Using tongs, lay the steak in the frying pan and set your timer for 2 minutes per side for rare, 3 minutes per side for medium-rare, or 4 minutes per side for well-done. When the steak is cooked, remove from the heat and set on a plate to rest for 5 minutes.

2. While the steak is resting, whisk together all of the dressing ingredients in a small bowl. Set aside.

3. In a large bowl, toss the rest of the salad ingredients together, then pile them on two or three plates, depending on your serving size.

4. Thinly slice the rested steak against the grain and lay the slices on top of the plated salad. If desired, top with the almonds and additional cilantro and mint. Drizzle with the dressing and serve immediately.

tips

• *If you prefer milder flavors, leave the seeds out of the chili pepper. If you really enjoy spicy foods, add a whole chili pepper (including the seeds) to the dressing.*

• *If you plan on having leftovers, I recommend dressing only the portions of salad that you will serve right away.*

SALAD

APPROXIMATE NUTRITION BREAKDOWN *(based on 1 of 3 servings)*	
CALORIES: 213	FAT: 12 g
PROTEIN: 23 g	CARBS: 4 g

DRESSING

APPROXIMATE NUTRITION BREAKDOWN *(based on 1 of 3 servings)*	
CALORIES: 54	FAT: 5 g
PROTEIN: 1 g	CARBS: 4 g

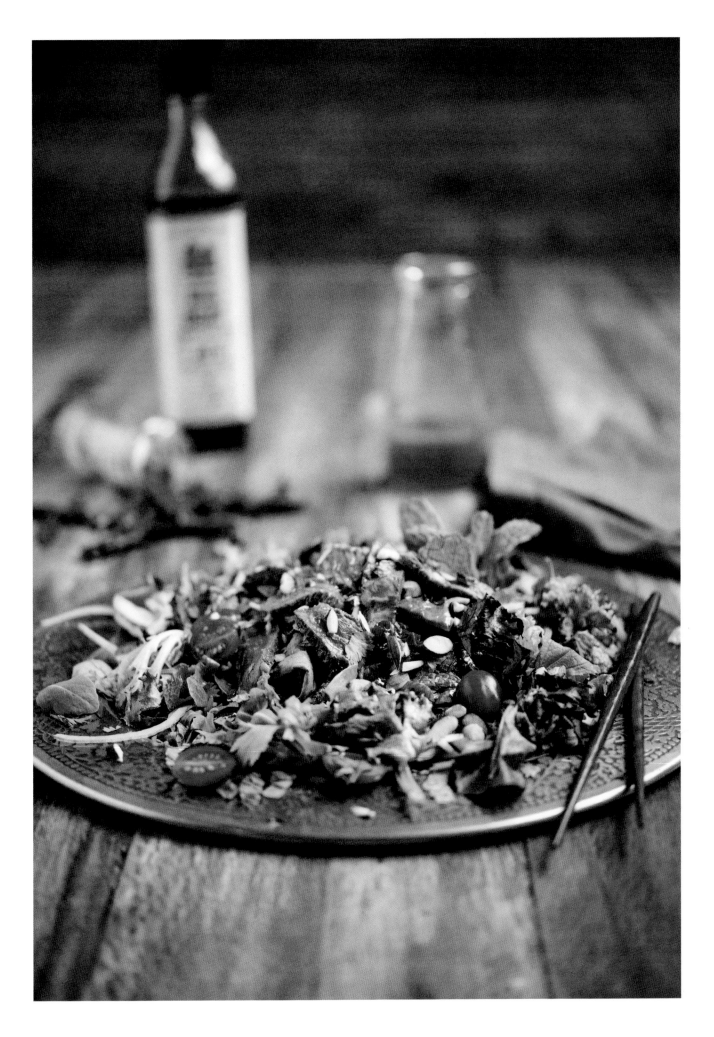

CHAPTER 4:

THINGS THAT ARE STUFFED

Download the Fed & Fit iPhone and Android app! You can scan the above QR codes directly in the app, which will then populate a consolidated grocery shopping list for the scanned recipes.

Olive-Stuffed Pork Tenderloin

Pork tenderloins are an "everyone wins" food in my house. My husband loves that they're delicious and more affordable than other cuts of meat. I love how they are incredibly simple to prepare and can be transformed with a flavorful stuffing. While this olive paste is delicious, think of this recipe as a method! Experiment with your own pork tenderloin stuffings and have fun with it.

OPTION

NUT-FREE · EGG-FREE · AIP · GAPS

prep time: 10 minutes | cook time: 20 minutes | yield: 3 to 5 servings

1 (1¼-pound) pork tenderloin, trimmed

½ cup pitted Kalamata olives

1 tablespoon extra-virgin olive oil

1 tablespoon fresh lemon juice (about ½ small lemon)

1 teaspoon Italian seasoning

½ teaspoon fine sea salt

¼ teaspoon ground black pepper

1 tablespoon salted butter (use EVOO for AIP)

SPECIAL EQUIPMENT
About 2 feet of kitchen twine

1. Butterfly the pork tenderloin: Keeping your knife parallel to the cutting board, make a cut down the middle of one side of the tenderloin, going only halfway through the circumference (do not cut all the way through). Open the tenderloin like a book with the cut side facing up.

2. Blend the olives, olive oil, lemon juice, and Italian seasoning until a paste forms. Spread this paste along the inside of the butterflied pork tenderloin.

3. Starting with one of the long sides, roll the tenderloin into a log, like a pinwheel. Using kitchen twine, tie the tenderloin together, knotting it at both ends. Season all sides of the tenderloin with the salt and pepper.

4. Preheat the oven to 375°F. Melt the butter in a large oven-safe frying pan over high heat. Once melted, add the tenderloin and sear for 2 minutes on one side, then turn it and sear for 2 minutes each on two more sides. Turn the tenderloin once more, then transfer the pan to the oven. Bake for 15 minutes, or until the juices run clear.

5. Let the tenderloin rest for at least 5 minutes. Cut away and discard the twine and slice the tenderloin into ½-inch pieces.

APPROXIMATE NUTRITION BREAKDOWN (based on 1 of 5 servings)			
CALORIES: 228		FAT:	11 g
PROTEIN: 30 g		CARBS:	1 g

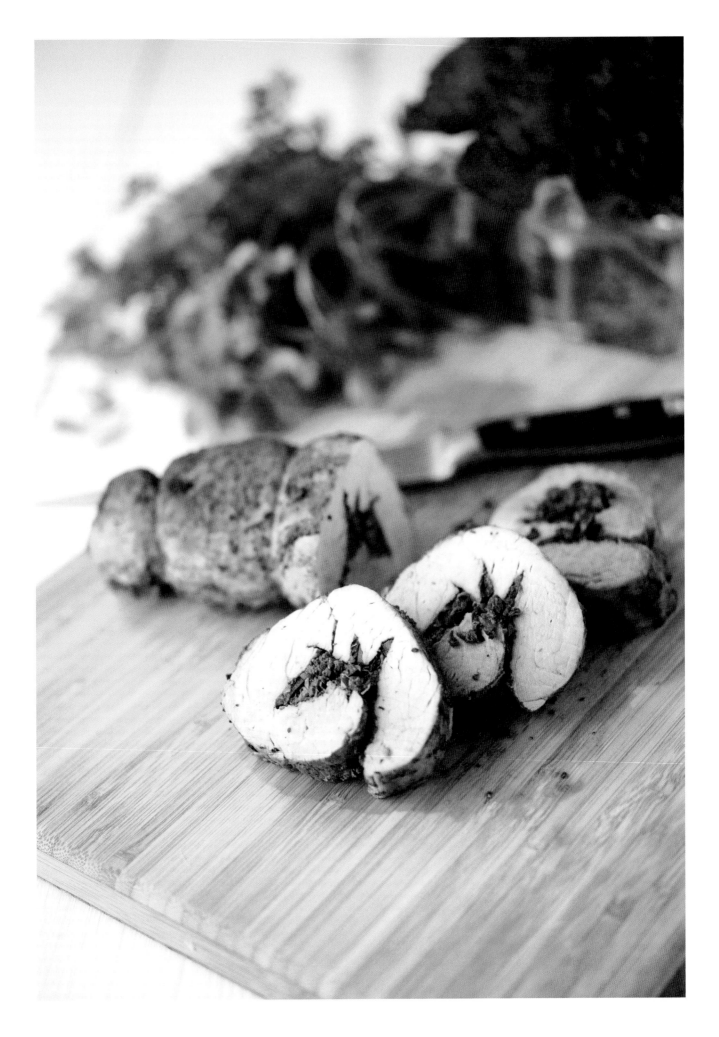

Chorizo-Stuffed Mushrooms

WITH AVOCADO MAYO

These stuffed mushrooms are straight from the heart. I whip them up when I want a special weeknight dinner with my honey or as a first course when we throw dinner parties for friends and family. Chorizo, avocado, and portabella mushrooms are a three-way match made in heaven. I just know you're going to love these.

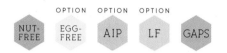

| prep time: 10 minutes | cook time: 1 hour | yield: 2 to 3 servings as a meal, 6 servings as an appetizer |

1 pound chorizo (bulk or link style) (use ground pork for AIP)

½ purple onion, finely chopped (about ½ cup) (omit for low-FODMAP)

¼ cup chopped fresh cilantro, plus more for garnish

6 portabella mushrooms, destemmed and hollowed out

Sliced jalapeño peppers, for garnish (optional)

AVOCADO MAYO
(omit for AIP and egg-free)

¼ cup mayo, store-bought or homemade (page 349)

½ avocado (omit for low-FODMAP)

2 tablespoons fresh lime juice (about 1 lime)

1. Preheat the oven to 375°F. If using link-style chorizo, squeeze the sausage out of its casings. In a medium-sized mixing bowl, using either your hands or a spoon, mix the chorizo with the onion and cilantro until both are evenly distributed in the meat.

2. Lay the portabella mushrooms in a baking dish with the hollowed-out cavities facing up. Spoon an equal amount of the chorizo stuffing into each mushroom. Bake for 45 minutes, or until the tops start to turn golden brown.

3. While the mushrooms are in the oven, blend the mayo, avocado, and lime juice together in a blender until smooth. When the mushrooms are finished cooking, drizzle the tops with the avocado mayo and garnish with the additional cilantro and jalapeño slices, if desired. Serve warm.

APPROXIMATE NUTRITION BREAKDOWN	
(based on 1 of 6 appetizer servings)	
CALORIES: 462	FAT: 38 g
PROTEIN: 21 g	CARBS: 9 g

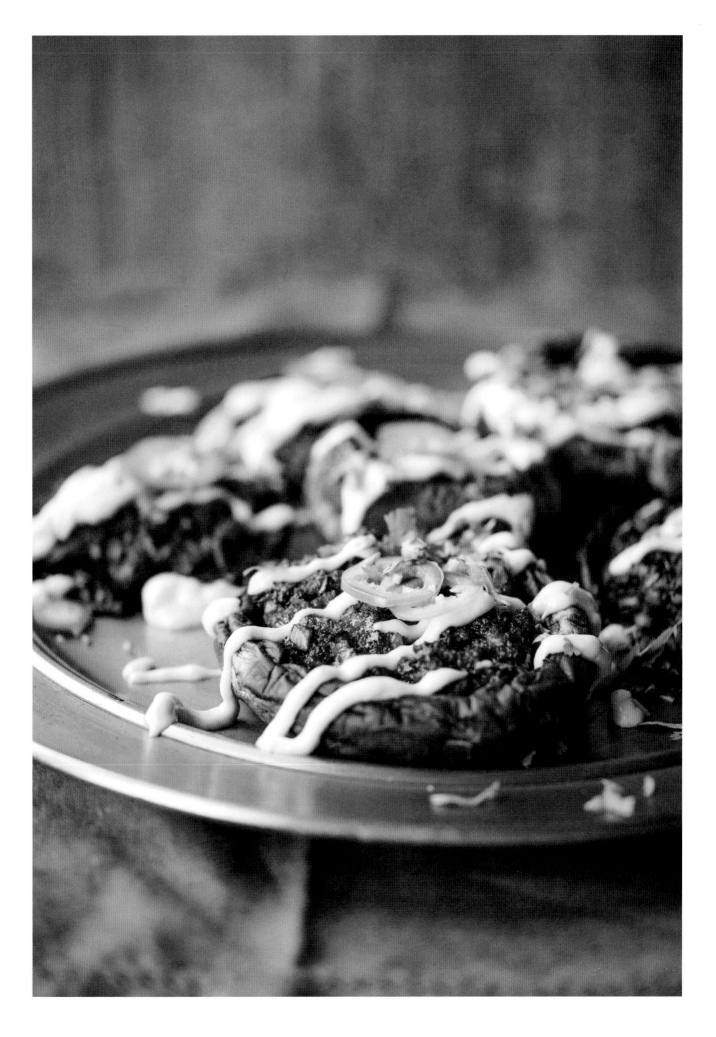

Curried Beef & Butternut Squash Stuffed Peppers

This recipe came to me one day when I was on a *major* curry kick. My handy little jar of curry powder had sat happily undisturbed in my spice drawer for months until I needed curry in everything. I adore stuffed peppers because they freeze and reheat exceptionally well. With a scoop of mashed butternut squash in the bottom of each pepper, these are a delicious balanced meal in one package!

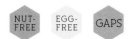

NUT-FREE · EGG-FREE · GAPS

| prep time: 15 minutes | cook time: 1 hour 25 minutes | yield: 6 servings |

1 small butternut squash (1½ to 2 pounds)

3 tablespoons salted butter, ghee, or coconut oil, divided

2 teaspoons fine sea salt, divided

½ yellow onion, diced

3 cloves garlic, minced

2 pounds ground beef

1 tablespoon curry powder

1 teaspoon paprika

¼ teaspoon ground black pepper

⅛ teaspoon cayenne pepper

¼ cup full-fat coconut milk

1 (4-ounce) jar Thai red curry paste

¼ cup fresh lime juice (about 2 limes)

6 large red bell peppers

2 tablespoons finely chopped fresh cilantro, for garnish (optional)

1. Preheat the oven to 400°F.

2. Cut the squash in half lengthwise and scrape out the seeds. Place the halves face up in a baking dish. Melt 1 tablespoon of the butter and rub it on the cut side of the squash. Sprinkle with ¼ teaspoon of the salt. Tent the baking dish with aluminum foil and bake for 1 hour, or until the flesh is easily pierced with a fork.

3. While the squash is baking, melt 1 tablespoon of the butter in a large frying pan over high heat. Add the onion and cook for about 5 minutes, until translucent and starting to brown, then add the garlic and cook for an additional 3 minutes, or until fragrant. Add the ground beef and cook for about 10 minutes, breaking it up with a spatula as it cooks, until it's evenly browned. Add the curry powder, paprika, black pepper, cayenne pepper, and 1 teaspoon of the salt. Stir and continue to brown until the meat is fully cooked. Add the coconut milk, curry paste, and lime juice, stir, and set aside.

4. To make the butternut squash mash, scrape all the flesh from the rind into a large bowl or food processor. Add the remaining tablespoon of butter and remaining ¾ teaspoon of salt and blend until well combined and smooth.

5. To prepare the peppers, cut off the tops and scrape out the seeds and membranes. Spoon about ¼ to ½ cup of the squash into the bottom of each pepper, then top it off with the ground beef.

6. Stand the peppers upright in a baking dish that is just large enough fit them all, but snugly. If you have trouble keeping them upright, wedge some crinkled aluminum foil between the peppers to create a more secure fit. Cover the tops of the peppers with a sheet of aluminum foil and bake for 20 minutes, then remove the foil and return to the oven to bake uncovered for 5 more minutes.

7. Serve warm garnished with the fresh cilantro (if using), or let cool and then individually wrap and freeze. To reheat, either place the frozen peppers (no need to defrost) in a preheated 350°F oven for 30 minutes or microwave on high for 3 to 4 minutes, until heated through.

APPROXIMATE NUTRITION BREAKDOWN (based on 1 of 6 servings)	
CALORIES: 569	FAT: 31 g
PROTEIN: 32 g	CARBS: 41 g

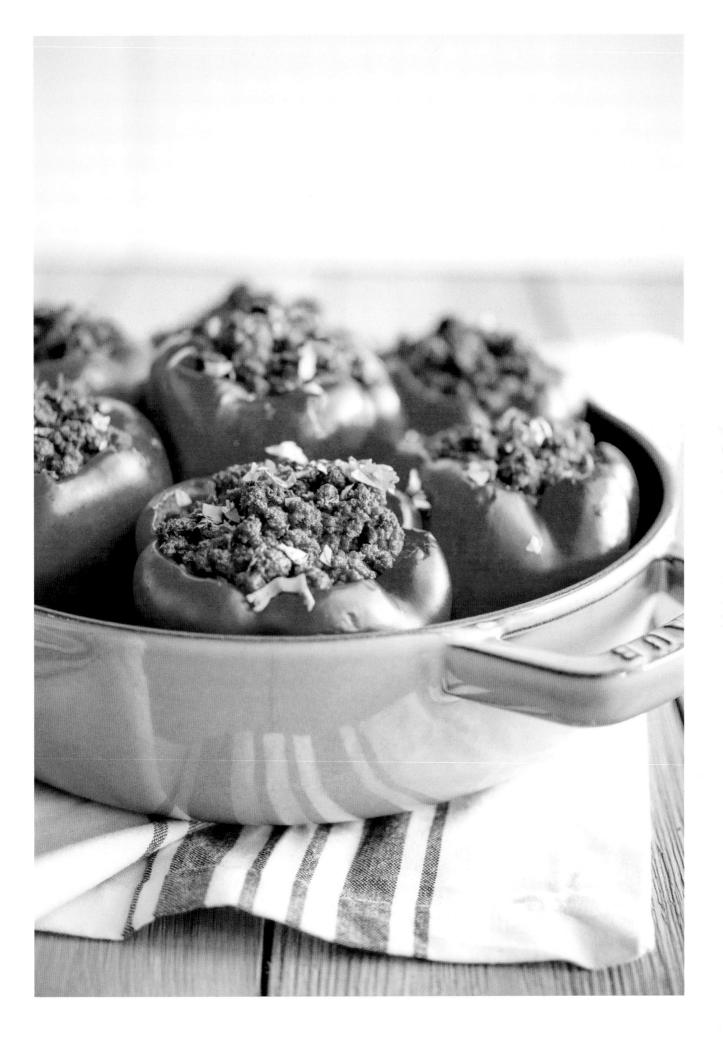

Italian Stuffed Eggplant

This meal ranks as a top-ten favorite in my house! It's been acclaimed by a dinner party of non-Paleo adults, by picky kids, and, best of all, by my comfort food–loving husband. Insanely satisfying and wonderfully nourishing, this dish will convince you that eggplant needs to be in regular rotation on your grocery list. Note that these stuffed eggplants reheat exceptionally well if you want to freeze the leftovers!

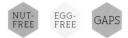

| prep time: 15 minutes | cook time: 1 hour 15 minutes | yield: 5 servings |

3 large eggplants (about 3 pounds)

1 tablespoon extra-virgin olive oil

2 tablespoons salted butter

1 small onion, chopped

4 cloves garlic, minced

1 pound hot Italian sausage, removed from casings if using links

1 (28-ounce) can diced tomatoes with juice

2 tablespoons Italian seasoning, plus additional for garnish

1 teaspoon fine sea salt

¼ teaspoon ground black pepper

1. Cut the eggplants in half lengthwise. Using a spoon or small knife, carve out the centers of five of the eggplant halves, leaving at least a 1-inch "wall" on all sides. Place the five hollowed-out eggplants in a baking dish, cut side up. Drizzle the tops with the olive oil and set aside.

2. Melt the butter in a large frying pan over high heat. Once melted, add the chopped onion, reduce the heat to medium, and cook for 10 minutes, or until golden brown. Add the garlic and cook for an additional 4 minutes, or until fragrant. Add the Italian sausage and, using a spoon or spatula to break it up into pieces, cook until browned and starting to become crispy.

3. While the sausage is cooking, cut the sixth eggplant half into ½-inch cubes. When the sausage is finished cooking, add the cubed eggplant, stir, and cook for at least 5 minutes, until the eggplant softens. Add the tomatoes, Italian seasoning, salt, and pepper. Stir to combine and bring to a simmer, then remove from the heat.

4. Preheat the oven to 350°F. Spoon an equal amount of the sausage filling into each eggplant half. Sprinkle the tops with additional Italian seasoning and bake for 45 minutes, or until the thickest part of the eggplant is easily pierced with a fork.

5. Enjoy warm!

tips

• *Leftovers will keep refrigerated for up to 5 days. This dish also freezes really well if you wrap each stuffed eggplant individually.*

• *Reheat either in the microwave for 4 to 5 minutes or in a preheated 350°F oven for 20 minutes.*

APPROXIMATE NUTRITION BREAKDOWN	
(based on 1 of 5 servings)	
CALORIES: 387	FAT: 25 g
PROTEIN: 18 g	CARBS: 25 g

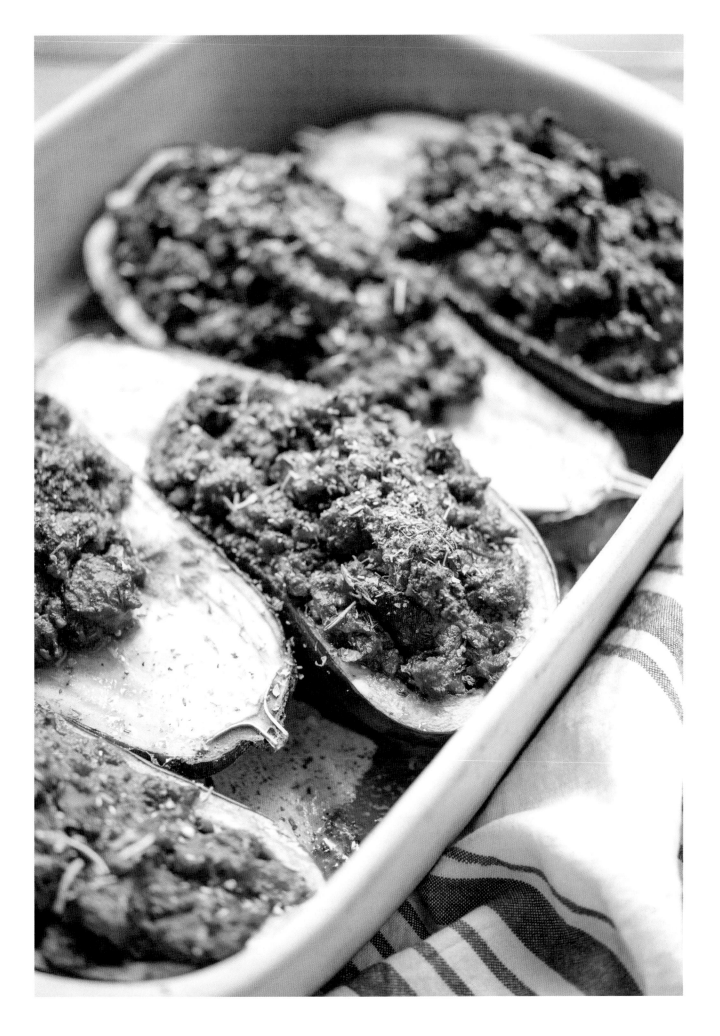

LOADED WHITE POTATOES:

Teriyaki Beef & Broccoli

Put down that Chinese takeout menu. We're going to make these loaded teriyaki potatoes instead! Just throw a couple potatoes in the oven and then get started on the filling. Before you know it, you'll have a satisfying *and* healthy Chinese-inspired dinner on your hands! Unlike that takeout you may have been eying, these will leave you feeling amazing.

OPTION

prep time: 5 minutes | *cook time: 45 minutes* | *yield: 4 servings*

4 medium white potatoes

SAUCE

2 teaspoons sesame oil (untoasted) (use EVOO for nut-free)

2 cloves garlic, minced

1 (½-inch) piece fresh ginger, minced (about 2 teaspoons)

¾ cup coconut aminos

1 teaspoon fish sauce

1 head broccoli, destemmed and cut into florets (about 3 cups)

1 tablespoon salted butter

1 pound wafer-thin sliced beef (see Tips)

½ teaspoon fine sea salt

1 tablespoon white sesame seeds, for garnish (omit for nut-free)

½ teaspoon red pepper flakes, for garnish

1. Preheat the oven to 450°F. Place the potatoes on a rimmed baking sheet and bake for 45 minutes, or until they give when squeezed with your hand, protected by an oven mitt or kitchen towel. When the potatoes are finished baking, set them aside to cool slightly.

2. While the potatoes are baking, prepare the sauce: Heat the sesame oil in a saucepan over medium heat. Add the garlic and sauté for about 4 minutes, until fragrant. Add the ginger and sauté for an additional 3 to 4 minutes, until fragrant. Stir in the coconut aminos and fish sauce. Bring to a simmer, uncovered, and let the sauce reduce for about 20 minutes. When it coats the back of a spoon, it's ready.

3. To cook the broccoli, place the florets in a steamer basket over a pot of boiling water. Place a lid on the pot and steam for 10 minutes, or until the broccoli is easily pierced with a fork. When finished, turn off the heat and set aside.

4. To cook the meat, melt the butter in a large frying pan over high heat. Cut the wafer-thin sliced beef in half into bite-sized pieces, then sprinkle with the salt. Add the meat to the hot butter and cook on one side for 2 to 3 minutes, until the beef starts to develop a slight char. Flip the pieces over and cook until they get the same color on the other side.

5. To assemble, cut the potatoes lengthwise along the top and use a fork to smash the thick flesh open. Place an equal amount of broccoli on each potato, then top with the beef. Drizzle with the sauce and garnish with the sesame seeds and red pepper flakes.

tips

• For convenience, I buy presliced beef for stir-fries that's labeled "wafer-thin beef." If you'd like to slice the beef yourself, purchase 1 pound of boneless sirloin steak and slice it wafer-thin against the grain. Then cut the slices in half to create bite-sized pieces.

APPROXIMATE NUTRITION BREAKDOWN *(based on 1 loaded potato)*		
CALORIES: 456		FAT: 17 g
PROTEIN: 31 g		CARBS: 48 g

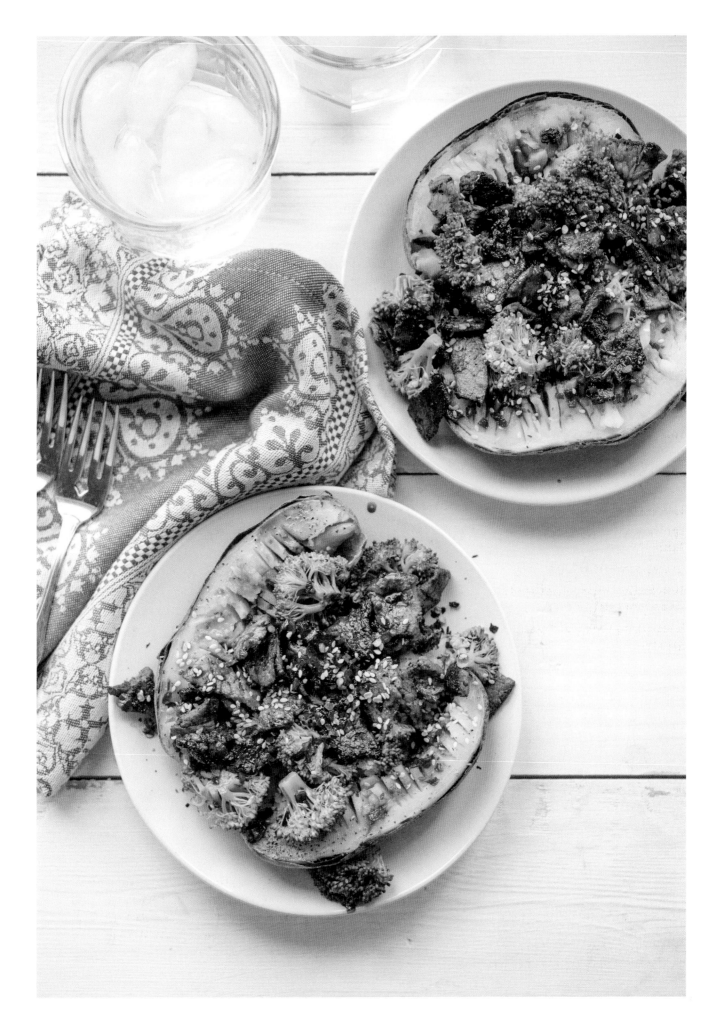

LOADED WHITE POTATOES:

Supreme Pizza

Okay, you get it. I *love* loaded potatoes! I also love pizza (who doesn't?), especially supreme pizza with a side of ranch dressing. When a pizza craving strikes, this is the healthiest and most satisfying remedy at my disposal. Make this recipe your own by adding your favorite pizza toppings!

OPTION

NUT-FREE   EGG-FREE

prep time: 10 minutes (not including the ranch) | *cook time: 1 hour 5 minutes* | *yield: 4 servings*

4 medium white potatoes

½ pound bulk Italian sausage or ground pork

SAUCE

1 (6-ounce) can tomato paste

2 tablespoons water

1 tablespoon fresh lemon juice (about ½ small lemon)

2 teaspoons Italian seasoning

½ teaspoon fine sea salt

¼ teaspoon ground black pepper

½ pound pepperoni, cut into bite-sized pieces

8 ounces sliced mushrooms

¼ cup sliced black olives

¼ cup 3-Ingredient Paleo Ranch (page 338) (omit for egg-free)

Chopped fresh basil or flat-leaf parsley, for garnish (optional)

1. Preheat the oven to 450°F. Place the potatoes on a rimmed baking sheet and bake for 45 minutes, or until they give when squeezed with your hand, protected by an oven mitt or kitchen towel. When the potatoes are finished baking, set them aside to cool slightly and reduce the oven temperature to 375°F.

2. While the potatoes are baking, brown the sausage in a large frying pan over high heat, using a spoon or spatula to break it up into pieces, for 10 minutes or until browned on all sides.

3. While the sausage is browning, make the sauce: In a small saucepan, whisk together the ingredients for the sauce until evenly combined. Bring to a simmer, then set aside.

4. When the sausage is browned, use a slotted spoon to transfer it to a separate bowl, then add the pepperoni to the hot pan. Sauté for 5 minutes, or until it starts to crisp. Transfer the pepperoni to a separate bowl, then add the mushrooms to the same pan. Sauté the mushrooms for 3 minutes per side, or until they darken in color.

5. To assemble, cut the potatoes lengthwise along the top and use a fork to smash the thick flesh open. Drizzle with the sauce, then top with the sausage crumbles, pepperoni, mushrooms, and olives. Return the stuffed potatoes to the 375°F oven to bake for 20 minutes.

6. Drizzle with the ranch dressing and serve warm. Garnish with basil or parsley, if desired.

APPROXIMATE NUTRITION BREAKDOWN	
(based on 1 loaded potato)	
CALORIES: 606	FAT: 38 g
PROTEIN: 23 g	CARBS: 47 g

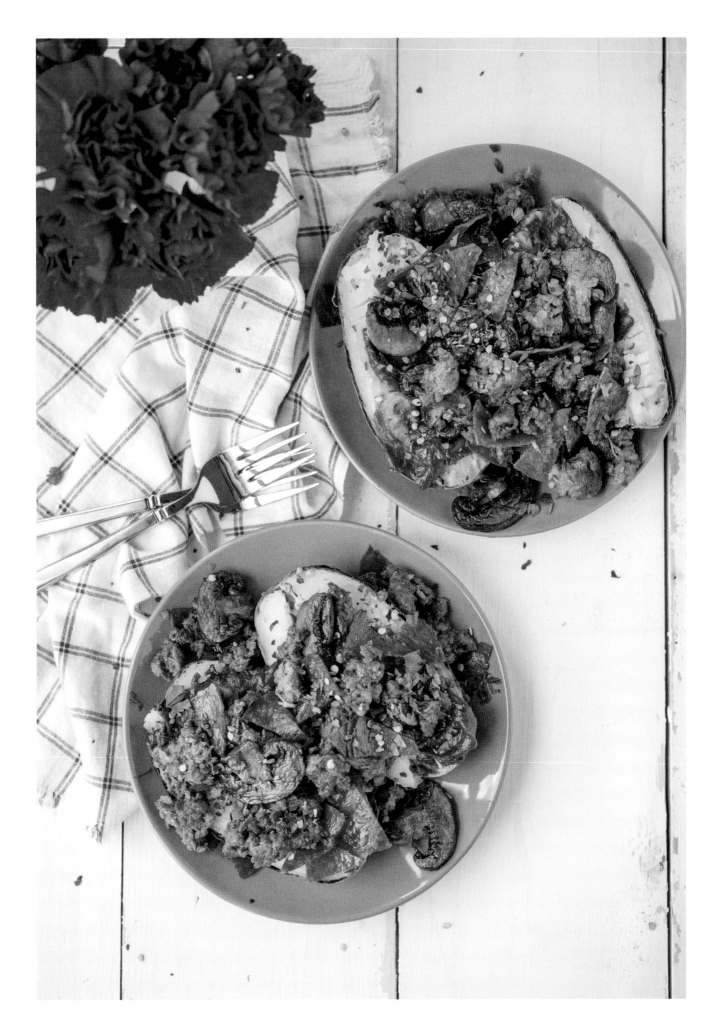

LOADED SWEET POTATOES:
Carnitas Street Taco

Street tacos and baked sweet potatoes—sounds like a match made in heaven to me! I like to plan these loaded potatoes for later in the week, after I've made some carnitas and need a new way to serve it up. Make these "tacos" your own with your favorite toppings! The sliced jalapeños and Paleo Sour Cream are what keep me coming back.

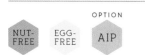

NUT-FREE   EGG-FREE   OPTION AIP

prep time: 10 minutes (not including the carnitas or sour cream) | *cook time: 45 minutes* | *yield: 4 servings*

4 medium sweet potatoes

2 cups Chipotle Carnitas (page 216), warmed

1 avocado, pitted and sliced

1 small jalapeño pepper, thinly sliced (omit for AIP)

¼ purple onion, finely chopped

¼ cup chopped fresh cilantro

¼ cup Paleo Sour Cream (page 341)

1. Preheat the oven to 450°F. Place the potatoes on a rimmed baking sheet and bake for 45 minutes, or until they give when squeezed with your hand, protected by an oven mitt or kitchen towel. When the potatoes are finished baking, set them aside to cool slightly.

2. To assemble, cut the potatoes lengthwise along the top and use a fork to smash the thick flesh open. Spoon an equal amount of the carnitas onto each potato and garnish with the avocado, jalapeño, onion, cilantro, and sour cream.

APPROXIMATE NUTRITION BREAKDOWN *(based on 1 loaded potato)*	
CALORIES: 566	FAT: 35 g
PROTEIN: 32 g	CARBS: 32 g

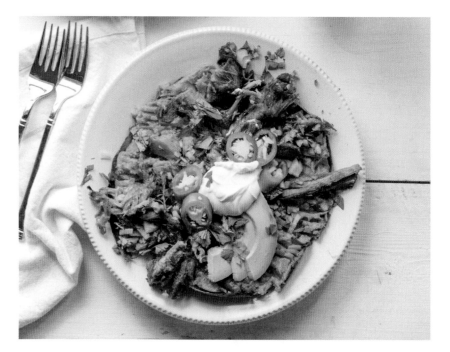

LOADED SWEET POTATOES:

Sausage & Kale

If you've been a longtime Fed & Fit follower, you've seen this dish before. It's my back pocket, go-to, and almost involuntary comfort food of choice. When I'm in need of a healthy dose of carbohydrates, these potatoes almost make themselves. The sweet potato, kale, sausage, and Paleo Sour Cream magically come together in a meal fit for a hungry queen.

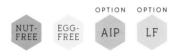

| | | OPTION | OPTION |
| NUT-FREE | EGG-FREE | AIP | LF |

prep time: 10 minutes (not including the sour cream) | *cook time: 45 minutes* | *yield: 4 servings*

4 medium sweet potatoes (low-FODMAP if tolerated)

1 pound bulk breakfast sausage (use ground pork for AIP)

1 bunch kale, destemmed and finely chopped

2 tablespoons fresh lemon juice (about 1 small lemon)

1 teaspoon fine sea salt

¼ cup Paleo Sour Cream (page 341) (low-FODMAP if tolerated)

¼ teaspoon ground black pepper (omit for AIP)

1. Preheat the oven to 450°F. Place the potatoes on a rimmed baking sheet and bake for 45 minutes, or until they give when squeezed with your hand, protected by an oven mitt or kitchen towel. When the potatoes are finished baking, set them aside to cool slightly.

2. While the potatoes are baking, prepare the filling: In a large frying pan over high heat, cook the sausage, using a spoon or spatula to break it up into small crumbles, until brown and crispy, about 10 minutes. Using a slotted spoon, transfer the cooked sausage to a bowl and set aside. Pour out the majority of the sausage grease, leaving enough behind to lightly grease the frying pan.

3. Add the kale, stir, and cover. Let the kale steam over medium heat for about 5 minutes, until it's wilted down. Add the lemon juice and salt. Stir to combine and remove from the heat.

4. To assemble, cut each potato along the top lengthwise and pinch them open, creating a well. Spoon an equal amount of sausage and then kale onto each potato. Add a dollop of sour cream and sprinkle with the pepper and additional salt, if desired.

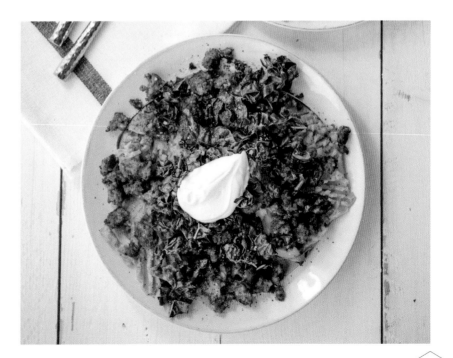

APPROXIMATE NUTRITION BREAKDOWN *(based on 1 loaded potato)*		
CALORIES: 445	FAT: 27 g
PROTEIN: 23 g	CARBS: 32 g

Sausage & Cranberry Stuffed Acorn Squash

WITH ROSEMARY ORANGE CREAM SAUCE

Goodness gracious, this stuffed squash is good! The crispy sausage, roasted cranberries, cream sauce, and perfectly baked squash result in a flavor combination that honestly blows me away. In fact, my not-Paleo father-in-law provided further validation by asking me for the recipe when he got a taste on the day I photographed this dish. So, if you're looking to treat yourself or impress your relatives, this one will not disappoint!

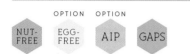

prep time: 15 minutes | *cook time: 1 hour 10 minutes* | *yield: 2 to 4 servings*

1 pound hot Italian sausage, removed from casings if using links (use ground pork for AIP)

1 acorn squash

2 teaspoons extra-virgin olive oil

½ teaspoon fine sea salt

⅛ teaspoon ground black pepper (omit for AIP)

1 cup fresh or frozen cranberries, coarsely chopped in a food processor

ROSEMARY ORANGE CREAM SAUCE
(omit for egg-free and AIP)

¼ cup mayo, store-bought or homemade (page 349)

2 teaspoons grated orange zest

1 tablespoon fresh orange juice

1 teaspoon chopped fresh rosemary

1. In a frying pan over medium heat, crumble and brown the sausage until it's beginning to get crispy. Remove from the heat and set aside.

2. Preheat the oven to 350°F. Using a sharp knife, cut the stem off the squash, then turn it upside-down so that it sits on the cut side. Cut the squash into four wedges and remove and discard the seeds. Rub the cut sides of each wedge with the olive oil and place them skin side down in a small baking dish or pie pan. Sprinkle the tops of the squash with the salt and pepper.

3. Mix the cranberries into the cooked Italian sausage, then spoon an equal amount of the mixture into each acorn squash wedge. It's okay if the sausage mixture spills over into the pan.

4. Tent the dish with aluminum foil and bake for 40 minutes, then remove the foil and return to the oven to bake uncovered for 20 more minutes, or until you can easily slide a fork into the flesh of one of the squash wedges.

5. While the stuffed squash is baking, whisk the sauce ingredients together in a small bowl. Set aside.

6. Let the squash cool for 5 to 10 minutes, then drizzle each piece with the rosemary orange cream sauce. Serve warm.

APPROXIMATE NUTRITION BREAKDOWN	
(based on 1 of 4 servings)	
CALORIES: 450	FAT: 35 g
PROTEIN: 19 g	CARBS: 16 g

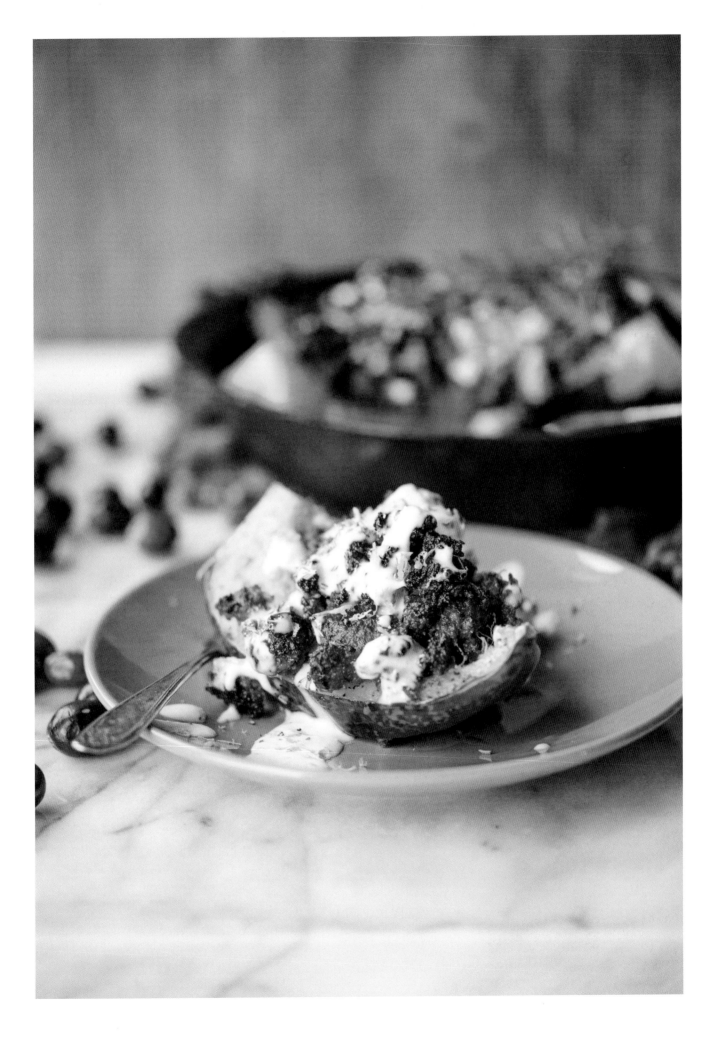

Sun-Dried Tomato Stuffed Chicken

WITH PECAN COATING

This incredibly flavorful chicken is inspired by one of the first recipes I ever posted on my blog. Like the stuffed pork tenderloin on page 186, think of this recipe as a new method! You can stuff, roll, and bake the chicken with a variety of flavors and textures. Have fun with it!

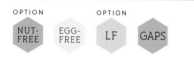

OPTION   NUT-FREE   EGG-FREE   OPTION   LF   GAPS

prep time: 10 minutes (not including time to reconstitute tomatoes) | *cook time: 25 minutes* | *yield: 2 to 4 servings*

½ packed cup sun-dried tomatoes, reconstituted in 1 cup boiling water for 1 hour or overnight, then drained

1 tablespoon lemon juice (about ½ small lemon)

2 tablespoons extra-virgin olive oil, divided

2 boneless, skinless chicken breast halves (1 pound), rinsed, patted dry, and pounded to ¼-inch thickness

1 teaspoon fine sea salt

¼ teaspoon ground black pepper

¾ cup finely chopped raw pecans (omit for nut-free and low-FODMAP)

Chopped fresh flat-leaf parsley, for garnish

SPECIAL EQUIPMENT

2 (2-foot) pieces kitchen twine

1. Preheat the oven to 400°F. Line a rimmed baking sheet with parchment paper.

2. Pulse the reconstituted tomatoes, lemon juice, and 1 tablespoon of the olive oil in a food processor until a paste forms.

3. Spread the tomato paste on one side of the chicken, evenly divided between the two breast halves. Roll up one breast half, creating a log, and tie it in place with the twine. Repeat with the other chicken breast half. Rub the remaining tablespoon of olive oil over the outside of the tied chicken and sprinkle with the salt and pepper.

4. Spread out the chopped pecans on a plate. Roll the tied chicken in the pecans so that all sides are coated. Place the coated chicken on the lined baking sheet.

5. Bake for 25 minutes, or until the juices run clear. If the pecans start to burn or get too dark, cover the pan with a sheet of aluminum foil while the chicken finishes baking. Serve garnished with the chopped parsley.

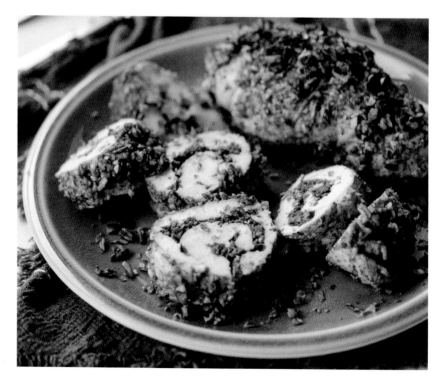

APPROXIMATE NUTRITION BREAKDOWN *(based on 1 of 4 servings)*	
CALORIES: 346	FAT: 22 g
PROTEIN: 29 g	CARBS: 10 g

Taco Squash Boats

My husband absolutely loves these Taco Squash Boats. Loves them! Maybe it's because the word *taco* is involved. They're wonderfully healthy, satisfying, and filling. After they come out of the oven, feel free to top them with your favorite salsa or Paleo Sour Cream (page 341)!

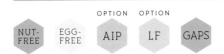

NUT-FREE · EGG-FREE · OPTION AIP · OPTION LF · GAPS

prep time: 15 minutes (not including the chicken) | *cook time: 45 minutes* | *yield: 3 to 6 servings*

3 yellow summer squash or zucchini, cut in half lengthwise

1 tablespoon extra-virgin olive oil

3 cups Simple Shredded Chicken (page 123)

2 tablespoons chili powder, plus more for sprinkling on top (omit for AIP)

2 tablespoons ground cumin

2 teaspoons garlic powder (omit for low-FODMAP)

1 teaspoon fine sea salt

½ teaspoon ground black pepper (omit for AIP)

Juice of 2 limes

¼ purple onion, finely chopped, for garnish (omit for low-FODMAP)

2 tablespoons chopped fresh cilantro, for garnish

1. Preheat the oven to 350°F. Hollow out each squash half, leaving a ½-inch wall of squash. Place the squash halves cut side up in a 9 by 13-inch baking dish. Sprinkle the cut sides with the olive oil.

2. In a large mixing bowl, mix the shredded chicken with the chili powder, cumin, garlic powder, salt, pepper, and lime juice until it's evenly coated. Spoon an equal amount of the chicken into each squash half.

3. Cover the baking dish with aluminum foil and bake for 30 minutes, then remove the foil and bake uncovered for an additional 15 minutes, or until the top of the chicken is starting to crisp.

4. Serve the stuffed squash garnished with the chopped purple onion and cilantro.

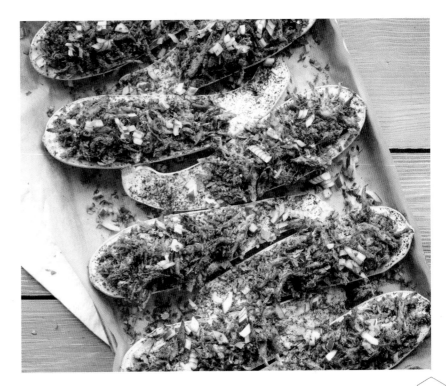

APPROXIMATE NUTRITION BREAKDOWN *(based on 1 of 6 servings)*			
CALORIES: 150		FAT: 8 g	
PROTEIN: 12 g		CARBS: 11 g	

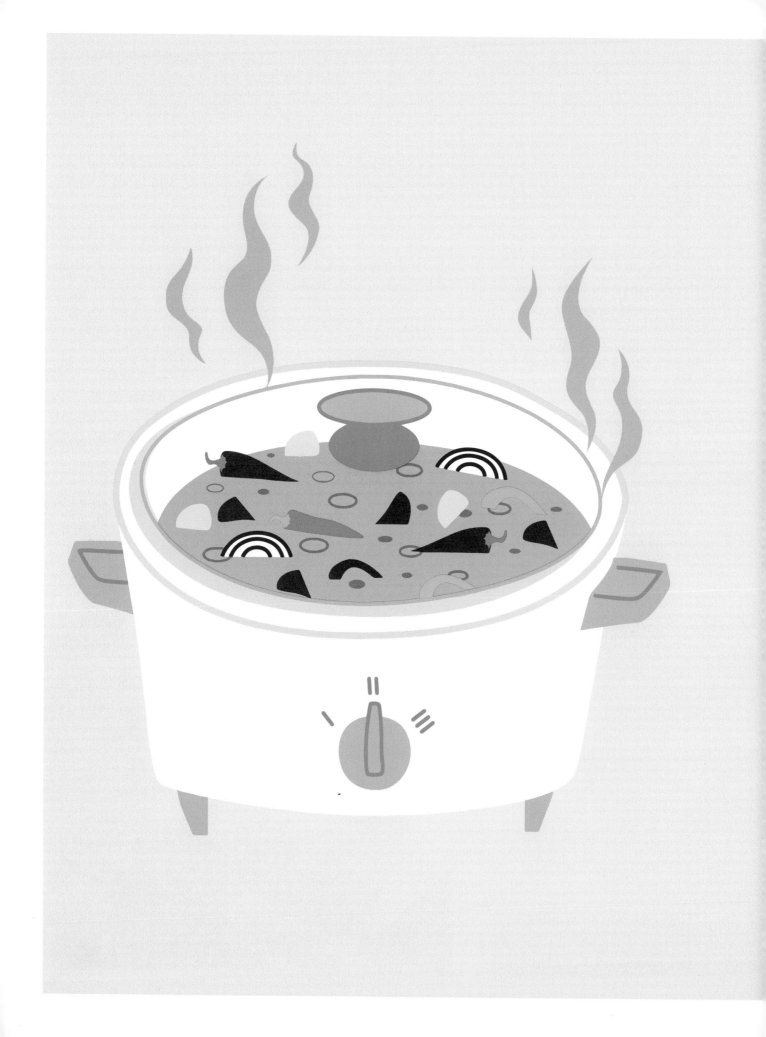

CHAPTER 5:

SET IT AND FORGET IT

 A Very Good Vegetable Beef Soup
206

 Garam Masala Beef & Butternut Stew
208

 Fork-Tender Balsamic Mustard Pork Chops
209

 Chicken Tikka Masala
210

 Lemon Thyme Chicken & Vegetables
212

 Brisket & Onions
213

 Barbacoa with Jicama Tortillas
214

 Chipotle Carnitas
216

Download the Fed & Fit iPhone and Android app! You can scan the above QR codes directly in the app, which will then populate a consolidated grocery shopping list for the scanned recipes.

A Very Good Vegetable Beef Soup

I adore this soup for many reasons, but most of all because the basic recipe can be personalized based on what vegetables are in season! This version is my favorite. I especially enjoy making this soup in a slow cooker so that the meat becomes extra tender, which is why it has found its way into this chapter of slow-cooked dishes. If you're pressed for time, you can use the stovetop method (see Tips). You can easily make this soup a low-carb meal by omitting the potatoes.

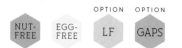

NUT-FREE · EGG-FREE · OPTION LF · OPTION GAPS

prep time: 25 minutes | *cook time: 4 to 10 hours (see Tips for faster stovetop method)* | *yield: 6 to 8 servings*

3 tablespoons salted butter, ghee, or coconut oil, divided

2 pounds beef stew meat

1 teaspoon fine sea salt

½ teaspoon ground black pepper

1 yellow onion, chopped

4 cloves garlic, minced (omit for low-FODMAP)

1½ cups peeled and diced carrots (7 small carrots or 3 large)

1½ cups diced celery (4 stalks)

6 ounces green beans, cut into 1-inch pieces (about 1½ cups)

1½ pounds russet potatoes, peeled and diced (about 4 small potatoes) (omit for GAPS)

1 (28-ounce) can diced tomatoes with juice

8 cups beef broth, store-bought or homemade (page 332) (or more if needed)

2 bay leaves

1 tablespoon fresh lemon juice (about ½ small lemon), or more if needed (optional)

¼ cup finely chopped fresh flat-leaf parsley, for garnish (optional)

1. Melt 1 tablespoon of the butter in a large sauté pan or frying pan over high heat. While the butter is melting, season the stew meat with the salt and pepper, then divide the meat into three batches. When the butter has stopped bubbling, add the first third of the meat. Cook for 1 to 2 minutes, until it has a nice brown color on two sides. Spoon the cooked meat out of the pan, blot up any liquid remaining with a paper towel, and repeat the process with the remaining 2 tablespoons of butter and remaining two batches of meat.

2. Place the browned meat and the rest of the ingredients, except for the lemon juice and parsley, in a slow cooker. Add enough broth to cover the meat and vegetables. Cook on high for 4 to 6 hours or on low for 8 to 10 hours, until the meat is tender.

3. Before serving, taste the soup. If it needs acid, add the lemon juice, and if it needs salt, add more salt to taste. Serve warm, garnished with the parsley.

tips

- *Browning the meat in batches helps ensure that you get a nice char (and more flavor) on each piece. If you crowd the pan with too many pieces, the run-off fluids will keep the neighboring pieces from crisping.*

- *Leftovers will keep refrigerated for up to 4 days or frozen for up to 5 months. To reheat, pull a container of soup from the freezer and place it in the refrigerator for at least 4 hours to partially defrost. Plop the slightly thawed soup in a soup pot, cover, and warm over medium heat until simmering.*

- *To make this soup on the stovetop, brown the meat as described in Step 1 in a soup pot or other large heavy-bottomed pot. Then add the rest of the ingredients, bring to a simmer over medium heat, and continue to simmer with the lid on for at least 1 hour, until the meat is tender.*

APPROXIMATE NUTRITION BREAKDOWN *(based on 1 of 8 servings)*	
CALORIES: 354	FAT: 12 g
PROTEIN: 30 g	CARBS: 28 g

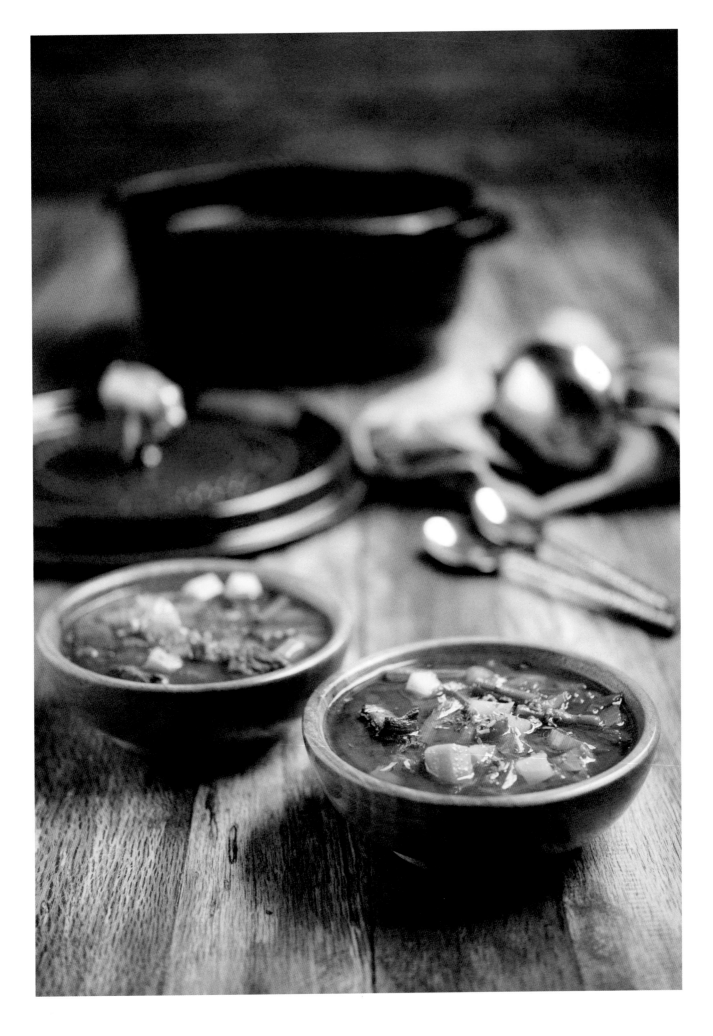

Garam Masala Beef & Butternut Stew

Flavor on flavor on flavor. I absolutely love this stew! I love the sweetness from the butternut squash, the charred note from the beef, the brightness from the lime juice, and the hat-tip to India. This is one of those dishes that tastes even better when reheated as leftovers.

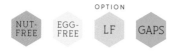

NUT-FREE   EGG-FREE   *OPTION* LF   GAPS

prep time: 15 minutes | *cook time: 3 or 6 hours* | *yield: 4 to 6 servings*

2 tablespoons salted butter

2 pounds beef stew meat, cut into ½-inch chunks

1 teaspoon fine sea salt

½ teaspoon ground black pepper

1 medium butternut squash (about 3 pounds), peeled, seeded, and cut into ½-inch cubes (omit for low-FODMAP)

6 cups beef broth, store-bought or homemade (page 332)

¼ cup fresh lime juice (about 2 limes)

2 tablespoons garam masala

¼ cup chopped fresh cilantro, for garnish

1 lime, cut into wedges, for garnish

1. Melt the butter in a large frying pan over high heat. Sprinkle the stew meat with the salt and pepper. Working in batches so that no two pieces touch each other, sear the meat on two sides for about 3 minutes per side, until it develops a nice brown char. Transfer the cooked beef to a slow cooker and repeat with the remaining batches.

2. Add the cubed squash to the slow cooker and stir together with the beef. Then add the broth, lime juice, and garam masala. Stir, cover, and cook on high for 3 hours or on low for 6 hours.

3. Serve garnished with the cilantro and lime wedges.

tips

• *Leftovers will keep refrigerated for up to 5 days or frozen for up to 5 months.*

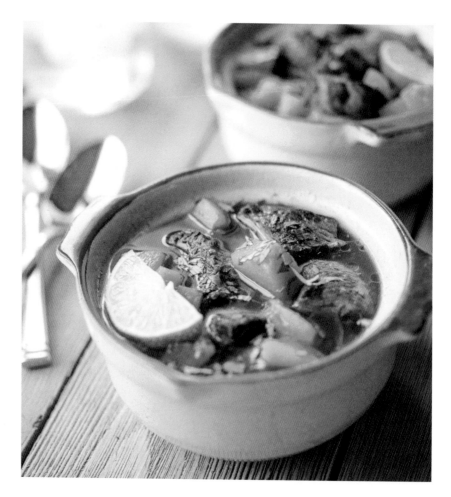

APPROXIMATE NUTRITION BREAKDOWN *(based on 1 of 6 servings)*	
CALORIES: 453	FAT: 15 g
PROTEIN: 54 g	CARBS: 30 g

Fork-Tender Balsamic Mustard Pork Chops

This is an ideal dish for a day when you want to maximize flavor and minimize effort. The browned onions, mustard, and balsamic vinegar work together to transform ordinary pork chops into the shining stars of your dinner table. To evolve the flavor of this dish, experiment with different kinds of mustard! I've made it with yellow mustard, whole-grain mustard, horseradish mustard, and other fun varieties.

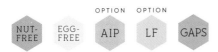

NUT-FREE   EGG-FREE   *OPTION* AIP   *OPTION* LF   GAPS

prep time: 10 minutes | *cook time: 3 to 7 hours* | *yield: 4 to 6 servings*

3 pounds boneless pork chops

1 teaspoon fine sea salt

½ teaspoon ground black pepper (omit for AIP)

4 tablespoons salted butter, ghee, or coconut oil, divided (use coconut oil for AIP)

1 yellow onion, finely chopped (about ½ cup) (omit for low-FODMAP)

¼ cup mustard of choice

¼ cup balsamic vinegar

Chopped fresh flat-leaf parsley, for garnish (optional)

1. Season both sides of the pork chops liberally with the salt and pepper. In a very hot frying pan, melt 2 tablespoons of the butter. Sear the pork chops for 2 to 3 minutes per side, until they have a nice brown color. Transfer the chops to a slow cooker.

2. Add the remaining 2 tablespoons of butter and the chopped onion to the pan. Sauté for 8 to 10 minutes, until the onion is translucent and slightly browned. Add the mustard and vinegar, whisking to incorporate and working to release the browned bits from the bottom of the pan so that they mix into the sauce. Pour the sauce over the pork chops in the slow cooker.

3. Cook on high for 3 hours or on low for 6 to 7 hours, until the chops are fork-tender. Serve garnished with fresh parsley, if desired.

Tips

- *Leftovers will keep refrigerated for up to 5 days or frozen for up to 5 months.*

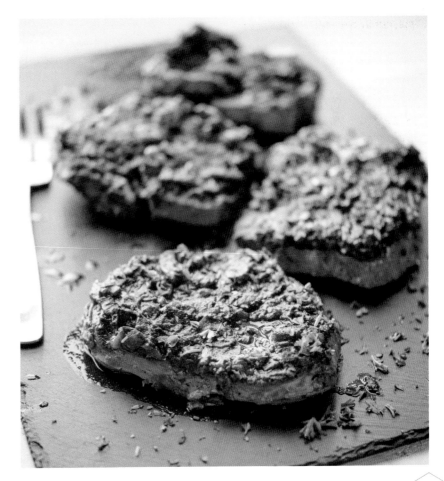

APPROXIMATE NUTRITION BREAKDOWN *(based on 1 of 6 servings)*	
CALORIES: 430	FAT: 24 g
PROTEIN: 49 g	CARBS: 5 g

Chicken Tikka Masala

This dish is at the tippy-top of my favorite foods list. In an effort to both tip my hat to tradition and keep the preparation relatively simple, I've blended methods here. You'll use high heat to bring out the roasted flavor of the spices, creating layers and a lot of depth. Then you'll turn to your beloved slow cooker to take care of the rest. Serve it over a big bowl of either Basic Cauliflower Rice or Cilantro Lime Cauliflower Rice (both on page 264) and top with jalapeños to your heart's desire.

NUT-FREE   **EGG-FREE**

prep time: 15 minutes | *cook time: 4 or 8 hours* | *yield: 4 to 6 servings*

SPICE BLEND

4 cloves garlic, grated

1 tablespoon grated fresh ginger (about ½-inch piece)

1 tablespoon garam masala

1 tablespoon turmeric powder

1 teaspoon ground coriander

1 teaspoon ground cumin

1 teaspoon fine sea salt

½ teaspoon red pepper flakes

3 tablespoons salted butter, divided

3 pounds boneless, skinless chicken breasts, rinsed, patted dry, and cut into 1-inch cubes

½ yellow onion, finely chopped

1 (6-ounce) can tomato paste

1 (28-ounce) can crushed tomatoes

1 (13½-ounce) can full-fat coconut milk

Cream scooped from the top of 1 (13½-ounce) can chilled full-fat coconut milk (about ½ cup)

¼ cup fresh lime juice (about 2 limes)

Jalapeño slices, for garnish

¼ cup coarsely chopped fresh cilantro, for garnish

1. In a small bowl, mix together the ingredients for the spice blend. Set aside.

2. Melt 2 tablespoons of the butter in a large frying pan over high heat. While the butter is melting, thoroughly coat the chicken on all sides with half of the spice blend. Working in batches so that no two pieces of chicken touch each other in the pan, add a portion of the seasoned chicken to the hot pan and sear for 2 to 3 minutes per side, just until the chicken develops a light brown crust. Transfer the browned chicken to a slow cooker and repeat the process with the remaining chicken.

3. When all of the chicken is cooked, melt the remaining tablespoon of butter in the hot pan. Add the rest of the spice blend and the chopped onion and cook, stirring, for 8 to 10 minutes, until the onion is browned but not burned. Add the tomato paste, whisk to incorporate, and cook for an additional 4 to 5 minutes, until the tomato paste develops a deep red color. Add the crushed tomatoes, coconut milk, coconut cream, and lime juice. Stir to incorporate and bring to a simmer. Simmer for 10 minutes, or until the sauce has thickened slightly and coats the back of a spoon.

4. Pour the sauce over the chicken in the slow cooker. Stir so that the chicken is coated on all sides. Cook on high for 4 hours or on low for 8 hours.

5. Serve garnished with the jalapeño slices and fresh cilantro.

tips

- *Leftovers will keep refrigerated for up to 5 days or frozen for up to 5 months.*

APPROXIMATE NUTRITION BREAKDOWN *(based on 1 of 6 per servings)*			
CALORIES: 498		FAT: 24 g	
PROTEIN: 55 g		CARBS: 17 g	

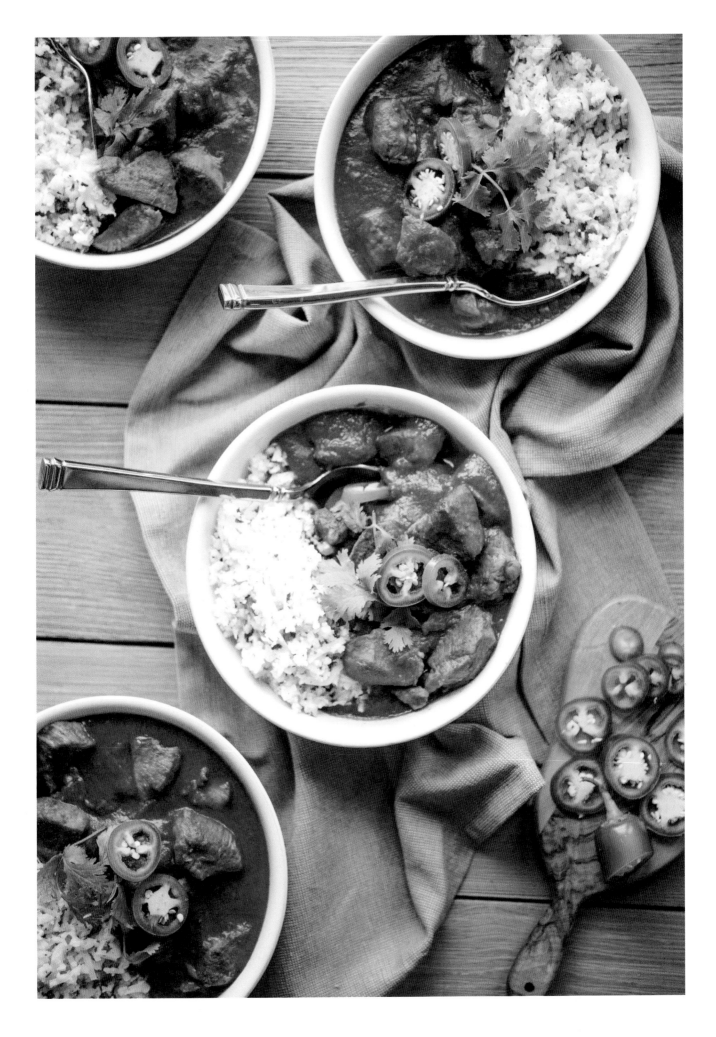

LEMON THYME

Chicken & Vegetables

All you need for this recipe are love, thyme, and time! The chicken comes out of the slow cooker fall-apart tender and bursting with fresh flavor. While this recipe calls for yellow potatoes and carrots, feel free to get creative! Parsnips, sweet potatoes, and beets would all be delicious additions.

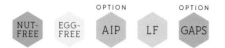

NUT-FREE · EGG-FREE · AIP (OPTION) · LF · GAPS (OPTION)

prep time: 10 minutes | *cook time: 4 or 6 hours* | *yield: 4 to 6 servings*

THYME RUB

1 tablespoon extra-virgin olive oil

1 tablespoon chopped fresh thyme

1 teaspoon fine sea salt

½ teaspoon ground black pepper (omit for AIP)

1 whole chicken (about 3 pounds), rinsed and patted dry

2 tablespoons chilled salted butter, cut into 8 pieces (use EVOO for AIP)

1½ pounds yellow potatoes, cut into roughly 2-inch pieces if large or left whole if small (see Tips) (omit for AIP and GAPS)

1 pound carrots, peeled and sliced on an angle into 2-inch-thick ovals

3 lemons, quartered

½ teaspoon fine sea salt

2 teaspoons fresh thyme leaves, chopped, for garnish

SPECIAL EQUIPMENT

6 inches kitchen twine

Tips

• *I prefer Baby Dutch potatoes for this recipe. They're small enough to leave whole.*

• *Leftovers will keep refrigerated for up to 5 days or frozen for up to 5 months.*

1. In a small bowl, whisk together the ingredients for the thyme rub. Set aside.

2. Separate the skin on the breast of the chicken from the meat by gently inserting your hand between the two. Place four pieces of the butter under the skin on one breast and the remaining four pieces under the skin on the other breast. Using your hands, massage the thyme rub all over the chicken. Insert two of the quartered lemons into the cavity of the chicken and, using the twine, tie the legs together.

3. Place the potatoes and carrots in a slow cooker. Place the prepared chicken on top of the vegetables. Cook on high for 4 hours or on low for 6 hours.

4. Serve warm, garnished with the ½ teaspoon salt, fresh thyme, and remaining lemon wedges.

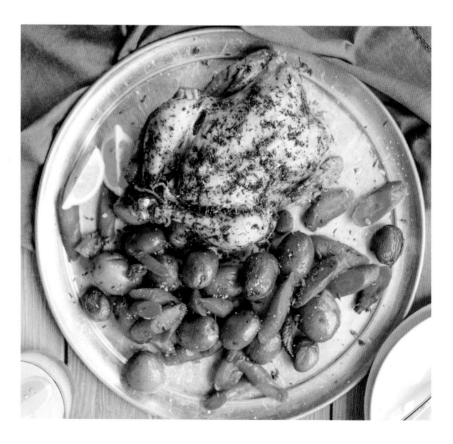

APPROXIMATE NUTRITION BREAKDOWN *(based on 1 of 6 servings)*	
CALORIES: 631	FAT: 35 g
PROTEIN: 51 g	CARBS: 30 g

Brisket & Onions

Oh man, I am proud of this recipe. Mostly because after every bite I involuntarily blurt out, "WOW, that's good." Not only is it perfectly tender and jaw-dropping delicious, but it's also as clean and healthful as it gets. This is a great protein to make for a week's worth of meals or for a big family get-together!

NUT-FREE   EGG-FREE   OPTION AIP   OPTION GAPS

prep time: 15 minutes | *cook time: 8 hours* | *yield: 10 to 15 servings*

2 tablespoons salted butter, ghee, or coconut oil (use coconut oil for AIP)

1 (5-pound) beef brisket, trimmed

2½ teaspoons fine sea salt, divided

1 teaspoon ground black pepper (omit for AIP)

1 yellow onion, cut into thin wedges

1 medium-sized purple onion, cut into thin wedges

4 cloves garlic, minced

2 cups beef broth, store-bought or homemade (page 332)

½ cup coconut aminos (omit for GAPS)

1. In a large heavy-bottomed pot, melt the butter over high heat. While the butter is melting, generously season both sides of the brisket with 2 teaspoons of the salt and the pepper. Place the brisket in the hot pan (make sure that your oven vent is turned on) and give each side a good sear. You're looking for a nice brown char on both sides. If you're unsure about the color, 5 minutes per side should suffice. Place the seared brisket in a slow cooker.

2. To the same pan that you used to sear the meat, add the onions and the remaining ½ teaspoon of salt. Sauté over medium heat until the onions are wilted and starting to brown, 10 to 15 minutes. Transfer the onions to the slow cooker over the brisket. Add the garlic, broth, and coconut aminos to the slow cooker.

3. Cook the brisket on low for 8 hours. Slice or shred the meat, season with more salt as needed, and serve warm, or place the entire pot in the refrigerator to chill overnight—this method will allow you to skim off the excess fat that cooked away from the brisket.

tips

• *Leftovers will keep refrigerated for up to 5 days or frozen for up to 5 months.*

• *To reheat, place the brisket (thawed, if previously frozen) in a baking dish with the onions and a few ladles of the remaining liquid and bake in a preheated 350°F oven for about 30 minutes.*

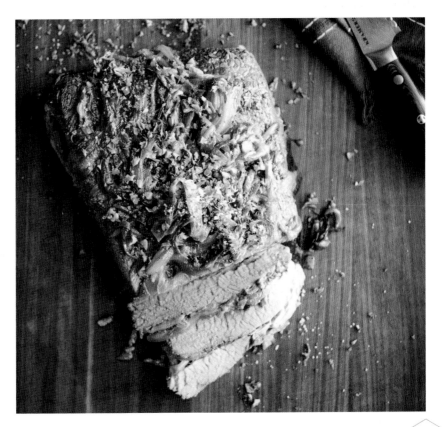

APPROXIMATE NUTRITION BREAKDOWN	
(based on 1 of 15 servings)	
CALORIES: 357	FAT: 28 g
PROTEIN: 27 g	CARBS: 4 g

Barbacoa with Jicama Tortillas

This barbacoa is *really* good. I've tasted and tested barbacoa like it's been my job for the past fifteen years, and I finally landed on what I believe to be the perfect recipe. It strikes a balance with maximum flavor and minimum effort. The leftovers are extremely versatile in that you can use them to make taco salads, scrambled eggs, or even stuffed peppers! That being said, barbacoa wrapped up in a warm jicama tortilla with some sliced avocado, cilantro, and a squeeze of fresh lime juice is pretty dang dreamy.

NUT-FREE · EGG-FREE · OPTION AIP · OPTION LF · OPTION GAPS

prep time: 10 minutes | *cook time: 4 hours 15 minutes* | *yield: 6 to 8 servings*

1 tablespoon chipotle chili powder (omit for AIP)

1 tablespoon ground cumin (omit for AIP)

1 tablespoon dried Mexican oregano leaves

1 teaspoon fine sea salt

½ teaspoon ground black pepper (omit for AIP)

½ teaspoon ground cloves

1 (3-pound) chuck roast, cut into 8 large chunks

2 tablespoons salted butter (use EVOO for AIP)

4 cloves garlic, minced (omit for low-FODMAP)

3 bay leaves

¼ cup apple cider vinegar

¼ cup fresh lime juice (about 2 limes)

JICAMA TORTILLAS

1 large jicama, peeled and sliced into thin discs (omit for low-FODMAP and GAPS)

1 avocado, sliced, for garnish (omit for low-FODMAP)

Chopped fresh cilantro, for garnish

1 lime, quartered, for serving

Salsa Verde (page 344), for serving (optional)

1. In a small bowl, mix together the chipotle powder, cumin, oregano, salt, pepper, and cloves. Dust the pieces of chuck roast with the spice mixture, making sure to coat all sides well.

2. Melt the butter in a large frying pan or sauté pan over high heat. Add the beef in batches so that the pan isn't overcrowded. Sear the beef for about 3 minutes per side, until it develops a nice char. Transfer the cooked beef to a slow cooker and repeat with the remaining meat.

3. Add the garlic and bay leaves to the cooked beef in the slow cooker. Pour in the vinegar and lime juice. Cook on high for 4 hours, or until the beef falls apart when tested with a fork.

4. Discard the bay leaves. Working in the slow cooker, use two forks to shred the beef. Stir it in the juices.

5. To make the jicama tortillas, either place the jicama discs in a steamer basket over a pot of boiling water for 3 minutes or place them in a microwave-safe bowl with 2 tablespoons water, cover, and microwave on high for 3 minutes. They're done when the texture goes from brittle to flexible. Let cool, then drain over paper towels.

6. Spoon the shredded beef into the tortillas and top with the avocado slices and cilantro. Serve with the lime wedges and Salsa Verde, if desired.

tips

• Leftover barbacoa and tortillas will keep refrigerated for up to 5 days. The barbacoa will keep frozen for up to 5 months.

• The jicama tortillas also go great with Chipotle Carnitas (page 216).

APPROXIMATE NUTRITION BREAKDOWN *(based on 1 of 8 servings)*	
CALORIES: 456	FAT: 32 g
PROTEIN: 40 g	CARBS: 9 g

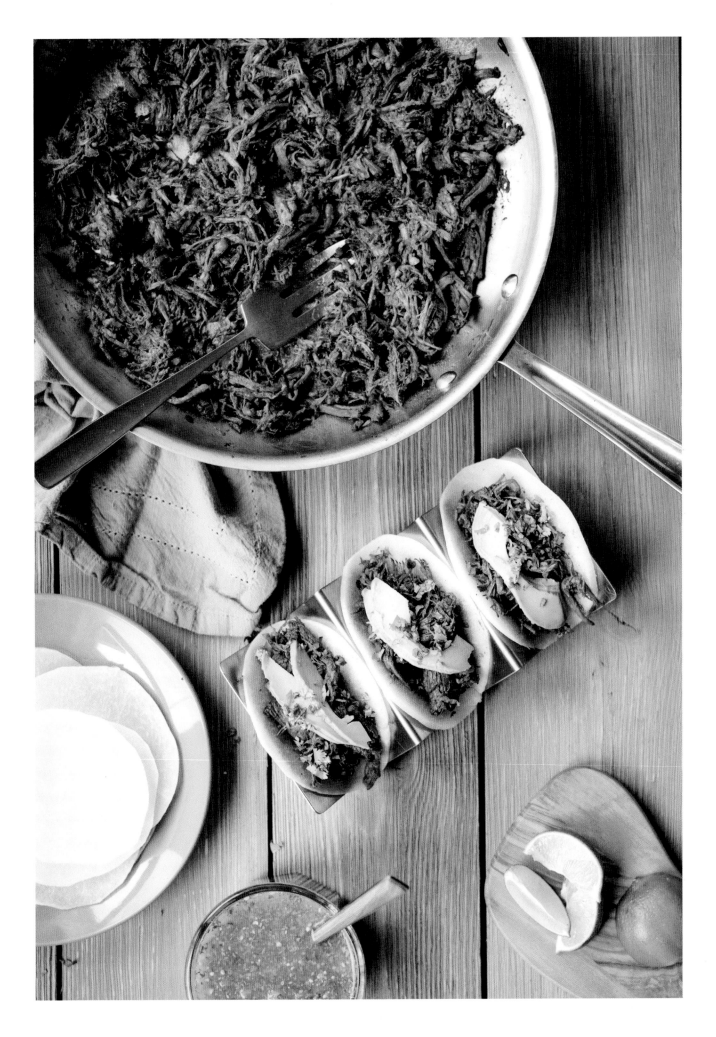

Chipotle Carnitas

I could eat carnitas every single day. Traditional carnitas, like the kind served in my favorite San Antonio restaurants, is braised for hours in lard (also known as a "confit"). The method I use is much easier and requires way less fat. Instead of braising in fat, I braise a seasoned pork shoulder in broth after browning it in a pan. The meat is then finished off in traditional carnitas style by tossing it in more fat and then roasting it to a slight crisp in the oven. You can enjoy this delicious dish alongside any vegetable, in some jicama tortillas (page 214) or lettuce wraps, or stuffed in a loaded sweet potato (page 198).

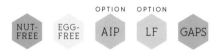

prep time: 15 minutes | *cook time: 4 to 10 hours* | *yield: 10 to 15 servings*

2 tablespoons plus 1 teaspoon fine sea salt, divided

2 tablespoons dried Mexican oregano

1 tablespoon chipotle chili powder (omit for AIP)

1 tablespoon garlic powder

1 tablespoon ground cumin (omit for AIP)

2 teaspoons ground black pepper (omit for AIP)

1 (4-pound) bone-in pork butt (aka shoulder), rinsed and patted dry

4 tablespoons salted butter, ghee, or coconut oil, divided (use coconut oil for AIP)

1 orange, cut into 4 wedges

1 yellow onion, cut into 4 wedges (omit for low-FODMAP)

2 cups chicken broth, store-bought or homemade (page 332)

Juice of 2 limes

¼ cup coarsely chopped fresh cilantro leaves, for garnish

1. Mix 2 tablespoons of the salt with the oregano, chipotle powder, garlic powder, cumin, and pepper. Rub the spice blend all over the pork.

2. Melt 2 tablespoons of the butter in either the stovetop-safe insert of your slow cooker or a large frying pan over high heat. Add the seasoned pork and sear on all four sides for 3 minutes per side, or until a crust starts to form.

3. Transfer the pork to the slow cooker and place the orange and onion wedges around it. Add the broth, cover, and cook for 8 to 10 hours on low or 4 to 6 hours on high. The pork is done when it falls apart easily when prodded with a fork.

4. Preheat the oven to 425°F. Transfer the cooked pork to a large mixing bowl and shred it into small chunks using two forks.

5. Melt the remaining 2 tablespoons of butter and pour it over the shredded pork. Spread out the pork on a rimmed baking sheet, sprinkle with the remaining teaspoon of salt, and roast for 10 to 15 minutes, until the tops are just starting to crisp. Remove from the oven and mix in the lime juice. Garnish with the cilantro and serve.

tips

• *Leftovers will keep refrigerated for up to 5 days or frozen for up to 5 months. If you plan to freeze leftovers, I recommend holding off on adding the fresh cilantro until the day you reheat and serve.*

APPROXIMATE NUTRITION BREAKDOWN	
(based on 1 of 15 servings)	
CALORIES: 370	FAT: 26 g
PROTEIN: 29 g	CARBS: 4 g

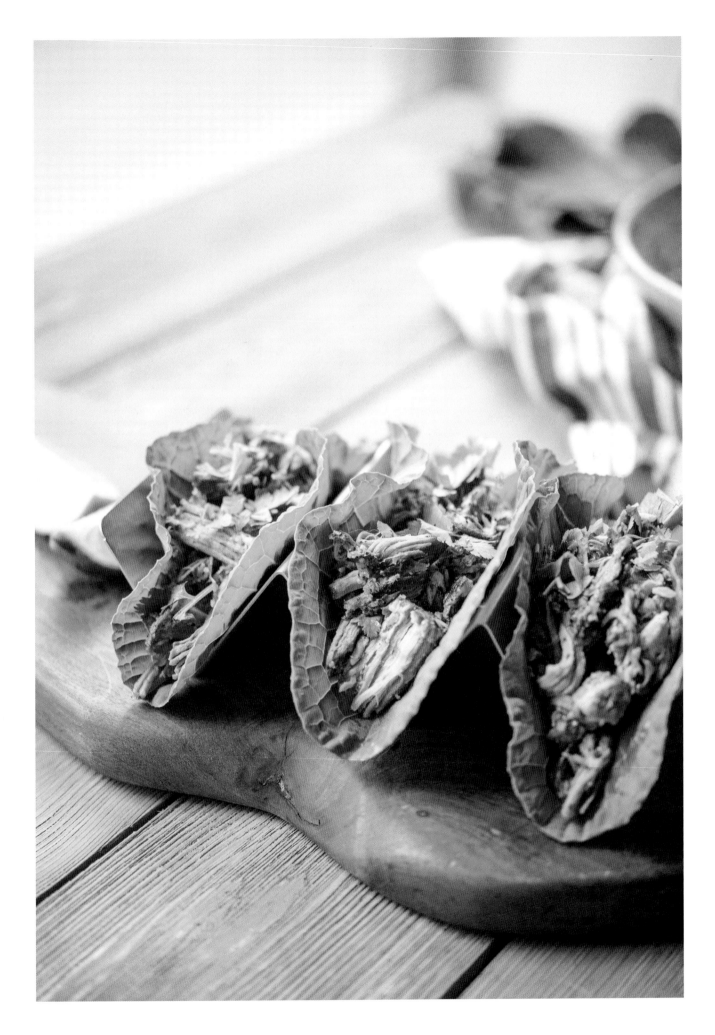

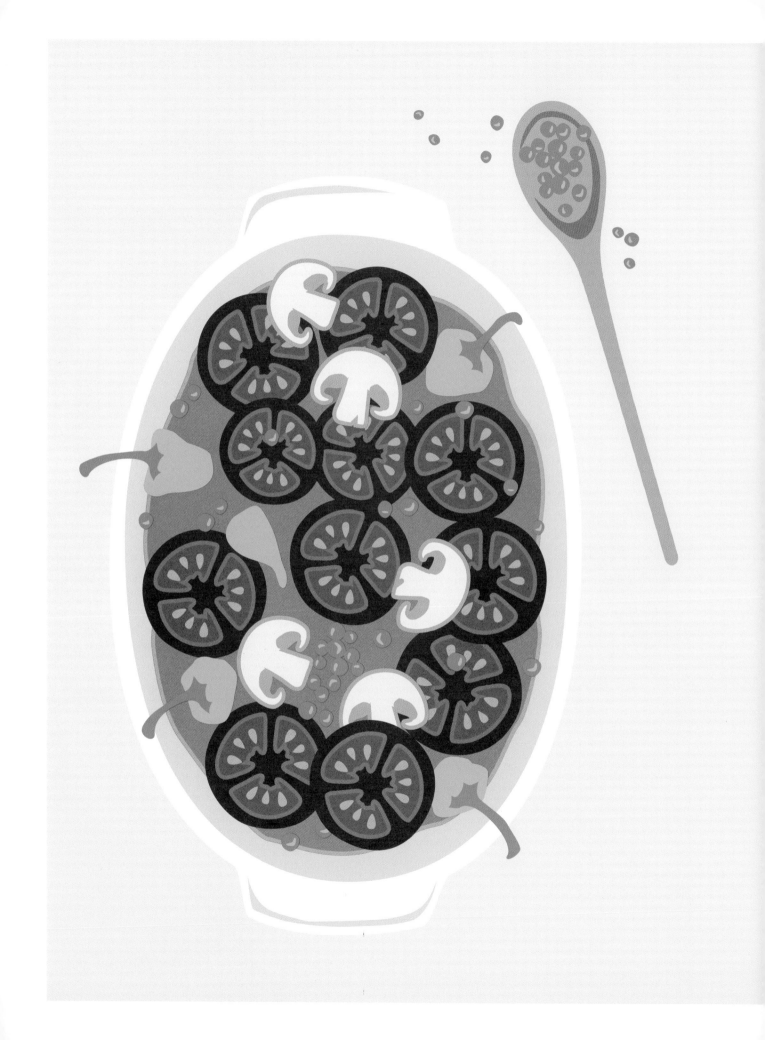

CHAPTER 6:
CASSEROLE IS MY FAVORITE FOOD

Download the Fed & Fit iPhone and Android app! You can scan the
above QR codes directly in the app, which will then populate a
consolidated grocery shopping list for the scanned recipes.

BBQ Chicken Potato Casserole

This dish reminds me of summer, sunshine, and family barbecues. Filling and delicious, this casserole is a real crowd-pleaser! Serve it up next to a fresh green salad and you'll have a complete meal. Note that this, like so many of my casserole recipes, freezes exceptionally well. You can either freeze the whole batch at once or spoon portions into individual serving–size bags for a quick defrost when you need a satisfying starchy meal.

OPTION

  LF

prep time: 15 minutes | *cook time: 1 hour or 3 to 8 hours, depending on method* | *yield: 6 to 8 servings*

3 pounds boneless, skinless chicken breasts, rinsed and patted dry

1½ teaspoons fine sea salt, divided

½ teaspoon ground black pepper, divided

4 tablespoons salted butter, ghee, or coconut oil, divided

3 pounds russet or other white potatoes (6 to 8 if they're small)

1 cup BBQ sauce, store-bought or homemade (page 336), divided (omit for low-FODMAP)

1 tablespoon plus 2 teaspoons apple cider vinegar

¼ cup diced purple onions, for garnish (omit for low-FODMAP)

¼ cup chopped fresh cilantro leaves, for garnish

tips

- *I like my mashed potatoes a little chunky, which is why the directions say to use a potato masher. If you prefer silky-smooth potatoes, you can blend the potatoes in a food processor or with an electric mixer instead.*

1. Season both sides of the chicken with ½ teaspoon of the salt and ¼ teaspoon of the pepper.

2. To sear the chicken, melt 1 tablespoon of the butter in a large sauté pan over high heat. When the butter is melted, add the chicken. Sear for 3 to 5 minutes per side, until lightly browned.

3. Cook the chicken using one of these two methods:

   Stovetop option: Pour enough water into the pan to cover the chicken, place the lid on the pan, and simmer over medium heat for 20 to 30 minutes, until cooked through. While the chicken is cooking, follow Step 4 to prepare the potatoes.

   Slow cooker option: Transfer the seared chicken to the slow cooker, add enough water to cover the chicken, and cook on high for 3 to 4 hours or on low for 6 to 8 hours. When the chicken has about 30 minutes left to cook, prepare the potatoes.

4. Prepare the potatoes: Peel the potatoes and cut them into 1-inch cubes. Place the potatoes in a large pot and cover with water. Place the pot over high heat and bring to a simmer. Cook for 20 to 30 minutes or until the potatoes are easily pierced with a fork. Drain and place the potatoes either in a large bowl or back in their cooking pot. Using a potato masher, mash the potatoes with the remaining 3 tablespoons butter, 1 teaspoon salt, and ¼ teaspoon pepper.

5. When the chicken is cooked, shred it using either the paddle attachment of a stand mixer or two forks. Toss the shredded chicken in ½ cup of the BBQ sauce.

6. Preheat the oven to 350°F. Spoon the seasoned mashed potatoes into a 9 by 13-inch baking dish, then layer the BBQ shredded chicken on top. Mix the remaining ½ cup BBQ sauce with the vinegar and drizzle it over the top of the chicken.

7. Bake for 30 minutes, until the top just starts to brown.

8. Let cool, then garnish with the onions and cilantro. Serve warm.

APPROXIMATE NUTRITION BREAKDOWN	
(based on 1 of 8 servings)	
CALORIES: 393	FAT: 8 g
PROTEIN: 43 g	CARBS: 37 g

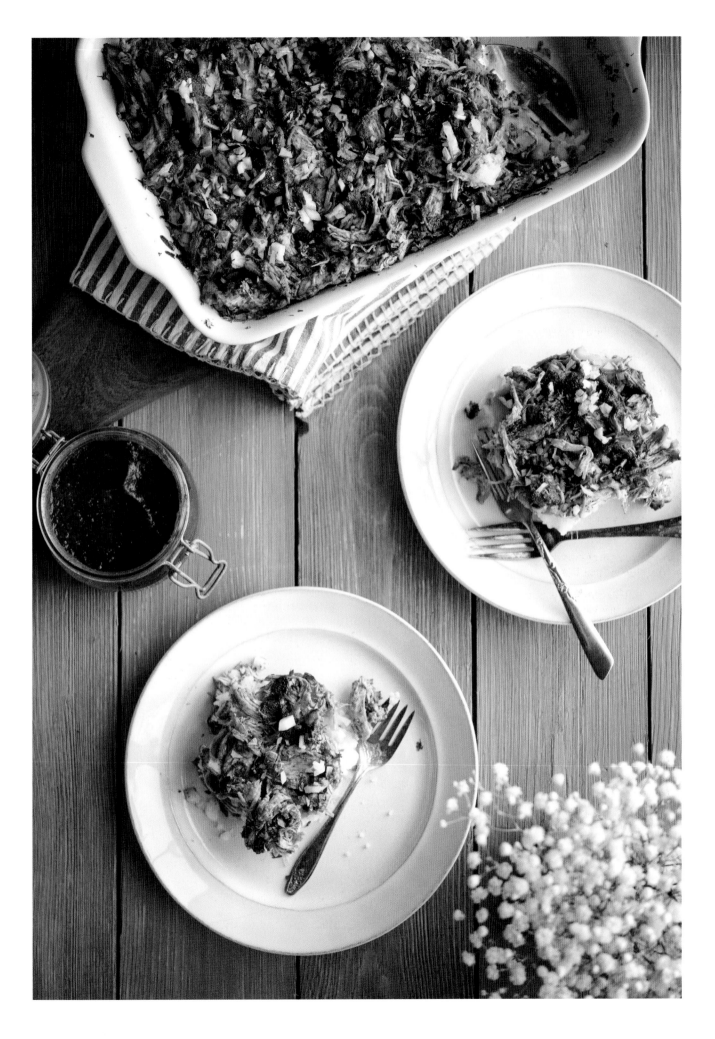

Buffalo Chicken Casserole

I always make this casserole with the intention of freezing half so that I can have healthy meals at the ready when a buffalo chicken craving strikes. Unfortunately, it never makes it to the freezer. Happily plating up servings for almost every meal of the day, my husband and I devour the whole thing in just a couple days. This one-pan dish is an incredibly delicious and balanced meal that will leave you feeling so satisfied. To make this dish more hands-off, you can cook the chicken in a slow cooker, if you like (see the tip below).

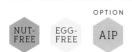

NUT-FREE   EGG-FREE   OPTION AIP

prep time: 20 minutes (not including the Buffalo sauce or ranch)	cook time: 1 hour 20 minutes	yield: 8 to 10 servings

4 sweet potatoes, cubed (about 8 cups)

1 tablespoon extra-virgin olive oil

1½ teaspoons fine sea salt, divided

2 tablespoons salted butter, divided (use EVOO for AIP)

4 pounds boneless, skinless chicken breasts, rinsed and patted dry

¼ teaspoon ground black pepper (omit for AIP)

¾ cup Buffalo Sauce (page 337), divided (omit for AIP)

6 packed cups destemmed and chopped kale (about 2 bunches)

2 tablespoons fresh lemon juice (about 1 small lemon), divided

¾ pound thick-cut bacon (about 8 strips), diced and cooked until crispy

⅓ cup 3-Ingredient Paleo Ranch (page 338) (omit for AIP)

¼ cup sliced green onions, for garnish

1. Preheat the oven to 375°F. Line a rimmed baking sheet with parchment paper.

2. Toss the sweet potato cubes in the olive oil and ½ teaspoon of the salt. Spread them out on the prepared baking sheet. Roast for 45 minutes, or until cooked all the way through. Remove the sweet potatoes from the oven and lower the oven temperature to 350°F for the casserole.

3. While the sweet potatoes are in the oven, cook the chicken: Melt 1 tablespoon of the butter in a large sauté pan that has a matching lid over high heat. Season the chicken with ½ teaspoon of the salt and the pepper. Once the butter is melted, sear the chicken on one side for 4 minutes, or until it browns slightly. Flip the chicken over and sear for an additional 3 minutes.

4. Cover the chicken with water, cover the pan with the lid, and simmer over medium heat for 20 to 30 minutes.

5. Pull the chicken from its cooking liquid and place the meat in a large bowl. Using two forks or an electric mixer, shred the chicken into small pieces. Pour in ½ cup of the Buffalo sauce and toss to combine. Set aside.

6. In a separate sauté pan, melt the remaining tablespoon of butter. Add the kale and sauté for about 8 minutes, until the color has deepened and each piece is wilted. Season with the remaining ½ teaspoon of salt and 1 tablespoon of the lemon juice.

7. Preheat the oven to 350°F. Spread out the roasted sweet potatoes evenly in a 9 by 13-inch baking dish or similar-sized ovenproof pan. Top with the kale and then with the Buffalo chicken. Drizzle the remaining ¼ cup of Buffalo sauce over the chicken and sprinkle the bacon over the top. Bake in the 350°F oven for 25 minutes, or until heated through.

8. Whisk the ranch dressing with the remaining tablespoon of lemon juice and drizzle it over the top. Garnish with the green onions and serve warm.

APPROXIMATE NUTRITION BREAKDOWN *(based on 1 of 10 servings)*			
CALORIES: 460		FAT: 24 g	
PROTEIN: 46 g		CARBS: 13 g	

• To cook the chicken in a slow cooker, approach the recipe this way: First, sear the chicken following Step 3, then transfer the seared chicken to a slow cooker, cover with water or broth, secure the lid, and cook on high for 3 to 4 hours or on low for 6 to 8 hours. When there is an hour of cooking time left, roast the sweet potatoes as directed in Steps 1 and 2. Then complete the rest of the recipe as written, following Steps 4 through 8.

• Leftovers will keep refrigerated for up to 5 days or frozen for up to 5 months.

• To defrost a whole frozen casserole, place the frozen casserole in a cold oven and turn the oven on to 350°F. Once the oven reaches temperature, bake for 30 minutes.

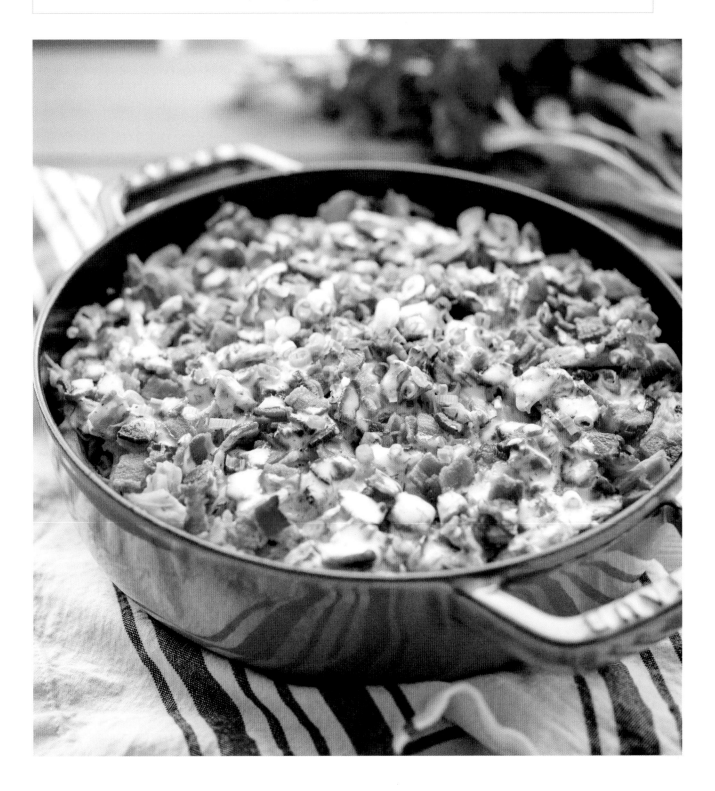

Chile Relleno Enchilada Casserole

The night I perfected this recipe, I served it up at a dinner party and people raved. Raved, I tell you! Packed with healthful Mexican-inspired flavors, this Paleo spin on a Tex-Mex favorite is a legitimate crowd-pleaser. The peppers, stuffed with a mixture of chorizo and ground beef and topped with a delicious red sauce, sit on top of an awesome Mexican Cauliflower Rice. And the cool Paleo Sour Cream and avocado really make this dish sing!

NUT-FREE · EGG-FREE · GAPS

prep time: 15 minutes (not including the cauli-rice or sour cream)	cook time: 1 hour	yield: 5 to 10 servings

10 poblano or hatch chili peppers

FILLING

1 tablespoon salted butter

½ yellow onion, finely chopped

1 pound chorizo (bulk or link style)

1 pound ground beef

2 teaspoons chili powder

2 teaspoons ground cumin

2 teaspoons dried Mexican oregano

1 teaspoon fine sea salt

RED SAUCE

1 tablespoon salted butter

½ yellow onion, finely chopped

2 cloves garlic

5 tomatoes, cut into 8 pieces each

2 tablespoons fresh lime juice (about 1 lime)

1 tablespoon chili powder

1 tablespoon ground cumin

1 tablespoon dried Mexican oregano

1 teaspoon fine sea salt

1 batch Mexican Cauliflower Rice (page 264)

FOR SERVING

½ batch Paleo Sour Cream (page 341)

1 avocado, sliced

¼ cup chopped fresh cilantro

APPROXIMATE NUTRITION BREAKDOWN (based on 1 of 10 servings)	
CALORIES: 494	FAT: 33 g
PROTEIN: 25 g	CARBS: 27 g

1. Place an oven rack in the top position and preheat the broiler to high. Line a rimmed baking sheet with parchment paper.

2. Place the peppers on the prepared baking sheet and set under the broiler for 10 minutes, turning them every 3 minutes. When charred and evenly blistered on all sides, remove from the oven, let cool, and then carefully peel the skin off of each pepper. Cut a 3-inch slit down the side of each pepper and scrape out the seeds and membrane.

3. While the peppers are cooling, prepare the filling: Melt the tablespoon of butter in a large frying pan over high heat. Add the onion and sauté for 10 minutes, or until translucent and starting to brown. If using link-style chorizo, squeeze the sausage out of its casings. Add the chorizo and ground beef to the pan and break it up with a spoon or rubber spatula. Continue to crumble the two meats together over medium heat for 12 to 15 minutes, or until cooked through and starting to crisp. Add the 2 teaspoons chili powder, 2 teaspoons cumin, 2 teaspoons oregano, and 1 teaspoon salt and stir to combine.

4. To make the sauce, melt the tablespoon of butter in a frying pan over high heat. Add the onion and sauté for 10 minutes, or until translucent and starting to brown. Add the garlic and sauté for another 4 minutes, or until fragrant. Stir in the tomatoes, lime juice, chili powder, cumin, oregano, and salt and sauté over medium heat for 10 minutes, or until the tomatoes are mostly broken down. Carefully pour the sauce into a blender and blend for 2 minutes, or until it has a smooth consistency.

5. Preheat the oven to 350°F. Spread out the cauliflower rice in a 9 by 13-inch or similar-sized baking dish. Place the prepared peppers on top of the rice. Spoon an equal amount of the meat stuffing into each pepper. Top the peppers with the red sauce.

6. Bake for 30 minutes, or until the top is bubbly.

7. Top with the sour cream, avocado slices, and cilantro, then cut into portions and serve.

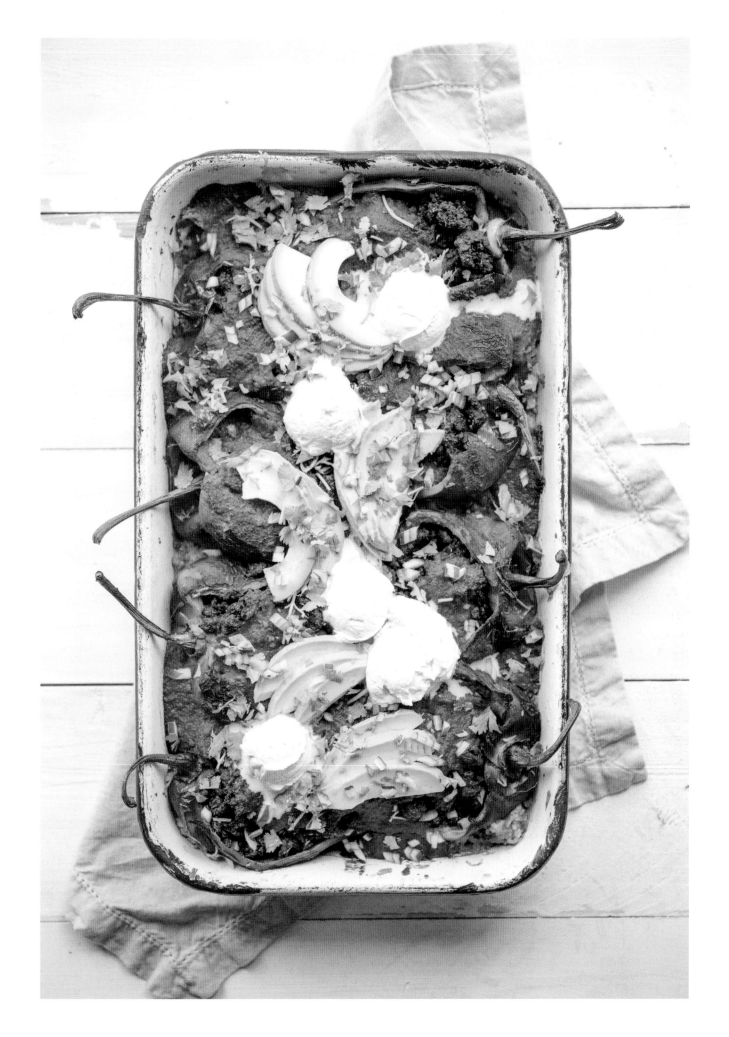

Creamy Chicken Piccata Casserole

This dish is a dream come true for me. A favorite restaurant of mine in San Antonio serves the dreamiest chicken piccata, but it is a traditional version, dredged in flour and served on pasta. I was determined to craft a Paleo-friendly version, and this one hits the spot. Flour-free and with the most amazing flavor, this casserole is going to delight you *and* your tummy.

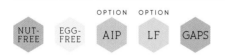

NUT-FREE   EGG-FREE   OPTION AIP   OPTION LF   GAPS

prep time: 10 minutes (not including the spaghetti squash) | *cook time: 50 minutes* | *yield: 4 to 6 servings*

1 batch Lemon Garlic Spaghetti Squash (page 267)

1 tablespoon salted butter, ghee, or coconut oil (use coconut oil for AIP)

4 cloves garlic, minced (omit for low-FODMAP)

2 pounds boneless, skinless chicken thighs, rinsed and patted dry

2 teaspoons fine sea salt

½ teaspoon ground black pepper (omit for AIP)

½ cup full-fat coconut milk (omit for low-FODMAP)

¼ cup fresh lemon juice (about 2 small lemons)

3 tablespoons capers

2 tablespoons white wine vinegar

1 tablespoon finely chopped fresh flat-leaf parsley

1. Place the Lemon Garlic Spaghetti Squash in a 9 by 13-inch baking dish. Preheat the oven to 350°F.

2. Melt the butter in a large frying pan over medium heat. Add the garlic and cook until it just starts to turn color, about 5 minutes.

3. Season the chicken thighs liberally on both sides with the salt and pepper. Working in two batches, add the chicken to the frying pan with the garlic butter. Sear for 5 minutes on one side, then turn over and sear for 2 minutes on the other side. Transfer the seared chicken thighs to the baking dish, placing them on top of the spaghetti squash.

4. Add the coconut milk, lemon juice, capers, and vinegar to the pan with the remaining garlic bits and butter. Stir until it starts to simmer, releasing any browned bits from the bottom of the pan. Pour over the chicken in the baking dish.

5. Bake for 30 minutes, until the top is bubbly. Let cool for 10 minutes, then garnish with the parsley and serve warm.

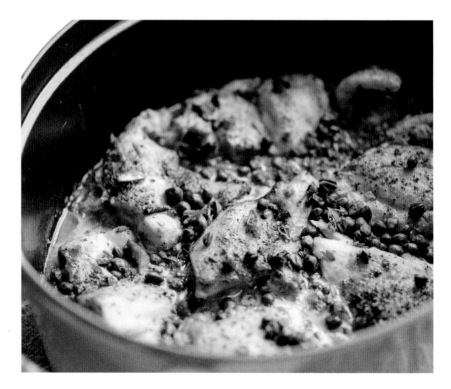

APPROXIMATE NUTRITION BREAKDOWN *(based on 1 of 6 servings)*			
CALORIES:	292	FAT:	15 g
PROTEIN:	31 g	CARBS:	11 g

Sauerkraut & Brat Bake

When it comes to the sweet spot between delicious and easy, this brat bake is right on target. It pretty much comes together in the time it takes to preheat your oven, and it freezes exceptionally well. I like to serve it with a generous dollop of mustard!

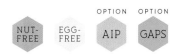

NUT-FREE · EGG-FREE · OPTION AIP · OPTION GAPS

prep time: 10 minutes | *cook time: 45 minutes* | *yield: 4 to 5 servings*

32 ounces sauerkraut, rinsed and drained

1½ pounds russet potatoes (about 4), peeled and shredded (omit for AIP and GAPS)

¼ teaspoon fine sea salt

⅛ teaspoon ground black pepper (omit for AIP)

2 pounds bratwursts (8 to 10 count)

½ teaspoon dried dill weed, plus more for optional garnish

Mustard of choice, for serving (optional)

1. Preheat the oven to 400°F.

2. Spread the rinsed and drained sauerkraut in an 8 by 10-inch baking dish. Spread the shredded potatoes evenly over the top. Sprinkle the tops of the potatoes with the salt and pepper. Place the bratwursts on the seasoned potatoes. Sprinkle the top of the bratwursts with the dill.

3. Bake for 30 to 35 minutes, until the tops of the bratwursts are browned.

4. Let cool for at least 5 minutes, then top with additional dill, if using. Serve warm with mustard, if desired.

tips

- *If you're looking for a low-carb meal, you can easily omit the potatoes from this recipe and follow the exact same directions!*

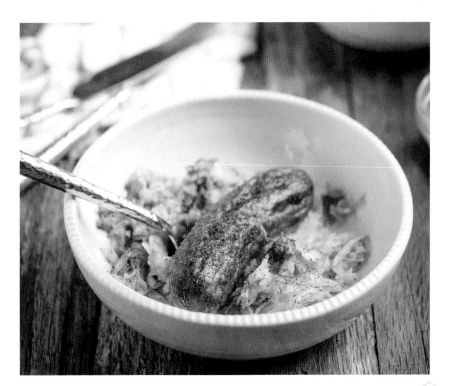

APPROXIMATE NUTRITION BREAKDOWN *(based on 1 of 5 servings)*	
CALORIES: 577	FAT: 42 g
PROTEIN: 44 g	CARBS: 29 g

Eggplant Lasagna

Well, it looks really good, but is it worth all the effort? YES. Yes, it is. Take my word for it. In fact, after you make this lasagna for the fifth time (because your family keeps requesting it), it's not going to feel like any effort at all. With eggplant slices for "noodles," the meaty Italian red sauce and creamy coconut milk "béchamel" make this one of the dishes I'm most proud of in the whole entire book. Enjoy!

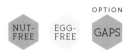

NUT-FREE   EGG-FREE   OPTION GAPS

| *prep time: 15 minutes* | *cook time: 1 hour 20 minutes* | *yield: 6 to 8 servings* |

RED SAUCE

1 tablespoon salted butter

½ small onion, diced (about ½ cup)

4 cloves garlic, minced

2 pounds hot Italian sausage, removed from casings if using links

1 (28-ounce) can diced tomatoes, drained*

12 ounces tomato puree or tomato sauce

2 tablespoons balsamic vinegar

2 tablespoons plus 2 teaspoons Italian seasoning, divided

1 teaspoon fine sea salt

BÉCHAMEL

1 tablespoon salted butter

1 (13½-ounce) can full-fat coconut milk, chilled*

½ cup unsweetened coconut butter

2 tablespoons fresh lemon juice (about 1 small lemon)

½ teaspoon fine sea salt

¼ teaspoon ground black pepper

2 large eggplants (about 2 pounds), peeled, and sliced lengthwise into ¼-inch-thick planks (for the "noodles")

5 medium tomatoes, sliced about ¼ inch thick

1 tablespoon chopped or very thinly sliced fresh basil, for garnish

1. To make the red sauce: Melt the tablespoon of butter in a large pot over medium heat. Add the onion and cook until translucent, about 10 minutes, then add the garlic and cook for 2 more minutes, until fragrant. Empty the onion and garlic mixture into a bowl.

2. Add the sausage to the pot, break it up with a spoon, and cook over high heat until the sausage starts to crisp, about 10 minutes. Drain the fat by pouring the sausage into a colander, then return the meat to the pot.

3. Return the onion and garlic mixture to the pot with the sausage. Add the drained diced tomatoes, tomato puree, balsamic vinegar, 2 tablespoons of the Italian seasoning, and 1 teaspoon salt. Stir to combine, bring to a simmer, and then cover and set aside over low heat while you make the béchamel.

4. To make the béchamel: Melt the tablespoon of butter in a sauté pan. Once melted, whisk in the coconut milk, coconut butter, lemon juice, salt, and pepper. Bring to a simmer over medium heat, whisking constantly, then set aside.

5. Preheat the oven to 350°F.

6. To assemble the lasagna: Place a layer of eggplant noodles in a 9 by 13-inch or similar-sized baking dish. Cover the noodles with about ¼ cup of the béchamel, followed by several full ladles of the red sauce. Repeat until all of the noodles are used up. For the final layer, place the sliced tomatoes across the top, then drizzle any remaining béchamel over the top. Sprinkle the top with the remaining 2 teaspoons of Italian seasoning.

7. Bake for 35 minutes, or until bubbly. Let the lasagna rest for at least 15 minutes so that the juices can settle back down. Serve warm, garnished with fresh basil.

If following a GAPS protocol, check the labels of the diced tomatoes and coconut milk carefully to confirm that they are free of additives.

APPROXIMATE NUTRITION BREAKDOWN *(based on 1 of 8 servings)*	
CALORIES: 684	FAT: 59 g
PROTEIN: 17 g	CARBS: 30 g

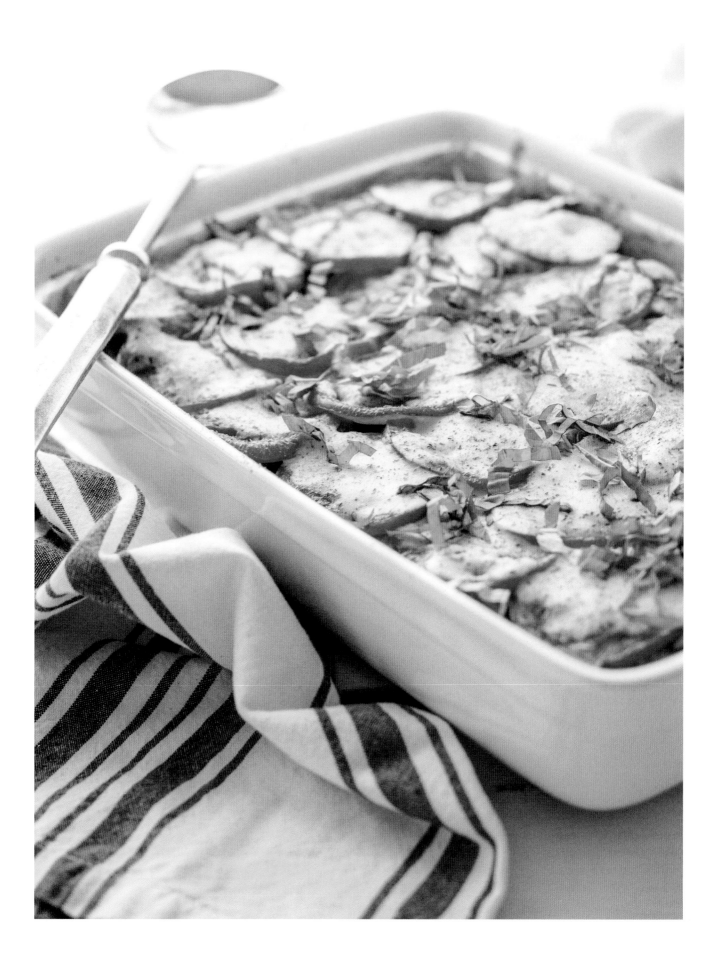

Roasted Garlic Cottage Pie

When I think of food that's "made with love," cottage pie immediately comes to mind. It's filling, nutritious, and comforting and tastes like family tradition—and it finds itself at that magical spot where comfort food and health food intersect. You and yours are going to love this meal! This recipe makes a pretty big batch, so it's perfect for a large family gathering or for a week's worth of meals.

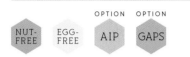

NUT-FREE | EGG-FREE | OPTION AIP | OPTION GAPS

prep time: 10 minutes (not including the cauliflower mash) | *cook time: 1 hour 10 minutes* | *yield: 6 to 8 servings*

2 tablespoons salted butter (use coconut oil for AIP)

1 yellow onion, chopped

4 cloves garlic, minced

2 pounds ground beef

1½ teaspoons rubbed dried sage

1 teaspoon dried rosemary leaves

1 teaspoon dried thyme leaves

1 teaspoon fine sea salt

½ teaspoon ground black pepper (omit for AIP)

½ teaspoon ground coriander

1 (6-ounce) can tomato paste (omit for AIP; choose additive-free for GAPS)

1 cup beef broth, store-bought or homemade (page 332)

16 ounces frozen crinkle-cut carrots

16 ounces frozen green peas (reserve ¼ cup for the top) (omit for AIP)

Double batch Roasted Garlic Cauliflower Mash (page 277)

2 tablespoons chopped fresh flat-leaf parsley, for garnish

1. Melt the butter in a large enameled cast-iron pot or frying pan over medium-high heat. Add the onion and cook for about 10 minutes, until translucent and just starting to brown. Add the garlic and cook for 2 to 3 more minutes, until fragrant.

2. Add the ground beef, sage, rosemary, thyme, salt, pepper, and coriander and cook over medium heat, stirring regularly to break up the meat, until all of the moisture has evaporated and some pieces are starting to develop a deeper brown color. Add the tomato paste, broth, carrots, and peas, reserving ¼ cup of the peas for the topping. Stir to combine, then set aside.

3. Preheat the oven 300°F. If working in a frying pan, transfer the meat mixture to a 9 by 13-inch or similar-sized baking dish. Spread the cauliflower mash over the meat mixture. Sprinkle the top with the leftover peas.

4. Cover with a sheet of aluminum foil and bake for 30 minutes, or until the edges start to look bubbly. Remove the foil and return to the oven. Increase the oven temperature to 425°F and bake for an additional 10 to 12 minutes, until the cauliflower topping just starts to brown.

5. Let the pie rest for at least 15 minutes before serving. Garnish with the fresh parsley and serve warm.

tips

- *Leftovers will keep refrigerated for up to 5 days or frozen for up to 5 months.*

APPROXIMATE NUTRITION BREAKDOWN *(based on 1 of 8 servings)*	
CALORIES: 612	FAT: 35 g
PROTEIN: 34 g	CARBS: 46 g

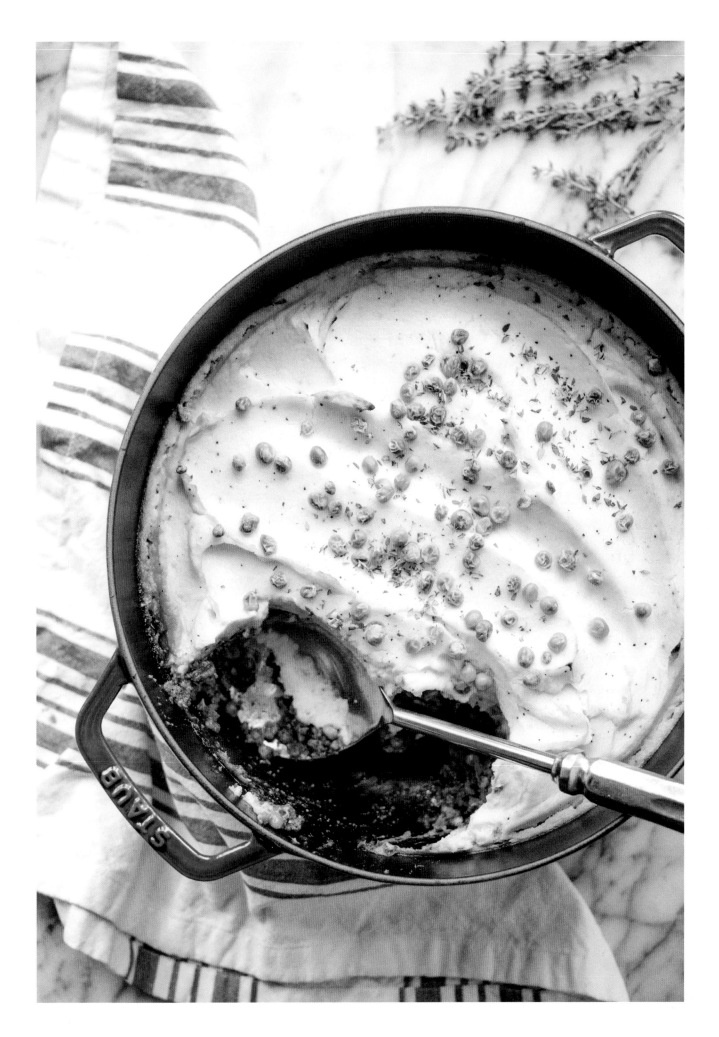

Turkey & Sweet Potato Casserole

This casserole was inspired by one of my most acclaimed blog recipes: Sweet Potato Cranberry Stuffing. The combination of sweet potato, sausage, and cranberries results in one seriously flavorful dish. In an effort to turn this über-popular side dish into a meal, I added turkey for protein, mashed the sweet potatoes, and crafted the tastiest sunflower seed crust! Though the flavors are especially great for fall, you can enjoy this dish any time of the year.

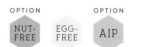

OPTION NUT-FREE · EGG-FREE · OPTION AIP

| prep time: 20 minutes | cook time: 1½ hours | yield: 8 to 10 servings |

1 (4-pound) boneless turkey breast, rinsed and patted dry

½ teaspoon fine sea salt

¼ teaspoon ground black pepper (omit for AIP)

1 pound bulk breakfast sausage or ground pork (use ground pork for AIP)

1 tablespoon salted butter (use coconut oil for AIP)

1 small yellow onion, finely chopped

4 cloves garlic, minced

2 cups chopped celery (about 6 stalks)

2 cups fresh or frozen cranberries

1 tablespoon Italian seasoning

SWEET POTATO MASH

4 pounds sweet potatoes, peeled and cut into 1-inch cubes

2 tablespoons salted butter (use coconut oil for AIP)

¼ cup full-fat coconut milk

2 tablespoons fresh lemon juice (about 1 small lemon)

1 teaspoon fine sea salt

½ teaspoon ground black pepper (omit for AIP)

SUNFLOWER SEED CRUST
(omit for nut-free and AIP)

1 tablespoon salted butter

1 cup hulled raw sunflower seeds

1 teaspoon fine sea salt

Sliced fresh chives, for garnish

1. Preheat the oven to 425°F and line a rimmed baking sheet with parchment paper.

2. Season the turkey breast with the salt and pepper. Place the turkey on the prepared baking sheet and bake for 18 to 20 minutes, until the juices run clear. Let the turkey rest for at least 10 minutes. Once it's cool enough to handle, cut it into bite-sized chunks and transfer the meat to a large mixing bowl.

3. To make the sweet potato mash: Place the cubed sweet potatoes in a pot, cover with water, and bring to a boil over high heat. Once boiling, cook for 10 to 15 minutes, until the sweet potatoes are easily pierced with a fork. Drain the sweet potatoes, then transfer them to a food processor. Blend with the butter, coconut milk, lemon juice, salt, and pepper until smooth.

4. While the sweet potatoes are cooking, brown the breakfast sausage in a large frying pan over high heat, breaking it up into small clumps as it cooks, about 10 minutes. Once cooked through and crispy, transfer the sausage to the mixing bowl with the turkey.

5. In the same frying pan, melt the tablespoon of butter over high heat. Add the onion and cook until translucent, about 5 minutes. Then add the garlic and celery and continue cooking for 10 minutes, or until the celery starts to wilt. Transfer the onion and celery to the bowl with the turkey and sausage. Add the cranberries and Italian seasoning and stir until well combined.

6. Preheat the oven to 350°F.

7. To make the sunflower seed crust, melt the tablespoon of butter in a small frying pan over medium heat. Add the sunflower seeds and stir constantly until they develop a golden color but do not burn, about 5 minutes. Season with the salt and set aside.

8. Spread out the turkey mixture in a 9 by 13-inch or similar-sized baking dish. Spread the mashed sweet potatoes on top. Finish with the toasted sunflower seeds, sprinkling them evenly across the top.

9. Bake for 30 minutes, or until the edges are bubbling.

10. Let rest for at least 10 minutes, then serve warm.

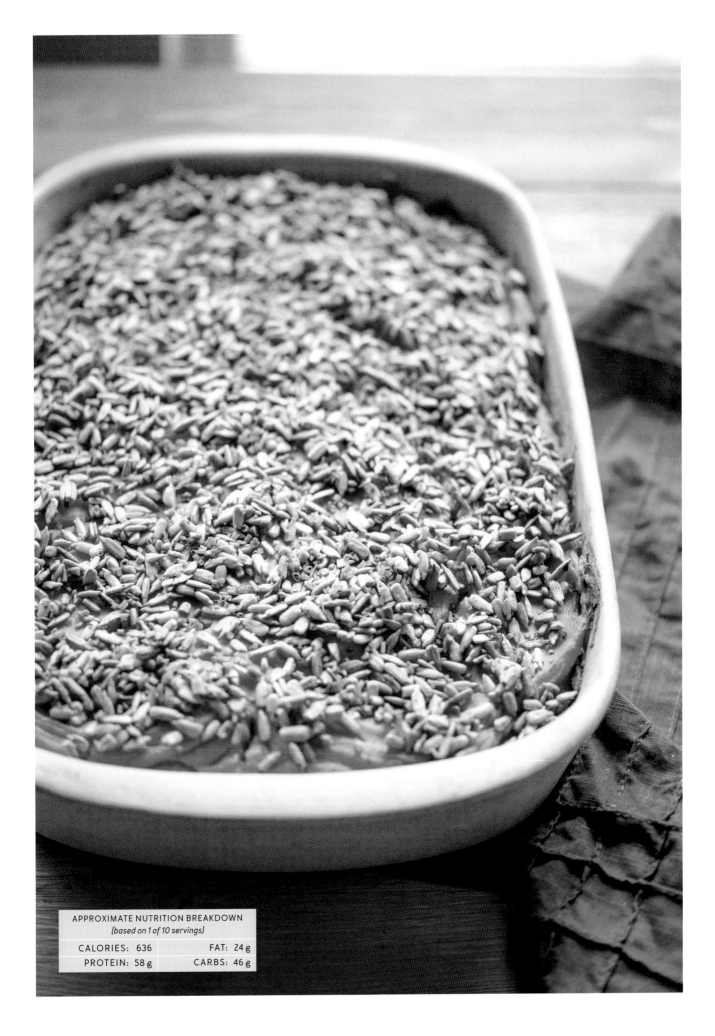

APPROXIMATE NUTRITION BREAKDOWN
(based on 1 of 10 servings)

CALORIES: 636	FAT: 24 g
PROTEIN: 58 g	CARBS: 46 g

Zucchini Pizza Casserole

I have cravings and stubbornness to thank for this gem of a recipe! It came into the world one day when I had a *major* craving for pepperoni pizza. My stubbornness is also to thank, because despite the convenience of ordering in gluten-free pizza, on that particular day I just didn't want to go there. Gluten-free crust, while a better choice than the wheat flour option, still doesn't make me feel great. So I put my thinking cap on and got to work with the foods I had on hand. Because zucchini tends to add a lot of unnecessary water to food, I dehydrated it with a short salt soak. The end product will totally "squash" the most serious pizza cravings.

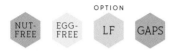

OPTION

NUT-FREE · EGG-FREE · LF · GAPS

prep time: 15 minutes, plus at least 30 minutes to disgorge the noodles | cook time: 25 minutes | yield: 2 to 4 servings

5 zucchini, shredded

1 tablespoon plus ½ teaspoon fine sea salt, divided

2 (6-ounce) jars tomato paste (omit for low-FODMAP)

2 tablespoons fresh lemon juice (about 1 small lemon)

1 tablespoon plus 1 teaspoon Italian seasoning, divided, plus more for the top*

¼ teaspoon ground black pepper

8 ounces sliced mushrooms

1 teaspoon extra-virgin olive oil

5 ounces pepperoni, sliced into bite-sized pieces

1 tablespoon finely chopped fresh parsley, for garnish

¼ teaspoon red pepper flakes, for garnish (optional)

If following a low-FODMAP protocol, be sure to use an Italian seasoning that does not include garlic or onion powder.

1. Place the shredded zucchini in a large bowl. Add 1 tablespoon of the salt and stir so that it's well combined. Set the bowl aside for at least 30 minutes or up to 2 hours. The salt will draw the water out of the zucchini. You'll know it's ready when the zucchini is sitting in a pool of water.

2. When the zucchini has released its water, preheat the oven to 350°F. Drain the water that has collected in the bottom of the bowl, then wring the excess water from the zucchini by placing it in a nut milk bag or cheesecloth and pressing firmly. Return the zucchini to the large bowl.

3. Add the tomato paste, lemon juice, 1 tablespoon of the Italian seasoning, the remaining ½ teaspoon of salt, and the pepper to the dehydrated zucchini. Mix until it's well combined and has an even texture. Spread out this zucchini "crust" in an 8-inch square or round baking dish.

4. In a separate bowl, toss the sliced mushrooms with the olive oil and remaining 1 teaspoon of Italian seasoning. Cover the zucchini mixture with the seasoned mushrooms and pepperoni slices. Sprinkle some extra Italian seasoning on top.

5. Bake for 25 minutes, or until the pepperoni starts to look crispy. Serve warm, garnished with fresh parsley and red pepper flakes, if desired.

tips

- *Most of the salt used to disgorge the zucchini stays in the water. I squeezed out 1½ cups of water!*

APPROXIMATE NUTRITION BREAKDOWN *(based on 1 of 4 servings)*	
CALORIES: 269	FAT: 11g
PROTEIN: 14g	CARBS: 34g

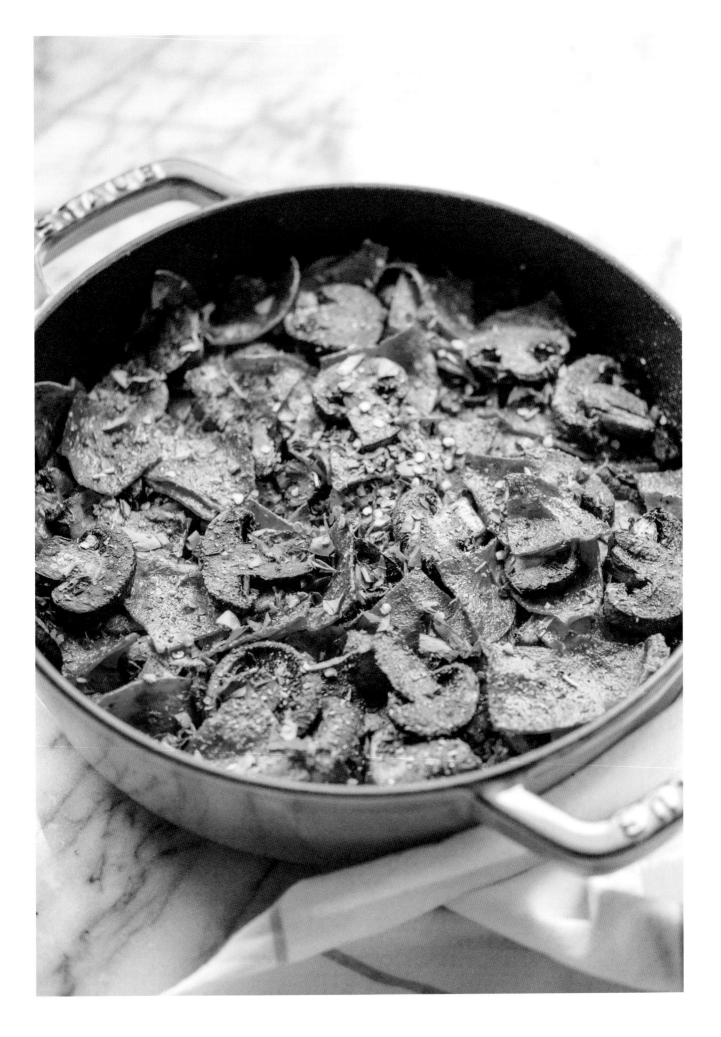

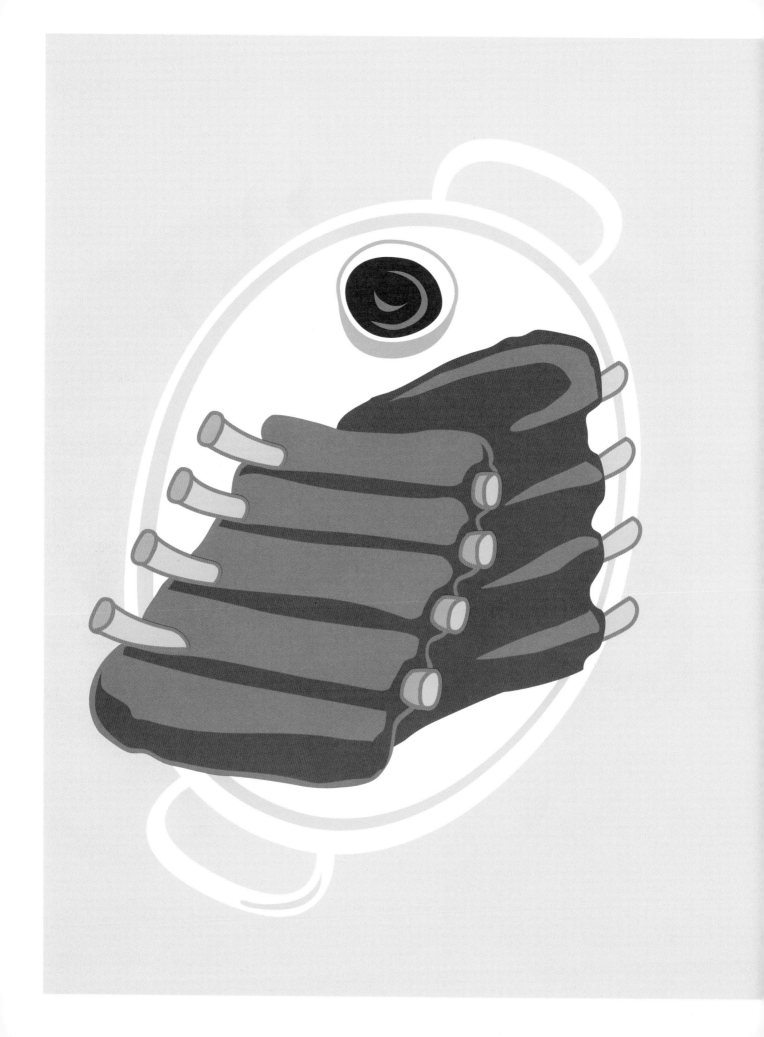

CHAPTER 7:

FAMILY FAVORITE PROTEINS & MEALS

Download the Fed & Fit iPhone and Android app! You can scan the above QR codes directly in the app, which will then populate a consolidated grocery shopping list for the scanned recipes.

Asian-Style Cabbage Rolls

WITH SAVORY ALMOND SAUCE

These cabbage rolls are my everything. I know the ingredient list looks long, but pulling them together is actually really straightforward! These are great for a crowd or a family dinner, or to prep for a week's worth of leftovers. Don't skip the sauce, either! It really takes these rolls to the next level and, if you're lucky enough to have some left over, is especially great over grilled chicken.

EGG-FREE   GAPS

prep time: 15 minutes | *cook time: 1 hour* | *yield: 6 to 8 servings*

1 large head napa cabbage

FILLING

2 tablespoons salted butter

1 (2-inch) piece fresh ginger, peeled and grated

5 cloves garlic, minced

2 carrots, peeled and shredded

2½ cups thinly sliced shiitake mushroom caps (about 8 ounces whole shiitakes)

2 pounds ground pork

3 green onions, sliced

½ cup fresh cilantro leaves and stems, chopped

½ to 1 teaspoon red pepper flakes

1 tablespoon coconut aminos

2 teaspoons fish sauce

1 teaspoon apple cider vinegar

1 teaspoon fine sea salt

SAVORY ALMOND SAUCE

1 tablespoon plus 1 teaspoon sesame oil (untoasted)

2 cloves garlic, minced

1 cup coconut aminos

½ cup smooth almond butter (unsweetened)

2 tablespoons apple cider vinegar

2 teaspoons fish sauce

1 teaspoon red pepper flakes

FOR GARNISH

2 tablespoons chopped fresh cilantro

1. Bring a large pot of water (ideally with a strainer insert) to a simmer. Submerge the head of cabbage in the water, stem side down. Reduce the heat to medium-low and let the cabbage poach for 10 minutes. Pull the cabbage from the water, drain, and set aside until it's cool enough to handle.

2. While the cabbage is cooling, prepare the filling: Melt the butter in a sauté pan over medium heat. Add the ginger, garlic, and carrots and sauté for about 10 minutes, until fragrant and the carrots are slightly wilted. Add the mushrooms and sauté for an additional 5 minutes, or until they're reduced in size and slightly brown.

3. Put the sautéed vegetables, along with the rest of the filling ingredients, in a large mixing bowl. Using your hands, mix the ingredients together until they're evenly incorporated.

4. Cut the root end off the cabbage head. Working very carefully because the leaves are delicate, gently separate the leaves and lay them out on paper towel–lined plates.

5. To fill the rolls, spoon about ¼ cup of the filling onto a cabbage leaf, over the stem, nearest the cut end. Carefully roll the cabbage toward the thinner uncut end, folding the sides over the center as you work. Place the stuffed roll seam side down in a parchment paper–lined 9 by 13-inch or similar-sized baking dish. Repeat this process with the rest of the filling mixture and cabbage leaves. Preheat the oven to 350°F.

6. To make the almond sauce, heat the sesame oil in a small saucepan over medium heat. Add the garlic and stir for about 5 minutes, until fragrant. Add the coconut aminos, almond butter, vinegar, fish sauce, and red pepper flakes. Whisk to combine and bring to a simmer.

7. Spoon about half of the almond sauce over the rolls.

8. Cover the baking dish with a sheet of aluminum foil. Bake for 30 minutes, then remove the foil and bake for an additional 15 minutes, or until the almond sauce on top starts to darken.

9. To serve, spoon additional almond sauce over the top of the rolls and garnish with a sprinkle of chopped cilantro.

APPROXIMATE NUTRITION BREAKDOWN *(based on 3 rolls per serving)*	
CALORIES: 333	FAT: 21 g
PROTEIN: 24 g	CARBS: 12 g

APPROXIMATE NUTRITION BREAKDOWN *(based on 2 Tbsp extra sauce per serving)*	
CALORIES: 159	FAT: 11 g
PROTEIN: 4 g	CARBS: 9 g

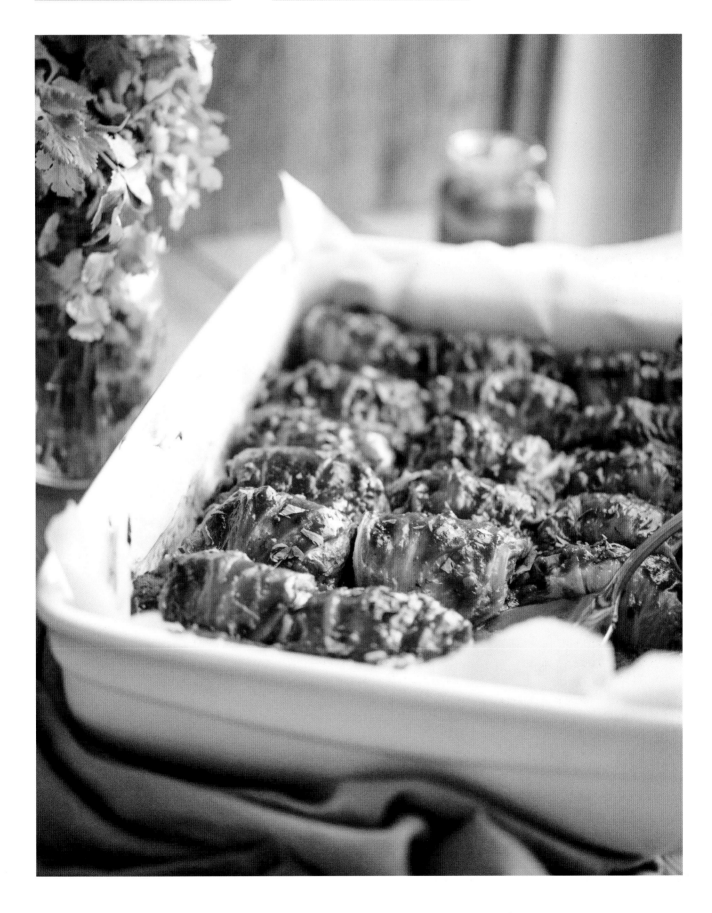

Beef Stroganoff

WITH TURNIP NOODLES

It's as good as it looks but five times as healthy. This beef stroganoff has an incredible flavor, and the noodles have a great texture. The trick to enjoying non-watery veggie-based noodles is to use salt to draw out some of the water before you start cooking. This recipe is easily doubled or even tripled!

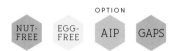

NUT-FREE EGG-FREE OPTION AIP GAPS

prep time: 15 minutes, plus at least 30 minutes to disgorge the noodles

cook time: 45 minutes

yield: 2 to 3 servings

NOODLES

4 turnips, peeled and spiral-sliced into noodles

2 tablespoons fine sea salt

2 tablespoons salted butter (use coconut oil for AIP)

2 tablespoons fresh lemon juice (about 1 small lemon)

STROGANOFF

3 tablespoons salted butter, divided (use coconut oil for AIP)

10 ounces boneless sirloin steak, cut into 1-inch cubes

1 teaspoon fine sea salt, divided

½ teaspoon ground black pepper divided (omit for AIP)

1 yellow onion, diced

3 cloves garlic, minced

1 pound button or crimini mushrooms, sliced

½ cup full-fat coconut milk

2 tablespoons whole-grain mustard or prepared yellow mustard

FOR GARNISH

2 tablespoons chopped fresh flat-leaf parsley

1. To disgorge the noodles: Working in a large bowl, toss the turnip noodles with the salt and set aside for at least 30 minutes. Then place the noodles in a nut milk bag, cheesecloth, or colander. Squeeze as much water out of the noodles as possible; keep squeezing until you have removed at least ¾ cup of water (this can take about 5 minutes).

2. While the noodles are sitting in the salt, prepare the stroganoff: Melt 1 tablespoon of the butter in a large frying pan over high heat. Sprinkle all sides of the steak cubes with about half of the salt and pepper. Place the steak cubes in the frying pan and sear each side for about 3 minutes, or until they develop a char. Transfer the meat to a separate bowl and set aside.

3. Melt the remaining 2 tablespoons of butter in the same pan over medium heat. Add the onion and sauté for about 10 minutes, until the onion is wilted and starting to develop a brown color. Add the garlic and cook for an additional 3 minutes, or until fragrant. Add the mushrooms and sauté for an additional 10 minutes, or until the mushrooms are reduced in size and starting to brown. Transfer the mushroom mixture to the bowl with the meat and set aside.

4. Add the coconut milk and mustard to the frying pan and whisk to incorporate. Bring to a simmer over medium heat, then return the meat and vegetables to the pan. Bring back to a simmer for an additional 5 minutes.

5. For the noodles, melt the 2 tablespoons of butter in a large frying pan with a tight-fitting lid. Add the noodles, stir to combine, and cover. Let steam for about 9 minutes, uncover, and then season with the lemon juice.

6. To serve, plate the noodles first, followed by the beef stroganoff, and then garnish with the parsley.

APPROXIMATE NUTRITION BREAKDOWN *(based on 1 of 3 servings)*	
CALORIES: 620	FAT: 40 g
PROTEIN: 34 g	CARBS: 40 g

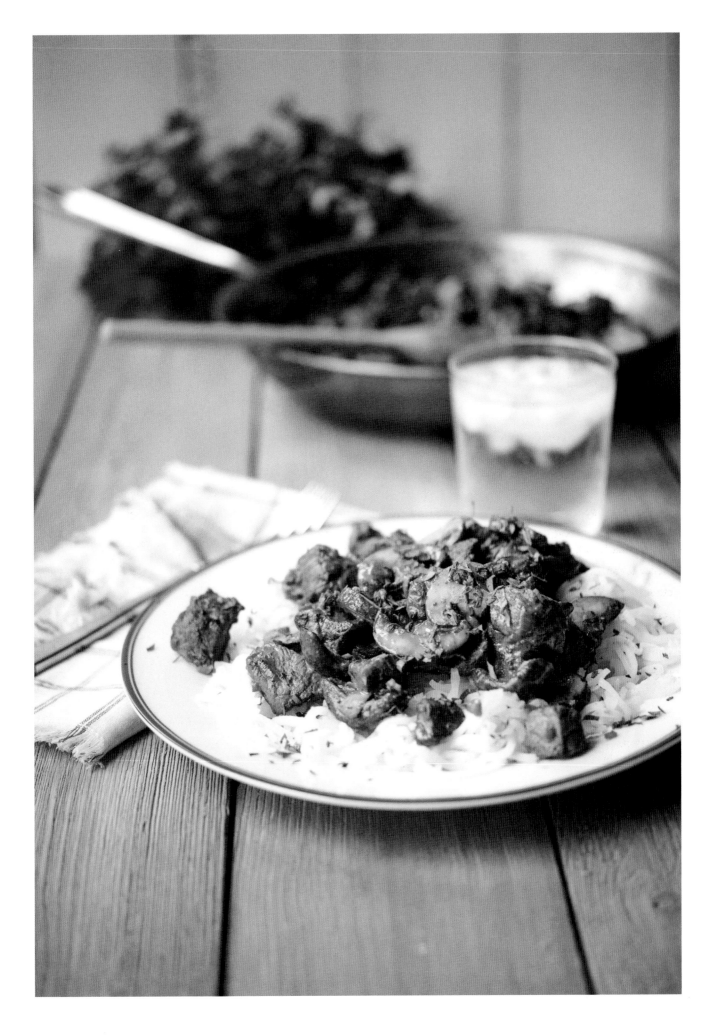

BURGERS:

Buffalo Ranch Bison

It *is* possible to enjoy a bunless burger and want for nothing. One of my tricks is to roll my favorite flavors right into the patty! So clearly I love Buffalo sauce and ranch dressing. The two come together here in a holy flavor union, resulting in the juiciest, most exciting burgers ever to grace my little kitchen. To serve, I recommend plating these burgers on top of some butter lettuce.

prep time: 5 minutes (not including the Buffalo sauce or ranch) | *cook time: 40 minutes* | *yield: 4 to 6 servings*

2 pounds ground bison

¼ cup Buffalo Sauce (page 337), plus more for serving

¼ cup 3-Ingredient Paleo Ranch (page 338), plus more for serving

½ purple onion, finely diced

1 tablespoon salted butter

¼ cup chopped fresh cilantro, for garnish

1. Place the ground bison, Buffalo sauce, ranch dressing, and onion in a large mixing bowl. Work the sauce and onions into the meat until they are evenly combined. Divide the meat into 4 to 6 even balls, then flatten those balls into ½-inch-thick patties.

2. Melt the butter in a large frying pan over high heat, then add about 3 patties to the pan. Cook the patties for about 5 minutes per side, until they start to develop a brown crust, for medium-done burgers. Repeat with the remaining patties.

3. Serve the burgers with a drizzle of Buffalo sauce and ranch and some fresh cilantro.

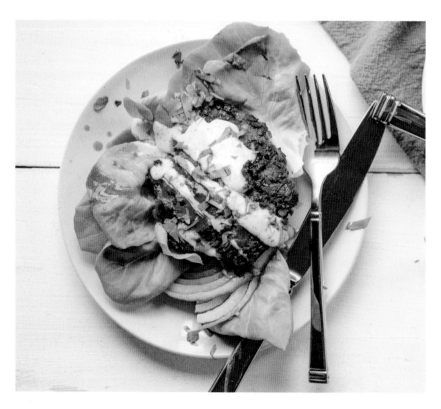

APPROXIMATE NUTRITION BREAKDOWN *(based on 1 of 6 servings)*			
CALORIES:	375	FAT:	27 g
PROTEIN:	31 g	CARBS:	2 g

BURGERS:

Salmon Cranberry

These burgers, fashioned after one of my favorite grab-and-go foods from my local grocery store, are always a huge hit. I especially love the fresh cranberry salsa! You get to enjoy it two ways—mixed right into the burgers and as a refreshing relish on top. To serve, I recommend plating these burgers with some peeled and sliced jicama.

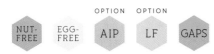

NUT-FREE | EGG-FREE | OPTION AIP | OPTION LF | GAPS

prep time: 10 minutes | *cook time: 10 minutes* | *yield: 4 to 5 servings*

¾ cup fresh or frozen cranberries

¼ cup fresh flat-leaf parsley leaves and stems

2 tablespoons fresh lemon juice (about 1 small lemon)

½ teaspoon fine sea salt

¼ teaspoon ground black pepper (omit for AIP)

2 tablespoons coconut aminos (omit for low-FODMAP)

1½ pounds salmon fillets, skinned, deboned, and cut into large pieces

1 tablespoon salted butter (use coconut oil for AIP)

1. Place the cranberries, parsley, lemon juice, salt, pepper, and coconut aminos in a food processor and pulse about 5 times, just until the cranberries are mostly broken up. Scrape the cranberry mixture into a mixing bowl and set aside.

2. Add the salmon pieces to the food processor and pulse about 10 times, until the salmon has an even "ground" texture.

3. Transfer the salmon to a large mixing bowl and add half of the cranberry mixture, reserving the rest for garnish. Work the cranberry mixture into the salmon until it has an even consistency. Divide the salmon into 4 or 5 even balls, then flatten those balls into ½-inch-thick patties.

4. Melt the butter in a large frying pan over high heat, then add about 3 patties to the pan. Cook the patties for about 4 minutes per side, until they start to develop a brown crust. Repeat with the remaining patties.

5. Serve the burgers topped with the remaining cranberry salsa.

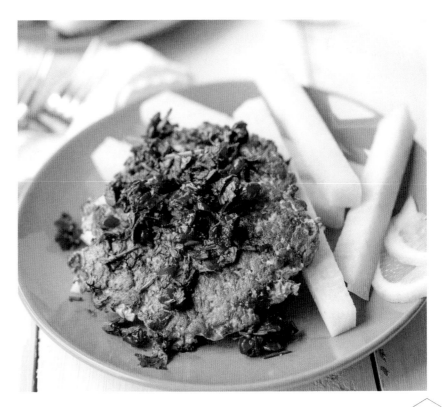

APPROXIMATE NUTRITION BREAKDOWN *(based on 1 of 5 servings)*	
CALORIES: 230	FAT: 10 g
PROTEIN: 29 g	CARBS: 4 g

BURGERS:

Caramelized Onion Balsamic Beef

Caramelized onions on top of a burger are always a hit. So I thought, what if I put caramelized onions *in* the burger, too? Long story short, it's an even bigger hit. These burgers are packed full of so much flavor, you're going to want to make them over and over again. To serve, I recommend plating these burgers on top of some fresh kale leaves.

NUT-FREE · EGG-FREE · AIP (OPTION) · GAPS

prep time: 10 minutes | *cook time: 1 hour* | *yield: 2 to 3 servings*

2 tablespoons salted butter, divided (use coconut oil for AIP)

3 yellow onions (about ¾ pound), finely diced

1 pound ground beef

¼ cup balsamic vinegar, plus more for drizzling

½ teaspoon fine sea salt

¼ teaspoon ground black pepper (omit for AIP)

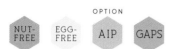 tips

- *To save time the day of, make the caramelized onions up to 2 days ahead.*

1. Melt 1 tablespoon of the butter in a large frying pan (preferably cast iron) over high heat. Add the onions, stir, and let caramelize over medium-low heat for about 40 minutes, stirring occasionally.

2. Place the ground beef in a large mixing bowl. Add about two-thirds of the caramelized onions, balsamic vinegar, salt, and pepper. Work the onions and seasonings into the meat until they are evenly combined. Divide the meat into 6 even balls, then flatten those balls into 1-inch-thick patties.

3. Melt the remaining tablespoon of butter in a large frying pan over high heat, then add about 3 patties to the pan. Cook the patties for about 5 minutes per side, or until they start to develop a brown crust, for medium-done burgers. Repeat with the remaining patties.

4. Serve with the remainder of the caramelized onions and an additional drizzle of balsamic vinegar.

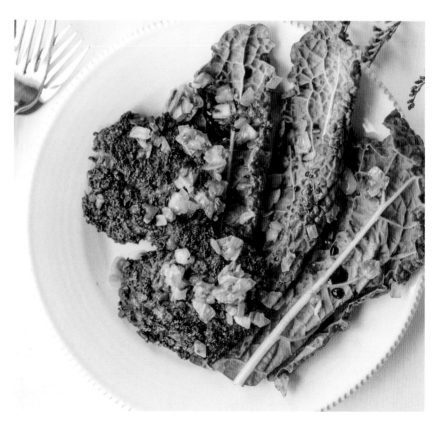

APPROXIMATE NUTRITION BREAKDOWN *(based on 1 of 3 servings)*	
CALORIES: 464	FAT: 30 g
PROTEIN: 29 g	CARBS: 19 g

BURGERS:

Tomatillo Turkey

These turkey burgers absolutely *burst* with bright flavor. If you like a little spice, you can throw a seeded jalapeño into the mix! Though optional, the avocado and sour cream garnishes make these burgers even more craveable. This recipe is easily doubled if you're feeding a crowd. To serve, I recommend plating these burgers on top of some fresh lettuce.

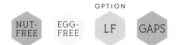

NUT-FREE   EGG-FREE   OPTION LF   GAPS

prep time: 10 minutes (not including the sour cream) | *cook time: 20 minutes* | *yield: 2 to 3 servings*

½ cup salsa verde, store-bought or homemade (page 344)

1 pound ground turkey

1 tablespoon salted butter

FOR GARNISH
(omit for low-FODMAP)

¼ cup Paleo Sour Cream (page 341)

1 avocado, sliced

2 tablespoons fresh cilantro leaves

1. Put the salsa verde and ground turkey in a large mixing bowl. Work the salsa into the meat until they are evenly combined. Divide the meat into 6 even balls, then flatten those balls into 1-inch-thick patties.

2. Melt the butter in a large frying pan over high heat, then add about 3 patties to the pan. Cook the patties for about 5 minutes per side, until they develop a slight char. Repeat with the remaining patties.

3. Plate the burgers with a dollop of sour cream, avocado slices, and cilantro leaves.

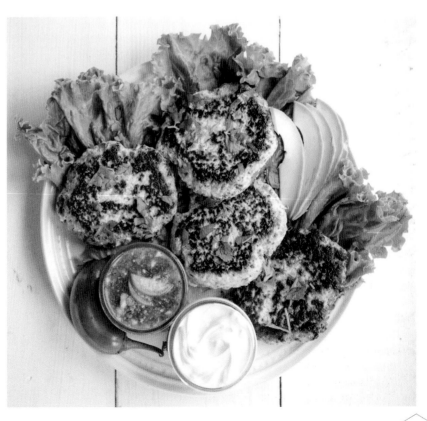

APPROXIMATE NUTRITION BREAKDOWN *(based on 1 of 3 servings)*	
CALORIES: 394	FAT: 26 g
PROTEIN: 30 g	CARBS: 8 g

Caramelized Onion Bacon Bison Meatloaf

WITH BALSAMIC MUSTARD GLAZE

I thought about naming this "Not Your Mom's Meatloaf." It is definitely not the meatloaf you grew up on, but I know it's going to knock your socks off. The flavors are bold and the method is simple. Remember not to rush the onions; the caramelized flavor they add to the meatloaf is well worth the wait.

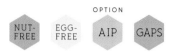

NUT-FREE EGG-FREE OPTION AIP GAPS

prep time: 15 minutes	cook time: 1 hour 45 minutes	yield: 6 to 9 servings

2 tablespoons salted butter (use coconut oil for AIP)

4 yellow onions (about 2 pounds), diced

2 pounds ground bison

¼ cup plus 3 tablespoons prepared yellow mustard or whole-grain mustard, divided

2 tablespoons plus 2 teaspoons balsamic vinegar, divided

1 teaspoon fine sea salt

½ teaspoon ground black pepper (omit for AIP)

½ pound thick-cut bacon

2 tablespoons chopped fresh flat-leaf parsley, for garnish

tips

- *You can make the caramelized onions a day or two in advance.*

- *Leftovers will keep refrigerated for up to 4 days or frozen for up to 4 months.*

1. In an enameled cast-iron or heavy-bottomed frying pan, melt the butter over medium heat. Add the onions, stir to coat in the butter, and slowly cook for about 45 minutes, stirring occasionally, until they're cooked down and develop a nice brown color. If the onions start to burn, lower the heat. *Note:* The longer you allow them to darken, the richer the flavor will be.

2. Scrape the caramelized onions into a large mixing bowl and preheat the oven to 350°F.

3. To the mixing bowl with the onions, add the ground bison, ¼ cup of the mustard, 2 tablespoons of the vinegar, salt, and pepper. Work the ingredients into the meat until the mixture has an even consistency. Press the meat mixture into a 9 by 5-inch loaf pan. Cut the bacon in half crosswise and lay it on top of the meatloaf in horizontal stripes that overlap slightly.

4. Bake for 40 minutes, or until the meatloaf is slightly reduced in size and grease is visible around the edges. Remove from the oven and increase the oven temperature to 450°F. Using a turkey baster, carefully suction out (and then discard) about ½ cup of liquid grease from the corners of the loaf pan.

5. In a small bowl, whisk together the remaining 3 tablespoons of mustard and the remaining 2 teaspoons of vinegar. Spoon the glaze over the top of the meatloaf and return the pan to the oven for an additional 15 minutes, or until the top starts to darken.

6. Let the meatloaf rest for 10 minutes. You can slice it directly in the pan and serve or, using kitchen tongs, remove the loaf from the pan and place it on a serving platter for slicing. Serve garnished with fresh parsley.

APPROXIMATE NUTRITION BREAKDOWN *(based on 1 of 9 servings)*	
CALORIES: 301	FAT: 20 g
PROTEIN: 22 g	CARBS: 8 g

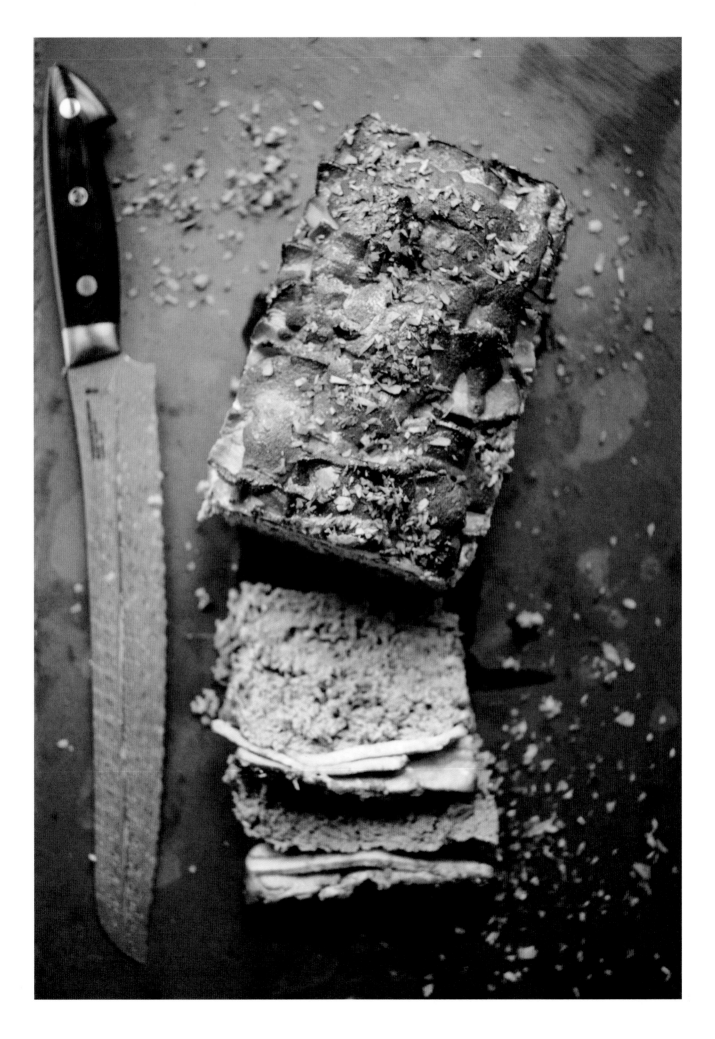

Creole Jambalaya

This dish is so satisfying. It's wonderfully filling and full of a variety of proteins, vegetables, and their accompanying nutrients. Feel free to customize the spice level to your taste, adding more cayenne if you like spicier foods or omitting the cayenne altogether. Jambalaya is a great dish to make for a crowd!

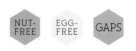

NUT-FREE   EGG-FREE   GAPS

prep time: 25 minutes (not including the cauliflower rice)

cook time: 50 minutes

yield: 9 to 12 servings

1 pound chorizo (bulk or link style)

1 pound shrimp, peeled and deveined

2 boneless, skinless chicken breast halves (about 1 pound), rinsed, patted dry, and cut into ½-inch pieces

1 tablespoon salted butter (if needed)

2 cups chopped celery (about 6 stalks)

1 small onion, chopped

1 red bell pepper, seeded and chopped

5 cloves garlic, minced

1 (28-ounce) can diced tomatoes

¾ cup chicken or beef broth, store-bought or homemade (page 332)

½ cup coconut aminos

½ cup Frank's RedHot Sauce

2 tablespoons fresh lemon juice (about 1 small lemon)

2 tablespoons dried oregano leaves

2 teaspoons fine sea salt

1 tablespoon onion powder

½ teaspoon ground black pepper

½ teaspoon cayenne pepper

Double batch Basic Cauliflower Rice (page 264)

¼ cup chopped fresh flat-leaf parsley, for garnish

1. If using link-style chorizo, remove the sausage from its casings. Cook the chorizo in an enameled cast-iron or other heavy-bottomed deep-sided sauté pan or Dutch oven over high heat, using a spoon or spatula to break it up into crumbles, for 10 minutes or until browned and starting to become crispy. Using a slotted spoon, remove the chorizo from the pan and place it in a large bowl, leaving the grease in the pan.

2. Reduce the heat to medium and add the shrimp to the pan with the sausage grease. Cook the shrimp for about 3 minutes per side, until pink and no longer opaque. Transfer the cooked shrimp to the bowl with the cooked chorizo.

3. Add the chicken to the pan and cook for about 3 minutes per side, until slightly browned. Transfer the cooked chicken to the bowl with the shrimp and chorizo and set aside.

4. If there isn't any grease left in the pan, add a tablespoon of butter. Turn the heat up to high and add the chopped celery, onion, and bell pepper. Sauté for about 10 minutes, until the onion is translucent and starting to brown and the bell pepper has softened. Add the garlic and cook for an additional 3 minutes, or until fragrant. Add the tomatoes, broth, coconut aminos, hot sauce, lemon juice, oregano, salt, onion powder, black pepper, and cayenne pepper. Stir to combine and bring to a simmer over medium heat.

5. Once the soup is bubbling, return the chorizo, shrimp, and chicken to the pan and add the cauliflower rice. Stir to combine and bring to a simmer once more. Season with more salt and cayenne pepper to taste.

6. Serve warm, garnished with fresh parsley.

tips

- *Leftovers will keep refrigerated for up to 3 days or frozen for up to 3 months.*

APPROXIMATE NUTRITION BREAKDOWN *(based on 1 of 12 servings)*	
CALORIES: 344	FAT: 19 g
PROTEIN: 28 g	CARBS: 16 g

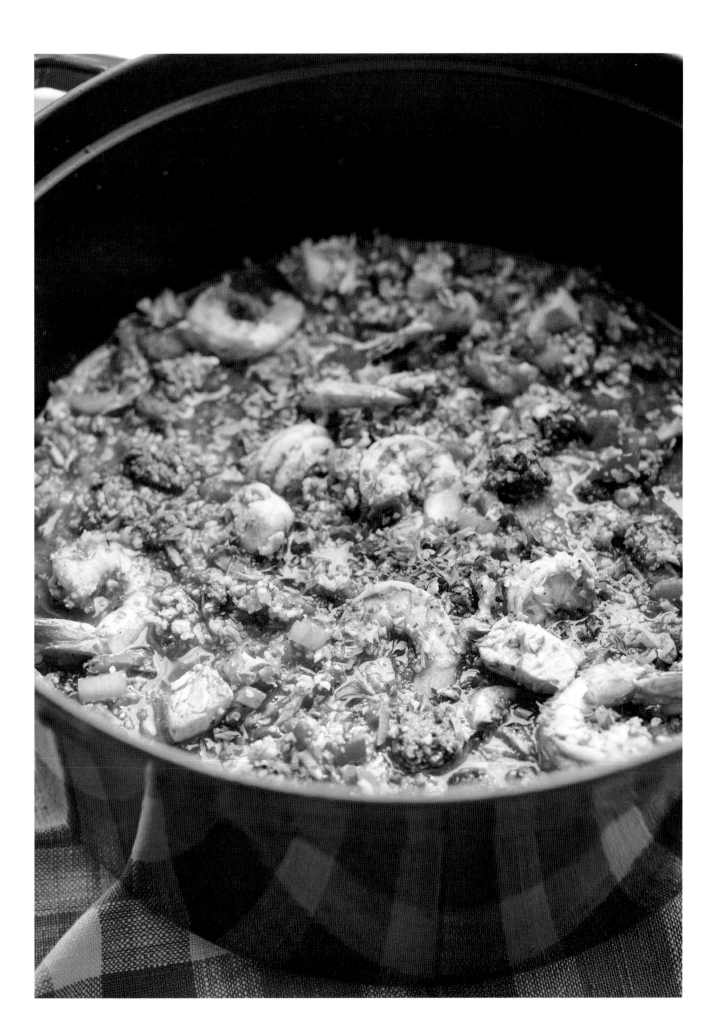

Oven Baby Back Ribs

These ribs make me feel like I'm totally winning at life. They're almost effortless to pull together and always blow people away. They're so darn delicious and have that perfect fall-off-the-bone *and* crispy texture combo from the final spell in the oven. Make these and wow your friends!

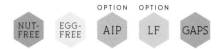

NUT-FREE • EGG-FREE • OPTION AIP • OPTION LF • GAPS

| prep time: 5 minutes | cook time: 2 hours 10 minutes | yield: 4 to 6 servings |

4 pounds baby back pork ribs (1 full rack or 2 half racks)

½ teaspoon fine sea salt

¼ teaspoon ground black pepper (omit for AIP)

1 cup BBQ sauce, store-bought or homemade (page 336), plus more for serving (omit for AIP and low-FODMAP)

1. Preheat the oven to 325°F. Rinse the ribs and pat them dry with a paper towel.

2. Sprinkle the salt and pepper over both sides of the rack(s), concentrating the seasoning on the top-facing (convex) side.

3. Place the ribs in a roasting pan or on a rimmed baking sheet. Using a basting brush or spoon, spread about three-quarters of the BBQ sauce over the ribs.

4. Bake for 2 hours, remove from the oven, and then turn the heat up to 450°F. Spread the remaining one-quarter of the BBQ sauce over the ribs and, once the oven is up to temperature, return the ribs to the oven for an additional 10 minutes, or until the tops start to develop a slight char.

5. Remove the ribs from the oven and let them rest for 10 minutes before serving. Cut the ribs apart and plate with extra BBQ sauce on the side.

APPROXIMATE NUTRITION BREAKDOWN (based on 1 of 6 servings)	
CALORIES: 607	FAT: 36 g
PROTEIN: 59 g	CARBS: 7 g

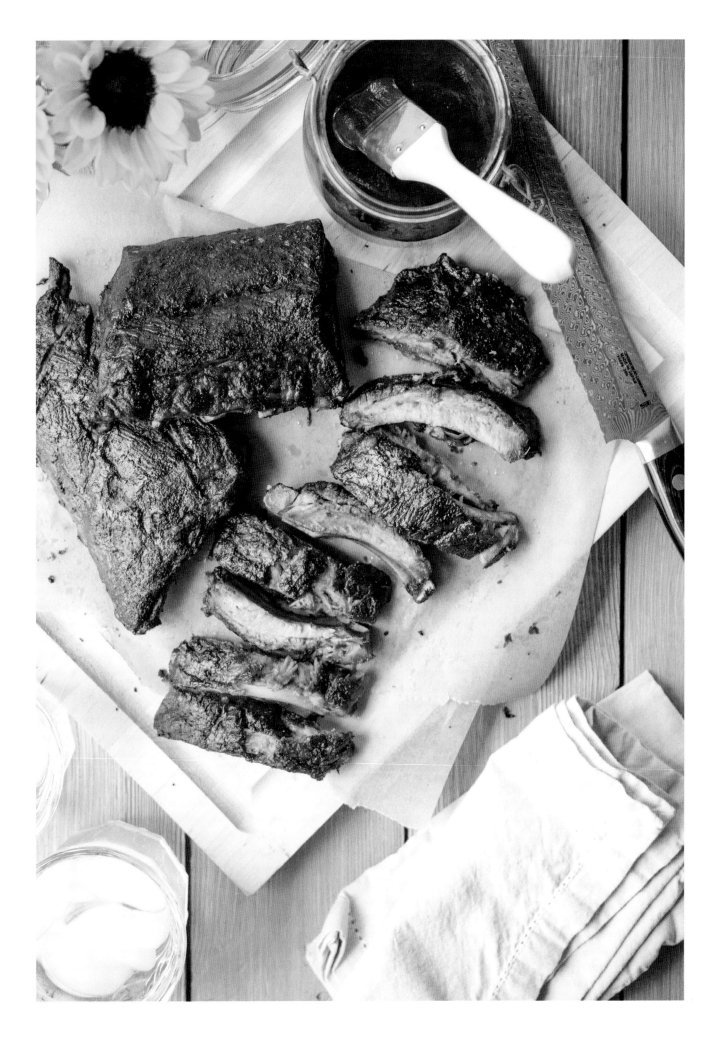

The Panang Curry My Husband Loves

My husband is a self-proclaimed panang curry savant. He's tasted and tested countless bowls in countless cities. One of the first projects I took on after we got married was to craft a panang curry that would win his vote as the "best *ever*." After dozens of attempts, I finally nailed it! I'm especially proud of this recipe because all of the ingredients can be found at most basic grocery stores.

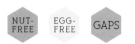

NUT-FREE   EGG-FREE   GAPS

prep time: 20 minutes (not including the cauliflower rice) | cook time: 40 minutes | yield: 6 to 8 servings

CURRY SAUCE

2 (13½-ounce) cans full-fat coconut milk

3 tablespoons Thai red curry paste

2 teaspoons grated lime zest (about 1 lime)

¼ cup lime juice (about 2 limes)

2 teaspoons fish sauce

½ teaspoon to 2 teaspoons red pepper flakes

1 onion, finely chopped

1 tablespoon salted butter, ghee, or coconut oil

2½ to 3 pounds boneless, skinless chicken breasts, rinsed, patted dry, and cut into ½-inch dice

2 red bell peppers, seeded and thinly sliced

¼ cup fresh basil leaves

FOR SERVING

Double batch Basic Cauliflower Rice (page 264)

Fresh basil leaves, cut into ribbons or left whole

8 lime wedges

1. Make the curry sauce: In a large sauté pan, whisk together the coconut milk, curry paste, lime zest, lime juice, fish sauce, and red pepper flakes (use ½ teaspoon for mild heat, 1 teaspoon for medium, or 2 teaspoons for hot). Simmer over medium-low heat, stirring often, until it is thick enough to coat the back of a spoon. This will take about 20 minutes.

2. While the sauce is simmering, prepare the rest of the ingredients: In a frying pan, cook the onion in the butter over medium heat until translucent and slightly brown. Add the chicken and cook on medium-high for about 5 minutes per side, or until each piece is completely white and cooked through. Transfer the chicken and most of the onions to a bowl. Add the bell peppers to the frying pan and cook over high heat for about 10 minutes, until they're wilted and slightly browned on a couple sides. Remove the pan from heat and set aside.

3. When the curry sauce has thickened, add the chicken, bell pepper, and onion mixture to it. Stir to incorporate and simmer for 5 minutes. Add the basil and simmer for 2 to 3 more minutes.

4. Serve warm over cauliflower rice. Garnish each serving with some fresh basil leaves and a lime wedge.

APPROXIMATE NUTRITION BREAKDOWN (based on 1 of 8 servings)	
CALORIES: 500	FAT: 28 g
PROTEIN: 45 g	CARBS: 20 g

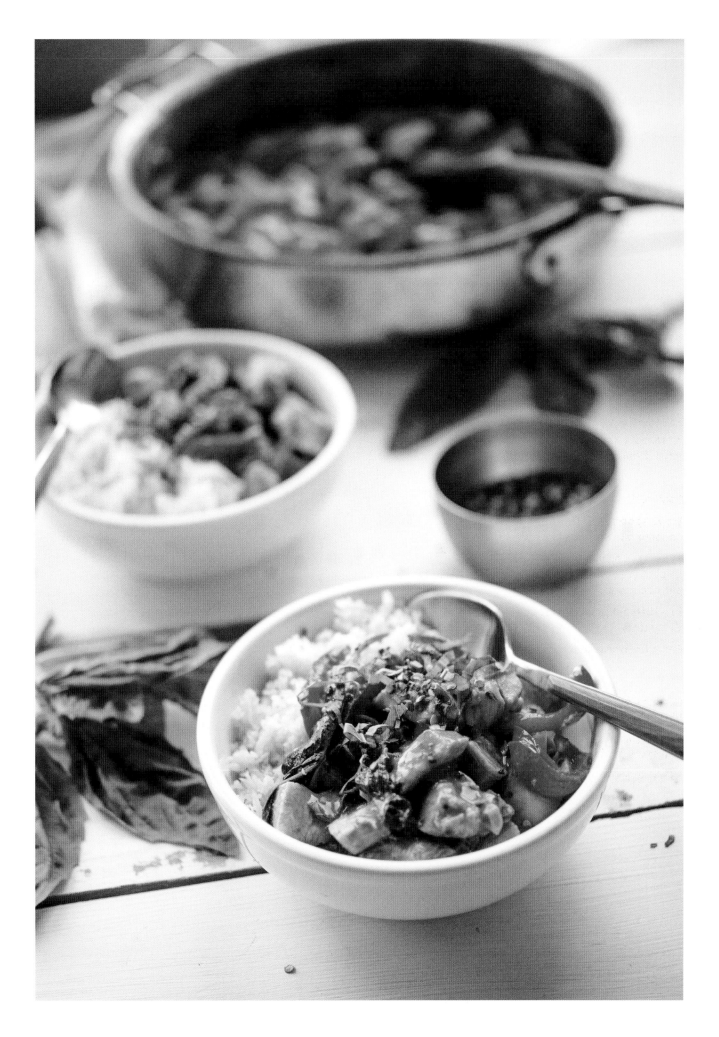

Rustic Pot Roast

This pot roast reminds me of home and a warm hug from my mom. If searing the meat and vegetables in advance is new to you, I encourage you to give it a go! It creates even more flavor and texture. This is a great meal to make for a hungry crowd. The recipe can be made in a slow cooker or in the oven. Because this makes so many servings, it's a great option to enjoy fresh and then freeze the leftovers for a healthy meal at another time!

NUT-FREE · EGG-FREE · OPTION AIP · OPTION LF · OPTION GAPS

prep time: 15 minutes | *cook time: 3½ to 6½ hours, depending on method* | *yield: 10 to 15 servings*

1 (5-pound) boneless chuck roast

1 teaspoon fine sea salt

½ teaspoon ground black pepper (omit for AIP)

3 tablespoons salted butter, divided (use coconut oil for AIP)

2 yellow onions (omit for low-FODMAP)

1 pound carrots, cut lengthwise into quarters

1 pound parsnips, cut lengthwise into quarters (omit for GAPS)

3 cups beef broth, store-bought or homemade (page 332), divided

2 teaspoons chopped fresh thyme (about 3 sprigs)

1 tablespoon chopped fresh rosemary (about 3 sprigs)

tips

- *Leftovers will keep refrigerated for up to 4 days or frozen for up to 5 months.*

- *To reheat on the stovetop, melt 1 tablespoon butter in a large frying pan over medium heat, then add the meat and vegetables and sauté for 4 to 5 minutes, until heated through. If frozen, place a lid on the frying pan and cook for an additional 4 to 5 minutes. To reheat in the microwave, cover with a paper towel and cook for 2 minutes if refrigerated or 4 to 5 minutes if frozen.*

1. Sprinkle all sides of the roast with the salt and pepper. Melt 2 tablespoons of the butter in a large heavy-bottomed pot, such as an enameled Dutch oven. (If planning to cook the roast in the oven, make sure to use an oven-safe pot.) Sear the roast over high heat for at least 4 minutes per side, until a brown crust appears. Once seared, transfer the roast to a slow cooker, or set aside on a rimmed baking sheet if using the oven cooking method.

2. While the meat is searing, prepare the onions: Cut the tips of the neck ends off the onions, leaving the root ends intact. From here, peel and then cut each onion into 4 wedges so that each piece has a corner of the root end still attached. (The root ends will help hold the wedges together.)

3. Over high heat, melt the remaining tablespoon of butter in the pot you used to sear the meat. Sear the onion wedges in the melted butter for 4 minutes per side, or until they develop a brown char. Transfer the seared onions to the slow cooker or to the baking sheet with the roast.

4. Working in batches, sear the carrots and parsnips in the pot for 4 minutes per side, or until they develop a brown char. Transfer the carrots and parsnips to the slow cooker or baking sheet.

5. Pour 2 cups of the broth into the now-empty pot. Using a whisk, stir up all of the browned bits on the bottom until they are incorporated into the broth.

6. Cook the roast using one of these two methods:

   Slow cooker option: Pour the broth in the pot over the meat and vegetables in the slow cooker. Add the remaining cup of broth and herbs. Cover and cook on high for 3 hours or on low for 6 hours.

   Oven option: Preheat the oven to 275°F. After deglazing the pot in Step 5, return the seared meat and vegetables to the pot and add the remaining cup of broth and herbs. Bake for 3 hours, or until the meat is tender.

APPROXIMATE NUTRITION BREAKDOWN	
(based on 1 of 15 servings)	
CALORIES: 387	FAT: 22 g
PROTEIN: 41 g	CARBS: 11 g

7. To serve, pull the roast from the broth and place it on a cutting board if you prefer to preslice it or on a platter for slicing at the table. Serve with the cooked vegetables and add additional salt as needed.

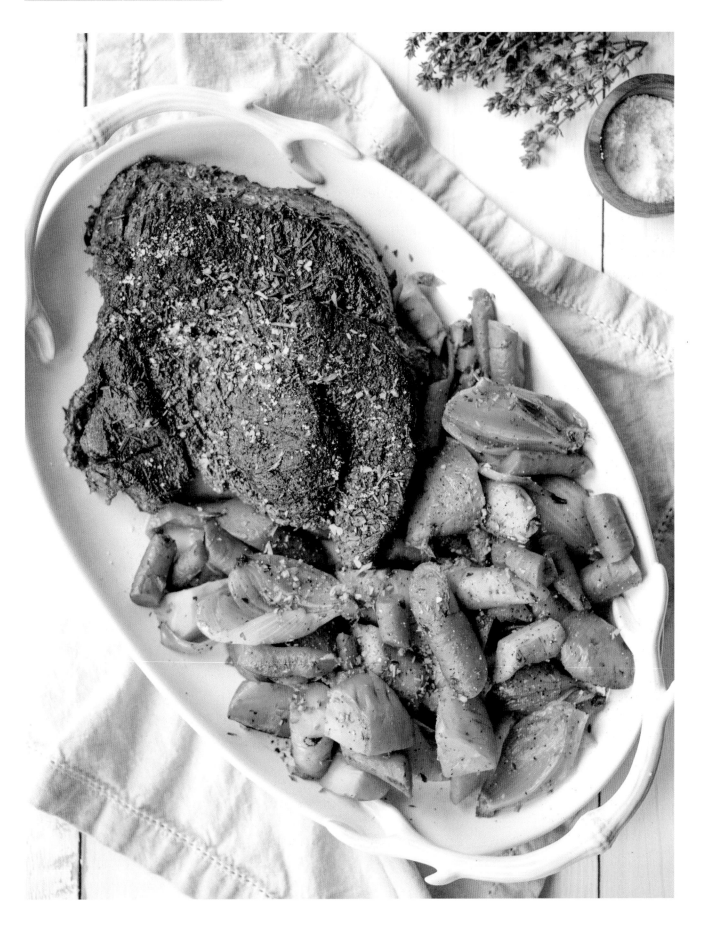

Shrimp Fried Rice

Sometimes a girl just needs a friggin' plate of shrimp fried rice, am I right? This dish is for you. It will squash that pesky Chinese takeout craving *and* leave you feeling healthy—I never met a Chinese takeout menu that could promise the same. Make it your own with extra coconut aminos or a squeeze of your favorite hot sauce.

OPTION

prep time: 15 minutes (not including the cauliflower rice)	*cook time: 20 minutes*	*yield: 2 to 4 servings*

3 tablespoons salted butter, divided

1 pound large shrimp, peeled, deveined, and patted dry

½ teaspoon fine sea salt

¼ teaspoon ground black pepper

½ teaspoon garlic powder

3 large eggs, lightly beaten

2 cups frozen peas

2 cups frozen sliced carrots

1 batch Basic Cauliflower Rice (page 130)

¼ cup fresh lemon juice (about 2 small lemons)

¼ cup coconut aminos

2 teaspoons sesame oil (untoasted) (use EVOO for nut-free)

1 teaspoon fish sauce

¼ cup sliced green onions (about 2 stalks)

2 tablespoons chopped fresh cilantro, for garnish

1. Melt 2 tablespoons of the butter in a large frying pan with a matching lid over medium-high heat. Sprinkle each side of the shrimp with the salt, pepper, and garlic powder. Once the butter is melted, add the shrimp and cook for 3 minutes per side, or until they turn pink. Remove the shrimp from the pan and place them in a bowl.

2. Melt the remaining tablespoon of butter in the pan over medium heat, then add the beaten eggs and cook until they are soft-scrambled, about 3 minutes. Transfer to the bowl with the shrimp.

3. Add the peas and carrots to the frying pan, cover, and allow to steam for 10 minutes. Once the carrots are easily pierced with a fork, add the cauliflower rice, lemon juice, coconut aminos, sesame oil, and fish sauce. Stir to combine, then return the shrimp and eggs to the pan. Stir in the green onions.

4. Plate, garnish with the cilantro, and enjoy warm.

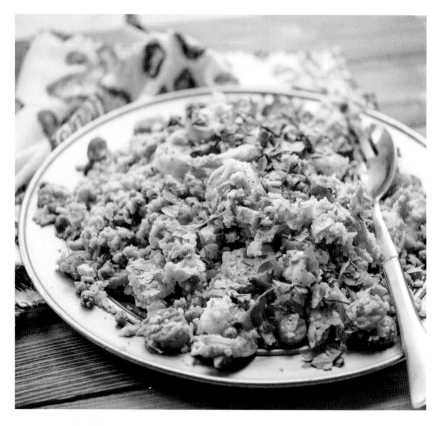

APPROXIMATE NUTRITION BREAKDOWN	
(based on 1 of 4 servings)	
CALORIES: 428	FAT: 18 g
PROTEIN: 33 g	CARBS: 35 g

The Frizzled Chicken Bake

This is the chicken that makes you want to call your mom to tell her about your amazing kitchen prowess. It's crispy, crunchy, filling, and flavorful. In other words, it's the best thing ever. Serve it alongside something that doesn't mind being overshadowed.

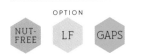

OPTION

NUT-FREE   LF   GAPS

½ cup mayo, store-bought or homemade (page 349)

1½ cups crushed pork rinds (see Tips)

1 teaspoon paprika

1 teaspoon garlic powder (omit for low-FODMAP)

2 pounds boneless, skinless chicken breast strips, rinsed and patted dry

½ teaspoon fine sea salt

tips

- *When choosing pork rinds, make sure that the ingredient list includes just two ingredients: pork skins and salt.*

prep time: 5 minutes (not including mayo) | *cook time: 25 minutes* | *yield: 4 to 6 servings*

1. Preheat the oven to 350°F. Line a rimmed baking sheet with parchment paper.

2. Place the mayo in a small bowl and the crushed pork rinds, paprika, and garlic powder in a separate bowl. Dip each chicken strip in the mayo and then in the pork rind mixture, patting it down so that the rinds form a crust on all sides.

3. Place the chicken on the prepared baking sheet, leaving at least 1 inch between the coated strips. Bake for 25 minutes, or until the juices run clear and the tops start to brown.

4. Remove from the oven, sprinkle with the salt, and serve warm.

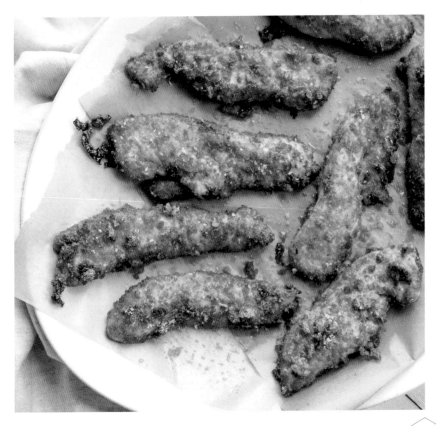

APPROXIMATE NUTRITION BREAKDOWN	
(based on 1 of 6 servings)	
CALORIES: 363	FAT: 21g
PROTEIN: 44g	CARBS: 1g

Tandoori Chicken Nuggets

WITH CILANTRO LIME YOGURT

These are the ultimate adult chicken nuggets. If you're having friends over for dinner, I suggest that you whip up a batch of these showstopping nuggets, open a bottle of wine, and bask in the glory of this Indian-inspired gourmet meal that makes the best leftovers. These nuggets are a regular feature in my make-then-freeze meal-prep routine for quick and delicious weeknight meals!

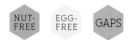

prep time: 10 minutes, plus at least 1 hour to marinate	*cook time: 25 minutes*	*yield: 6 to 8 servings*

2 pounds boneless, skinless chicken breasts, rinsed, patted dry, and cut into 2-inch cubes

TANDOORI MARINADE

Cream scooped from the top of 1 (13½-ounce) can chilled full-fat coconut milk (about ½ cup)

1 tablespoon liquid remaining in the can of coconut milk (from above)

3 tablespoons fresh lime juice (about 1½ limes)

3 cloves garlic, minced

1 (1-inch) piece fresh ginger, peeled and grated

1½ teaspoons fine sea salt

1 teaspoon garam masala

1 teaspoon ginger powder

1 teaspoon ground coriander

1 teaspoon ground cumin

1 teaspoon paprika

1 teaspoon turmeric powder

½ teaspoon cayenne pepper (see Tips)

CILANTRO LIME YOGURT

Cream scooped from the top of 1 (13½-ounce) can chilled full-fat coconut milk (about ½ cup)

1 tablespoon plus 1 teaspoon fresh lime juice (about 1 lime)

2 tablespoons chopped fresh cilantro, plus ½ teaspoon for garnish

1. Place the chicken in a large bowl.

2. In a food processor or blender, combine all of the ingredients for the marinade until smooth. Pour the marinade over the chicken and stir so that each piece is evenly coated. Cover and refrigerate for at least 1 hour or up to 8 hours.

Alternatively, you can put the chicken and marinade ingredients in a gallon-size resealable plastic bag and seal the bag closed. Gently shake the bag to combine the marinade ingredients until it's an even color. Place in the refrigerator for at least 1 hour or up to 8 hours.

3. To make the cilantro lime yogurt: Place the coconut cream, lime juice, and cilantro in a bowl. Whisk to combine until no lumps remain. Let the yogurt come to room temperature while the chicken marinates or refrigerate it until about 1 hour before you bake the chicken.

4. Preheat the oven to 400°F and line two baking sheets with parchment paper or aluminum foil. Remove the chicken pieces from the marinade, letting the excess marinade drip off. Place the chicken on the baking sheet, not letting any pieces touch. Bake for 15 minutes, then flip each piece over and bake for an additional 10 minutes.

5. Plate the chicken next to the yogurt, garnish with cilantro, and serve warm.

NUGGETS

APPROXIMATE NUTRITION BREAKDOWN *(based on 1 of 8 servings)*		
CALORIES: 173		FAT: 6g
PROTEIN: 26g		CARBS: 2g

YOGURT

APPROXIMATE NUTRITION BREAKDOWN *(based on 1 of 8 servings)*		
CALORIES: 27		FAT: 3g
PROTEIN: 0g		CARBS: 1g

• If you're sensitive to spice or want more or less heat, feel free to omit the cayenne pepper or adjust the amount to your liking. The yogurt will help take any unwanted heat off the tongue.

• When the chicken nuggets are finished cooking, the marinade will start to char on the paper or foil. This is normal!

• Leftovers will keep refrigerated for up to 4 days or frozen for up to 5 months.

• To defrost and reheat, place the nuggets in a preheated 370°F oven for 20 minutes if frozen or 15 minutes if refrigerated, or microwave on high for 4 to 5 minutes if frozen or 2 minutes if refrigerated.

• The yogurt will be firm when chilled. I recommend letting it come to room temperature before serving.

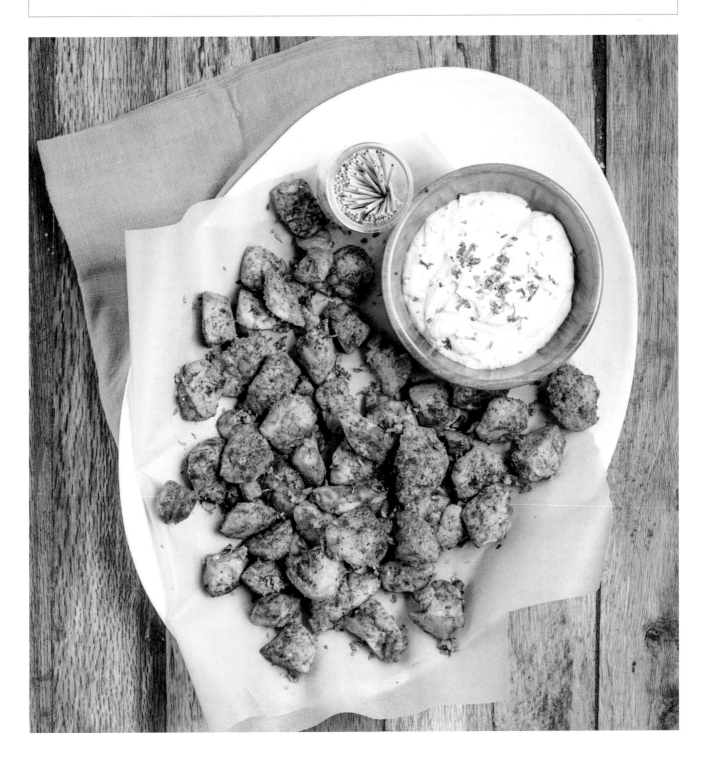

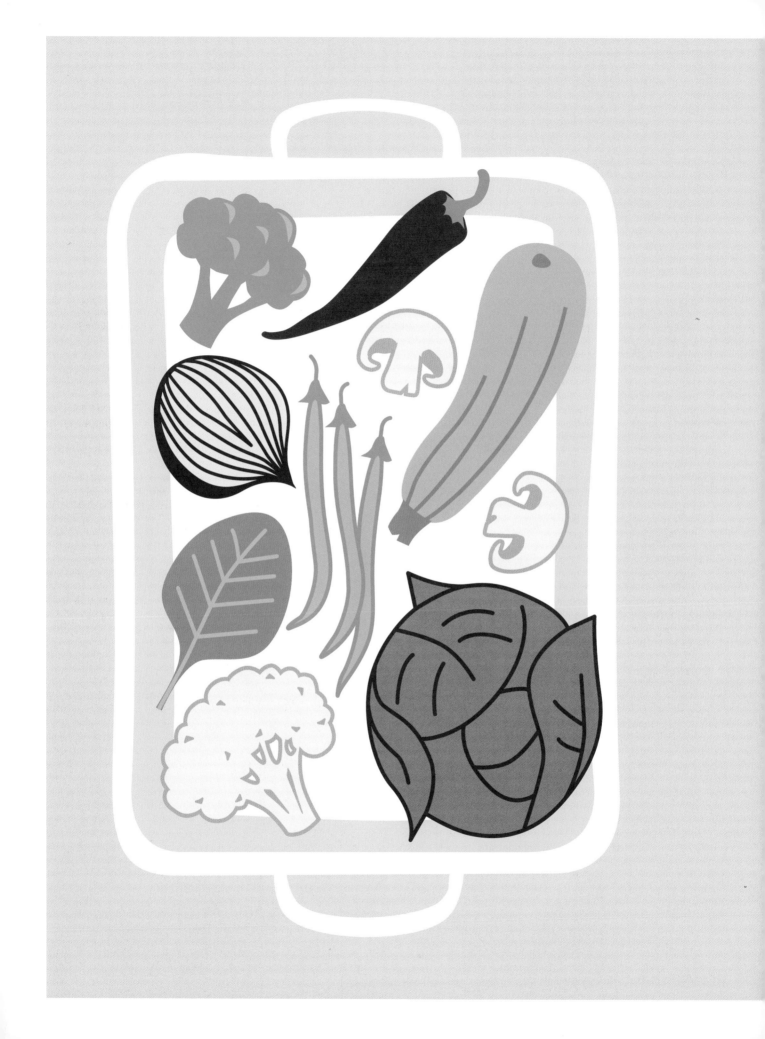

CHAPTER 8
VIBRANT VEGGIES

 Cauliflower "Potato" Salad
262

 Dirty Cauliflower Rice
264

 Mexican Cauliflower Rice
264

 Lemon Garlic Cauliflower Rice
264

 Cilantro Lime Cauliflower Rice
264

 Crispy Garlic Green Beans
266

 Lemon Garlic Spaghetti Squash
267

 Sautéed Lemon Garlic Spinach
268

 Lemony Bacon Super Greens
269

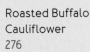 Loaded Cauliflower Mac & Cheese
270

 Mushroom Risotto
272

 N'Orzo Salad
274

 Roasted Buffalo Cauliflower
276

 Roasted Garlic Cauliflower Mash
277

 Scout Cabbage
278

 Summer Squash Casserole
280

 Tangy New-Fashioned Coleslaw
281

 Whole Brussels Bake
282

Zesty Okra Fries
283

Download the Fed & Fit iPhone and Android app! You can scan the above QR codes directly in the app, which will then populate a consolidated grocery shopping list for the scanned recipes.

Cauliflower "Potato" Salad

I can't even begin to tell you how many unsuspecting potluck BBQ attendees have been fooled by this "potato" salad. Along with a raw veggie tray, this salad is a great way to balance out the usual BBQ plate starches and breads with a flavorful bonus side dish. It also stores really well, so it's an ideal dish to make in advance!

prep time: 15 minutes (not including the ranch) | *cook time: 45 minutes* | *yield: 8 servings*

1 large head cauliflower, cut into florets and then into ½-inch dice (about 4 cups)

2 teaspoons extra-virgin olive oil

½ teaspoon fine sea salt

¼ teaspoon ground black pepper

½ teaspoon garlic powder

1 cup 3-Ingredient Paleo Ranch (page 338)

3 stalks celery, chopped (about 1 cup)

½ cup finely chopped dill pickles or dill relish

1 bunch green onions, chopped

3 tablespoons prepared yellow mustard

6 hard-boiled eggs, sliced into rounds

½ teaspoon paprika

1. Preheat the oven to 375°F. Line a rimmed baking sheet with parchment paper.

2. Toss the cauliflower florets in the olive oil, then spread them out on the prepared baking sheet so that no pieces are touching. Sprinkle the tops with the salt, pepper, and garlic powder. Bake for 45 minutes, or until the tops are starting to turn golden brown. Let cool completely before assembling the salad.

3. When the cauliflower is cool, place it in a large mixing bowl. Add the ranch dressing, celery, pickles, green onions, and mustard. Stir until everything is well mixed and evenly coated with the dressing.

4. To serve, spoon the salad into a serving bowl. Top with the hard-boiled egg slices, then sprinkle the paprika over the top. Serve at room temperature or chilled. Leftovers will keep in the refrigerator for up to 5 days.

tips

• If I'm using a powdered seasoning (other than salt and pepper) to flavor a veggie or protein headed to the oven, I like to sprinkle it on last. I've found that salt and pepper have a harder time finding a place to stick if the food is already coated in another fine powder (like garlic powder, in this instance).

• This is a great dish to make for a party! Make it the day before so you can just pull it out of the chiller before your guests arrive.

APPROXIMATE NUTRITION BREAKDOWN *(per serving)*		
CALORIES: 329		FAT: 29 g
PROTEIN: 7 g		CARBS: 9 g

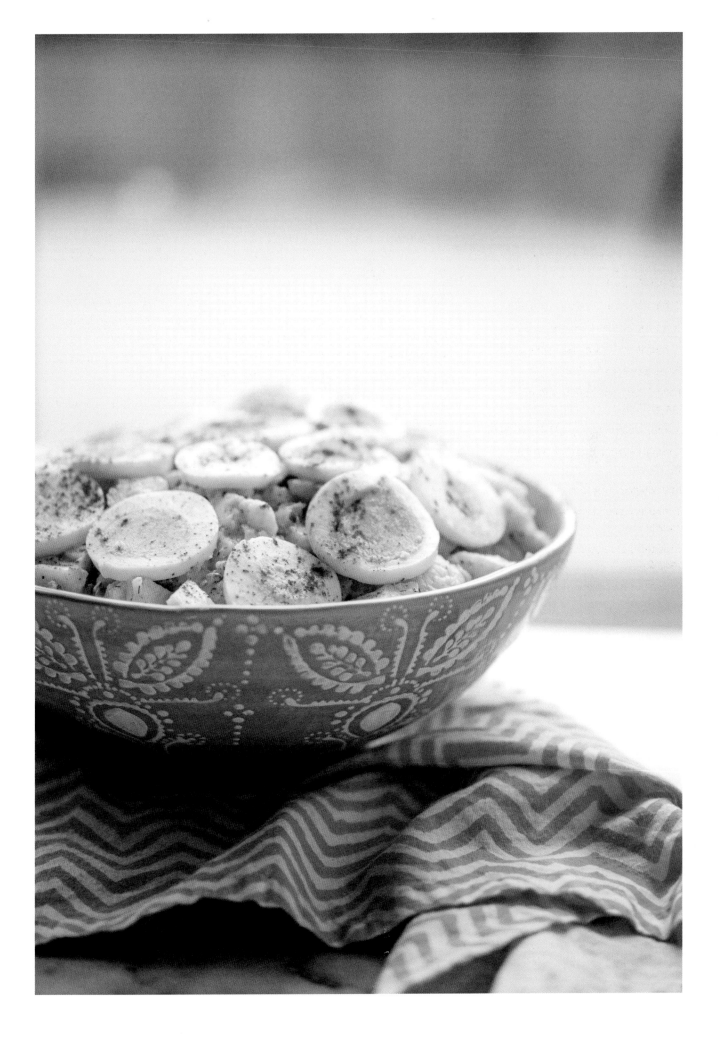

Cauliflower Rice

4 Ways

Oh, the possibilities! Rice made from cauliflower isn't as strange as it may sound. Trust me on this. Once you cook it up and add your flavorings of choice, you'll have a magical vegetable vehicle ready to fill the bowl underneath your favorite protein. It's a great meal component to make in advance. This "rice" freezes exceptionally well and can add a versatile, healthy dose of vegetable to any meal. Don't know which variety to try first? I am a true Garcia, so the Mexican Rice is probably my favorite. If you're looking for a plain cauli-rice that will accept the flavor of anything it's paired with, stop after Step 1.

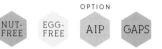

NUT-FREE · EGG-FREE · OPTION AIP · GAPS

prep time: 5 to 10 minutes

cook time: 15 to 30 minutes

yield: 4 servings

FOR ALL RECIPES

1 large head cauliflower, riced (about 3 cups)

1 tablespoon salted butter (use coconut oil for AIP)

DIRTY RICE

½ pound hot Italian sausage (use ground pork for AIP)

½ cup chopped white onions (about ½ medium onion)

½ cup chopped celery (1 to 2 stalks)

1 green bell pepper, seeded and finely chopped (omit for AIP)

4 cloves garlic, minced

2 tablespoons fresh lemon juice (about 1 small lemon)

¼ cup chopped fresh parsley

1 teaspoon fine sea salt

¼ teaspoon ground black pepper (omit for AIP)

LEMON GARLIC RICE

2 tablespoons fresh lemon juice (about 1 small lemon)

½ teaspoon garlic powder

½ teaspoon fine sea salt

¼ teaspoon ground black pepper (omit for AIP)

CILANTRO LIME RICE

½ cup finely chopped fresh cilantro

⅓ cup fresh lime juice (about 3 limes)

½ teaspoon fine sea salt

¼ teaspoon ground black pepper (omit for AIP)

MEXICAN RICE (NOT AIP FRIENDLY)

1 tablespoon salted butter

½ cup chopped white onions (about ½ medium onion)

1 (28-ounce) can diced tomatoes, thoroughly drained

1 (7-ounce) can diced green chilies, drained

2 tablespoons lime juice (about 1 lime)

1 teaspoon ground cumin

½ teaspoon fine sea salt

¼ teaspoon ground black pepper

DIRTY RICE

APPROXIMATE NUTRITION BREAKDOWN (per serving)	
CALORIES: 283	FAT: 18 g
PROTEIN: 14 g	CARBS: 18 g

LEMON GARLIC RICE

APPROXIMATE NUTRITION BREAKDOWN (per serving)	
CALORIES: 81	FAT: 3 g
PROTEIN: 4 g	CARBS: 11 g

CILANTRO LIME RICE

APPROXIMATE NUTRITION BREAKDOWN (per serving)	
CALORIES: 90	FAT: 3 g
PROTEIN: 4 g	CARBS: 12 g

MEXICAN RICE

APPROXIMATE NUTRITION BREAKDOWN (per serving)	
CALORIES: 177	FAT: 6 g
PROTEIN: 6 g	CARBS: 26 g

tips

• To "rice" cauliflower, either grate the cauliflower by hand using the largest holes on a box grater or affix the grating attachment to a food processor and let it do the work for you.

1. Steam the riced cauliflower using one of these two methods:

Microwave option: Place the riced cauliflower in a microwave-safe bowl with ¼ cup water. Cover and microwave on high for 10 minutes, until cooked through. Let cool slightly, then drain. Add the butter and toss to combine.

Stovetop option: Melt the butter in a large frying pan or sauté pan with a tight-fitting lid over medium heat, then add the riced cauliflower. Stir to incorporate, then cover the pan. Let steam over medium-low heat for 12 to 15 minutes, until the cauliflower is cooked through.

For Dirty Rice: In a large frying pan or sauté pan over high heat, cook the sausage for about 10 minutes, until browned and crispy, using a spatula to break it up as it cooks. Using a slotted spoon, transfer the sausage to a bowl, leaving the grease behind. To the grease, add the onions and cook for about 5 minutes, until translucent. Add the celery, bell pepper, and garlic. Stir and cook until the celery and bell pepper have softened,

about 5 minutes. Return the sausage to the pan and add the cooked cauliflower rice. Add the lemon juice, parsley, salt, and pepper and stir to combine. Leave on the heat for about 5 minutes, until the rice is hot. Serve warm.

For Mexican Rice: Melt the butter in a large frying pan or sauté pan over high heat. Add the onions, stir, and cook for 10 minutes, or until translucent and starting to brown. Add the cooked cauliflower rice, tomatoes, chilies, lime juice, cumin, salt, and pepper and stir to combine. Leave on the heat for about 5 minutes, until the rice is hot. Serve warm.

For Lemon Garlic Rice: Combine the cooked cauliflower rice, lemon juice, garlic powder, salt, and pepper in a large mixing bowl. Stir to combine and enjoy!

For Cilantro Lime Rice: Combine the cooked cauliflower rice with the cilantro, lime juice, salt, and pepper in a large mixing bowl. Stir to combine and enjoy!

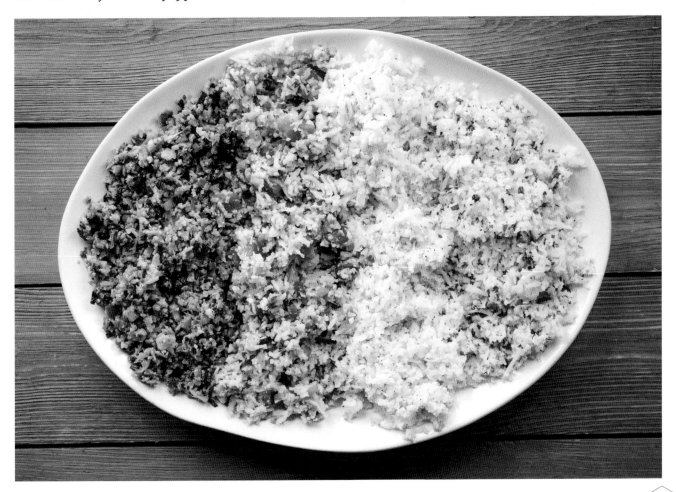

Crispy Garlic Green Beans

Steamed green beans are delicate and lovely, but I prefer mine with a sprinkle of garlic and sea salt and that fresh-out-of-the-oven crunch. When they're prepared like this, I find myself wanting a heaping helping next to an impressive bunless burger on my plate. If you serve them like French fries, consider doubling the batch—they go quick!

NUT-FREE · EGG-FREE · OPTION AIP · OPTION LF · GAPS

prep time: 5 minutes | *cook time: 30 minutes* | *yield: 4 servings*

1 pound fresh green beans

1 tablespoon extra-virgin olive oil

½ teaspoon fine sea salt

¼ teaspoon ground black pepper (omit for AIP)

½ teaspoon garlic powder (omit for low-FODMAP)

1. Preheat the oven to 400°F. Line a rimmed baking sheet with parchment paper.

2. Toss the green beans in the olive oil and spread them out evenly on the prepared baking sheet. Sprinkle the tops with the salt, pepper, and garlic powder. Bake for 30 minutes, or until the tops are starting to turn brown but before the ends burn. Serve warm!

3. These green beans freeze and reheat really well. I recommend freezing them on a baking sheet until solid, then transferring them to freezer bags for up to 5 months of storage. Reheat the frozen beans (no need to defrost) either in the microwave on high for 3 to 4 minutes or in a preheated 350°F oven for 25 minutes.

tips

- *If you want even more flavor, try adding a squeeze of fresh lemon juice to the crispy green beans before serving. This is a great way to brighten the flavor without having to add more salt.*

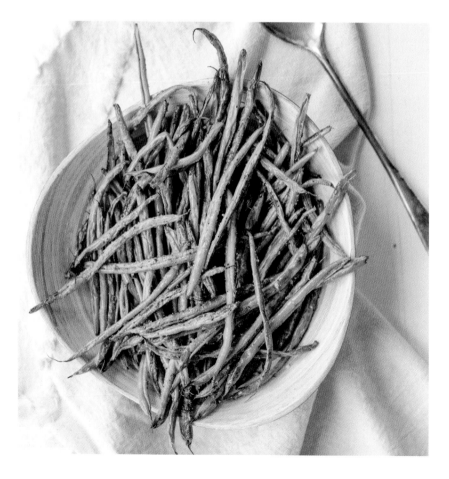

APPROXIMATE NUTRITION BREAKDOWN *(per serving)*			
CALORIES:	65	FAT:	3 g
PROTEIN:	3 g	CARBS:	8 g

Lemon Garlic Spaghetti Squash

I'm a lemon garlic spaghetti girl. Back in my pre-Paleo days, lemon garlic angel hair pasta was an occasional indulgence that always left me feeling bloated and sick. Now I can have this much healthier lemon garlic "spaghetti" as often as I like, and it makes me feel like a million bucks. This dish is a great base for a lot of proteins and casseroles—get creative!

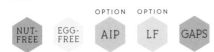

NUT-FREE | EGG-FREE | OPTION AIP | OPTION LF | GAPS

| *prep time: 5 minutes* | *cook time: 1 hour 10 minutes* | *yield: 6 servings* |

1 medium spaghetti squash (about 5 pounds)

2 tablespoons salted butter (use coconut oil for AIP)

3 cloves garlic, minced (omit for low-FODMAP)

¼ cup fresh lemon juice (about 2 small lemons)

1 teaspoon fine sea salt

¼ teaspoon ground black pepper (omit for AIP)

1 tablespoon chopped fresh flat-leaf parsley, for garnish (optional)

tips

• *This squash will keep refrigerated for up to 5 days or frozen for up to 5 months.*

1. Preheat the oven to 375°F.

2. Using a sharp knife and working carefully, pierce the squash four or five times through the flesh and into the center. Place on a rimmed baking sheet and bake for 1 hour, or until the squash gives when gently poked with a large spoon or pressed with your hand in an oven mitt. Let cool for at least 30 minutes.

3. When the squash is cool enough to handle, use a serrated or really sharp knife to cut it in half lengthwise. Use a large spoon to scrape out and dispose of the seeds.

4. In a large frying pan or sauté pan, melt the butter over medium-high heat. Once the butter is melted, add the garlic and cook for about 4 minutes, until fragrant but not brown. Add the cooked spaghetti squash to the pan and stir to combine. Add the lemon juice, salt, and pepper and stir until any remaining clumps of squash are broken up into individual strands. Leave on the heat for about 5 minutes, until the squash is hot and bubbling. Transfer to a serving bowl, top with the parsley, and enjoy!

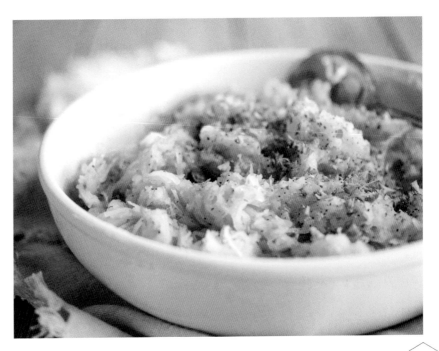

APPROXIMATE NUTRITION BREAKDOWN	
(per serving)	
CALORIES: 66	FAT: 4g
PROTEIN: 1g	CARBS: 8g

Sautéed Lemon Garlic Spinach

Spinach made this way goes fast in my house. Like, really fast. In fact, I've been known to cook up a pound of raw spinach for each person at the dinner table. I feel confident that Popeye would've ditched the cans if he'd known about this flavorful version of his favorite green.

NUT-FREE · EGG-FREE · OPTION AIP · OPTION LF · GAPS

prep time: 3 minutes | *cook time: 15 minutes* | *yield: 4 servings*

1 tablespoon salted butter (use coconut oil for AIP)

4 cloves garlic, minced (omit for low-FODMAP)

1 pound fresh spinach (about 6 heaping cups)

1 tablespoon fresh lemon juice (about ½ small lemon)

¼ teaspoon fine sea salt

⅛ teaspoon ground black pepper (omit for AIP)

1. In a medium-sized saucepan or frying pan with a tight-fitting lid, melt the butter over high heat. Add the garlic and cook for about 5 minutes, until fragrant. Add the spinach, stir, cover, and cook for 4 minutes, or until all of the spinach is cooked down.

2. Add the lemon juice, salt, and pepper and stir to combine. Serve warm.

tips

• *Leftovers will keep refrigerated for up to 5 days.*

• *This recipe is easily doubled or tripled (or quadrupled!). Just cook the spinach in batches if it won't all fit in the pan at one time.*

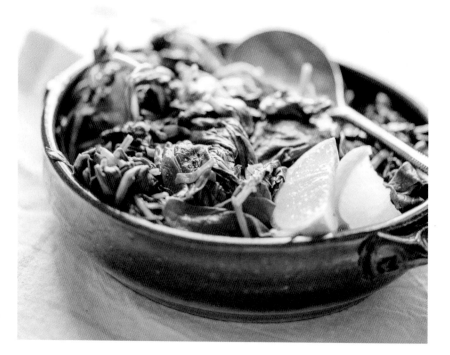

APPROXIMATE NUTRITION BREAKDOWN *(per serving)*			
CALORIES:	57	FAT:	3 g
PROTEIN:	3 g	CARBS:	5 g

Lemony Bacon Super Greens

Super greens! How many times have you heard that you need to eat more leafy greens? It's been said so often that it's beginning to sound like white noise. While the advice is sage, chewing on tough, thick greens isn't everyone's jam. That's where these greens come to the rescue! The lemon and bacon (and the process of wilting the greens) make this a truly craveable side dish packed with necessary vitamins, minerals, and fiber. Feel free to get creative with the greens you add!

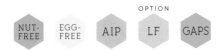

prep time: 10 minutes | *cook time: 20 minutes* | *yield: 6 servings*

1 pound bacon, chopped

4 cloves garlic, minced (omit for low-FODMAP)

1 bunch collard greens, destemmed and chopped

1 bunch kale, destemmed and chopped

¼ cup fresh lemon juice (about 2 small lemons)

1 teaspoon fine sea salt

1. In a large saucepan or frying pan with a lid, cook the bacon over medium heat for about 10 minutes, until crispy. Transfer the bacon to a bowl, leaving the fat in the pan. Add the garlic to the bacon fat and cook for 5 minutes, or until fragrant.

2. Add the chopped greens and toss them in the fat. Place the lid on the pan and let steam over medium heat for about 5 minutes, until the greens are wilted. (The exact timing will depend on the toughness of the greens.) If the pan won't hold all of the greens at once, wilt the greens in batches, adding more as space becomes available.

3. Once all of the greens are cooked down and wilted, add the lemon juice and salt and stir to combine. Serve warm.

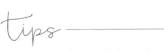

Tips

• *This recipe calls for collards and kale, but you can definitely toss in Swiss chard, spinach, or whatever else is in season. Cooking times will vary depending on the type of greens you use (chard and spinach, for example, are more tender than kale and collards and will cook more quickly) and the size and age of the greens (large, mature leaves are tougher than their young, tender counterparts).*

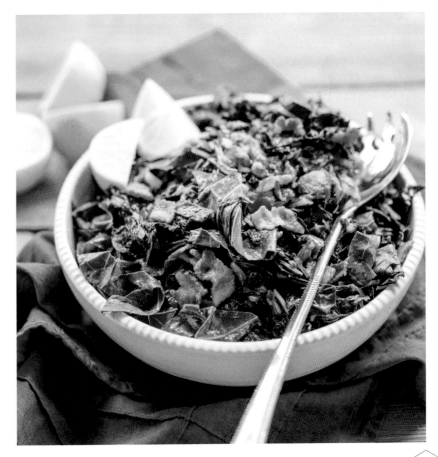

APPROXIMATE NUTRITION BREAKDOWN *(per serving)*			
CALORIES:	174	FAT:	13 g
PROTEIN:	7 g	CARBS:	10 g

Loaded Cauliflower Mac & Cheese

I've waited years to share this recipe. Years! Back in my brief days of following a vegan template, nutritional yeast was my go-to when I had a craving for anything cheesy. This combination of cheesy nutritional yeast, tender cauliflower, and bacon makes for a seemingly decadent treat that sneaks a lot of healthy nutrients onto your plate.

NUT-FREE · EGG-FREE · AIP (OPTION) · GAPS

prep time: 15 minutes | *cook time: 30 minutes* | *yield: 4 to 6 servings*

½ pound bacon, thinly sliced crosswise

2 heads cauliflower

½ cup full-fat coconut milk

½ cup nutritional yeast

½ teaspoon fine sea salt

¼ teaspoon ground black pepper (omit for AIP)

1 teaspoon finely chopped fresh chives, for garnish

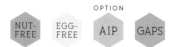

tips

• *Nutritional yeast is an excellent source of B vitamins. You can find this yellow powder in the natural foods aisle of your local grocery or at a natural foods store.*

1. In a wide soup pot or heavy-bottomed saucepan, cook the bacon over medium-high heat until crispy. Using a slotted spoon, scoop the bacon into a bowl. Drain off most of the fat remaining in the pan, but don't wipe the pan down.

2. While the bacon is cooking, cut the cauliflower florets away from the stems. (You should have 6 cups of florets.) Steam the cauliflower using one of these two methods:

   Stovetop method: Bring about 4 inches of water to a boil in a large pot. Place the cauliflower in a colander or steamer basket that sits above the water and steam for 10 to 15 minutes, until the cauliflower gives easily when poked with a fork.

   Microwave method: Place the cauliflower in a large microwaveable bowl with ¼ cup water. Cover and microwave on high for 10 minutes, or until the cauliflower gives easily when poked with a fork.

3. Transfer the steamed cauliflower to the pot you used to cook the bacon. Add the remaining ingredients, except the chives, and stir to combine. Cook over medium heat for about 5 minutes, then remove from the heat. Stir in half of the bacon and transfer to a serving dish. Garnish with the remaining half of the bacon and the chives. Serve warm.

APPROXIMATE NUTRITION BREAKDOWN *(based on 1 of 6 servings)*	
CALORIES: 175	FAT: 10 g
PROTEIN: 9 g	CARBS: 16 g

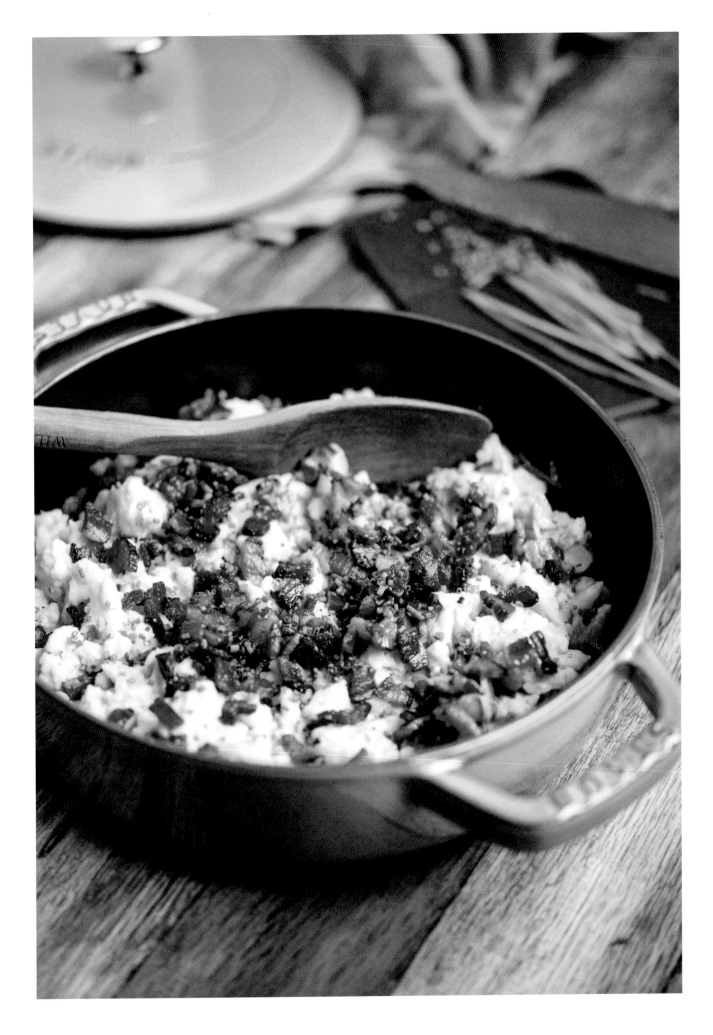

Mushroom Risotto

This dish is brought to you by the part of my brain that's completely enamored of Ina Garten. Whenever I make risotto, roasted chicken, or bright salads worthy of friends and fresh floral arrangements, I think to myself, "How easy was that?" and daydream about our imaginary house in East Hampton.

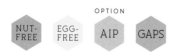

OPTION

NUT-FREE | EGG-FREE | AIP | GAPS

prep time: 15 minutes | *cook time: 50 minutes* | *yield: 8 servings*

4 slices thick-cut bacon (about ¾ pound), chopped

½ medium onion, finely chopped

4 cloves garlic, minced

1 pound crimini mushrooms, sliced

2 tablespoons salted butter (use coconut oil for AIP)

2 heads cauliflower, riced (about 6 cups)

Cream scooped from the top of 1 chilled (13½-ounce) can full-fat coconut milk (about ½ cup)

¼ cup fresh lemon juice (about 2 small lemons)

1 teaspoon fine sea salt

¼ teaspoon ground black pepper (omit for AIP)

2 tablespoons chopped fresh flat-leaf parsley, for garnish

1. In a large sauté pan with a matching lid, cook the bacon over high heat until crispy, about 10 minutes. Using a slotted spoon, transfer the cooked bacon to a bowl, leaving the fat in the pan.

2. Add the chopped onion to the pan, toss to coat, and cook for 10 minutes, or until the onion is starting to brown. Reduce the heat to medium, stir in the garlic, and cook for another 5 minutes, or until fragrant. Add the mushrooms, toss, and cook until they have reduced in size and are starting to brown, about 10 minutes. Transfer the mixture to the bowl with the bacon and set aside.

3. In the same pan, melt the butter over medium heat. Add the riced cauliflower and toss to coat. Cover with the lid and let steam for 5 minutes, stirring occasionally to make sure that the rice doesn't burn. Remove the lid and let the rice cook for an additional 5 minutes, or until slightly softened.

4. Add the coconut cream, lemon juice, salt, and pepper to the rice. Stir until the coconut milk is melted and the ingredients are well combined. Bring to a simmer over medium heat, then return the bacon and mushroom mixture to the pan. Stir to combine, bring back up to a simmer, and then remove from the heat. Serve warm, garnished with fresh parsley.

tips

- *Leftovers will keep in the refrigerator for up to 5 days or in the freezer for up to 5 months.*

APPROXIMATE NUTRITION BREAKDOWN (per serving)			
CALORIES:	213	FAT:	15 g
PROTEIN:	7 g	CARBS:	15 g

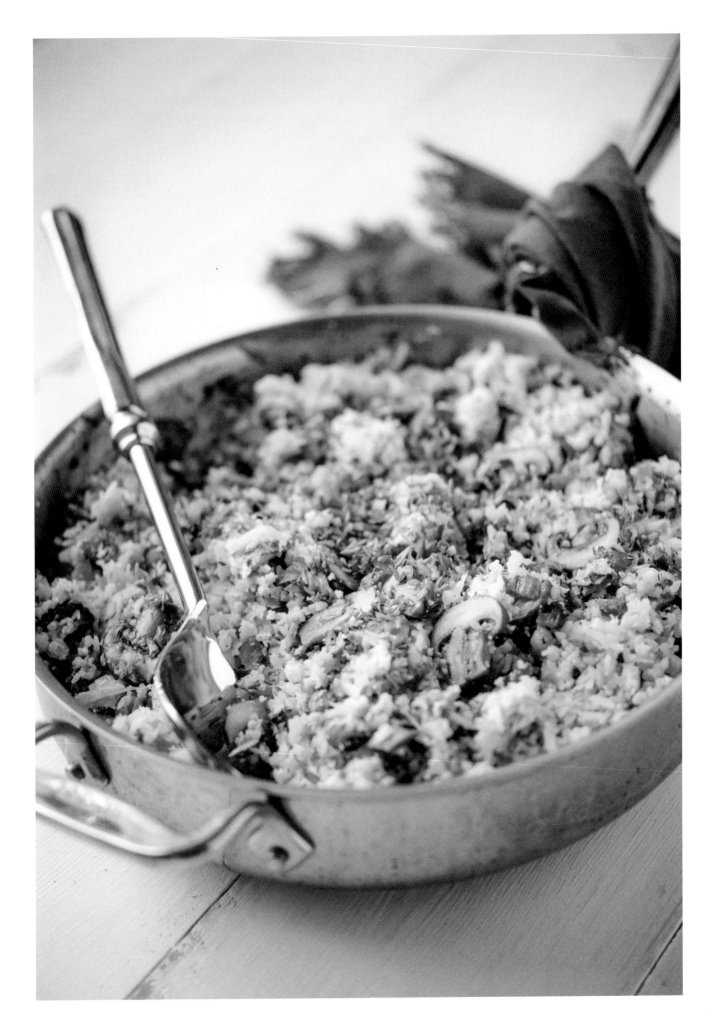

N'Orzo Salad

I could eat orzo salad by the bucketful. It's not the pasta itself that I love so much, but the roasted veggies and the bright lemony dressing. This extremely healthy version is a great replacement for my beloved orzo salad! With cauliflower rice as a stand-in for the orzo, you can get really creative with the roasted veggies. Feel free to roast whatever veggies you have on hand.

OPTION

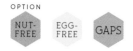

prep time: 15 minutes, plus 1 hour to cool the rice and roasted veggies | *cook time: 45 minutes* | *yield: 8 servings*

ROASTED VEGGIES

2 pints cherry tomatoes

1 yellow bell pepper, seeded, destemmed, and cut into 1-inch cubes

1 red bell pepper, seeded, destemmed, and cut into 1-inch cubes

2 medium carrots, peeled and cut into 1-inch discs

1 large red onion, roughly chopped

3 tablespoons extra-virgin olive oil

1 teaspoon fine sea salt

½ teaspoon ground black pepper

"ORZO"

1 head cauliflower, riced (about 3 cups)

1 tablespoon salted butter (for stovetop option)

½ cup chopped fresh cilantro leaves and stems

4 green onions, finely chopped

½ cup fresh lemon juice (about 4 small lemons)

1 teaspoon fine sea salt

¼ teaspoon ground black pepper

⅓ cup pine nuts, toasted, for garnish (omit for nut-free)

1. Prepare the roasted veggies: Preheat the oven to 375°F. Line two rimmed baking sheets with parchment paper. Toss the veggies in the olive oil. Spread them out in the prepared baking sheets so that no two pieces overlap. Sprinkle the tops with the salt and pepper. Bake for 45 minutes, or until the tops start to turn brown. Allow the veggies to cool before using.

2. While the veggies are in the oven, steam the riced cauliflower using one of these two methods:

   Microwave option: Place the riced cauliflower in a microwave-safe bowl with ¼ cup water. Cover and microwave on high for 10 minutes, until cooked through. Let cool slightly, then drain. Add the butter and toss to combine.

   Stovetop option: Melt the butter in a large frying pan or sauté pan over medium heat. When the butter is melted, add the riced cauliflower. Stir to incorporate, then cover the pan. Let steam over medium-low heat for 12 to 15 minutes, until the cauliflower is cooked through.

3. Let the cauliflower rice cool completely by spreading it out on a baking sheet and leaving it at room temperature or transferring it to the refrigerator for about 1 hour.

4. Once the rice is cool, place it in a large mixing bowl. Add the cooled roasted veggies, green onions, cilantro, lemon juice, salt, and pepper and toss to combine. Serve chilled, with the pine nuts on top.

tips

- *Save yourself some time the day of and roast the veggies or cook the cauliflower rice the day before!*

- *Boost the flavor of the pine nuts by carefully roasting them in a dry frying pan over medium heat for 3 to 4 minutes, until fragrant but not burnt.*

APPROXIMATE NUTRITION BREAKDOWN *(per serving)*			
CALORIES:	165	FAT:	11 g
PROTEIN:	4 g	CARBS:	16 g

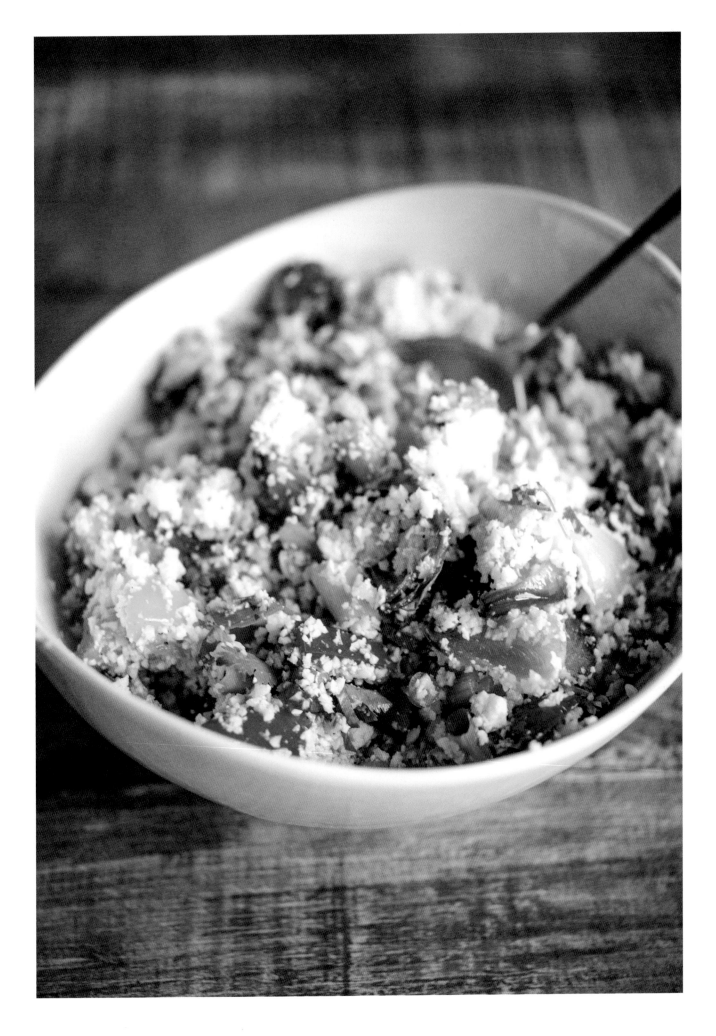

Roasted Buffalo Cauliflower

This may be my favorite recipe in the entire book. I know this is a strange declaration; we're talking about a cauliflower side dish, after all. It's just that good. This dish will make a cauliflower believer out of anyone, mark my words. Serve it alongside some simple proteins or in a bowl topped with barbacoa (page 214) or carnitas (page 216).

prep time: 10 minutes (not including the Buffalo sauce) | *cook time: 40 minutes* | *yield: 6 servings*

2 heads cauliflower, trimmed and cut into florets (about 6 cups)

2 teaspoons extra-virgin olive oil

¼ teaspoon fine sea salt

¼ cup mayo, store-bought or homemade (page 349)

2 tablespoons Buffalo Sauce (page 337)

Sliced fresh chives, for garnish (optional)

1. Preheat the oven to 375°F. Line a rimmed baking sheet with parchment paper.

2. Toss the cauliflower florets in the olive oil. Lay them out on the prepared baking sheet, then sprinkle the tops with the salt. Bake for 30 minutes, or until the tops are just starting to turn golden brown.

3. While the cauliflower is baking, whisk the mayo and Buffalo sauce together in a large mixing bowl.

4. Pull the cauliflower from the oven and pour it into the mixing bowl with the Buffalo sauce. Toss so that each piece is evenly coated, then place the cauliflower back on the baking sheet.

5. Increase the oven temperature to 400°F. Return the cauliflower to the oven and bake for 8 to 10 minutes, until the tops have started to brown slightly and the sauce has formed a light crust.

6. Serve warm, garnished with chives, if desired.

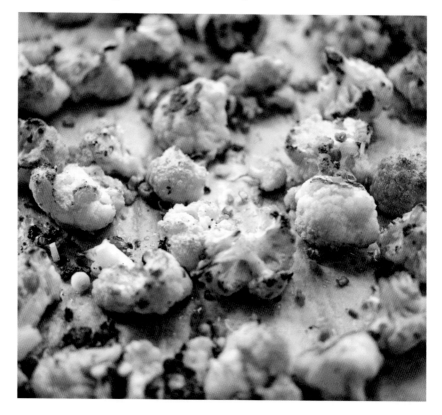

APPROXIMATE NUTRITION BREAKDOWN *(per serving)*			
CALORIES:	167	FAT:	12 g
PROTEIN:	5 g	CARBS:	14 g

Roasted Garlic Cauliflower Mash

All I can say is, you've never had a cauliflower mash like this. The roasted garlic adds a serious depth of flavor, the coconut milk provides a delectable creaminess, and the lemon juice delivers the brightness that we often seek when we add sour cream to mashed potatoes. This is vegetable side heaven, and I can't wait for you to try it.

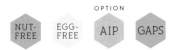

NUT-FREE   EGG-FREE   OPTION AIP   GAPS

prep time: 10 minutes (not including the roasted garlic)	cook time: 20 minutes	yield: 6 servings

2 heads cauliflower, trimmed and cut into florets (about 6 cups)

1 tablespoon salted butter (use coconut oil for AIP)

1 bulb roasted garlic (page 346)

Cream scooped from the top of 1 chilled (13½-ounce) can full-fat coconut milk (about ½ cup)

2 tablespoons salted butter (use coconut oil for AIP)

1 tablespoon fresh lemon juice (about ½ small lemon)

1 teaspoon fine sea salt

¼ teaspoon ground black pepper (omit for AIP)

1 tablespoon chopped fresh chives, for garnish

1. Steam the cauliflower by using one of these two methods:

   Microwave option: Place the cauliflower in a microwave-safe bowl with ¼ cup water. Cover and microwave on high for 10 minutes, until cooked through. Let cool slightly, then drain. Add the butter and toss to combine.

   Stovetop option: Melt the butter in a large frying pan or sauté pan over medium heat. When the butter is melted, add the riced cauliflower. Stir to incorporate, then cover the pan. Let steam over medium-low heat for 12 to 15 minutes, until the cauliflower is cooked through.

2. Place the cooked cauliflower in a food processor or large mixing bowl. Squeeze the roasted garlic from the cloves into the bowl, then add the rest of the ingredients, except the chives. Blend until smooth. Transfer to a serving bowl, garnish with the chives, and serve warm.

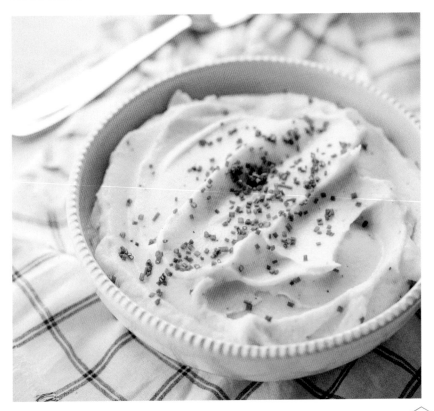

APPROXIMATE NUTRITION BREAKDOWN *(per serving)*	
CALORIES: 162	FAT: 10 g
PROTEIN: 6 g	CARBS: 17 g

Scout Cabbage

This recipe takes me all the way back to my days as a Girl Scout. In fact, this is probably the only recipe in my Girl Scout recipe Rolodex that would qualify for this book! Anyhoo, this is the cabbage recipe that launched a thousand middle school camping girls' smiles. I've elevated the dish a bit, but the principle is the same: upside-down cabbage is flavored at each layer with bacon filling. Although we used to toss the whole thing in the fire, you can achieve the same tasty effect with your oven. Enjoy!

OPTION

NUT-FREE · EGG-FREE · AIP · GAPS

| prep time: 10 minutes | cook time: 1½ hours | yield: 4 servings |

½ pound bacon, cut into ½-inch pieces

½ medium onion, chopped

2 tablespoons fresh lemon juice (about 1 small lemon)

1 head green cabbage

1 lemon, quartered

2 tablespoons chopped fresh flat-leaf parsley, for garnish

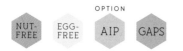

tips

- Leftovers will keep refrigerated for up to 5 days or frozen for up to 5 months.

1. Preheat the oven to 375°F.

2. Cook the bacon in a large frying pan over medium heat for about 5 minutes, until it is beginning to release some fat. Add the chopped onion to the pan, increase the heat to high, and sauté for 5 minutes, or until the onion is translucent and the bacon is crispy. Remove from the heat, add the lemon juice, and stir to combine.

3. To core the cabbage, slide a paring knife around the core so that you're able to remove a cone-shaped piece. A 3-inch-diameter opening should give you enough room to add the filling. You can always trim out more cabbage if you think the space is too small.

4. Place the cored cabbage top side down (so that the hole faces up) in a baking dish or oven-safe pot that is small enough to hold it upright (I like to use a 3-quart pot). Pour the bacon and onion filling inside the cabbage, then place the lemon wedges in the cavity. Loosely cover the top with a piece of aluminum foil.

5. Bake for 1 hour, then uncover and bake for an additional 15 minutes. Let cool for about 5 minutes.

6. When it's cool enough to handle, transfer the cabbage to a cutting board and use a large sharp knife to divide it into 4 large wedges.

7. Garnish with fresh parsley and serve with the lemon wedges.

APPROXIMATE NUTRITION BREAKDOWN (per serving)	
CALORIES: 190	FAT: 12 g
PROTEIN: 5 g	CARBS: 17 g

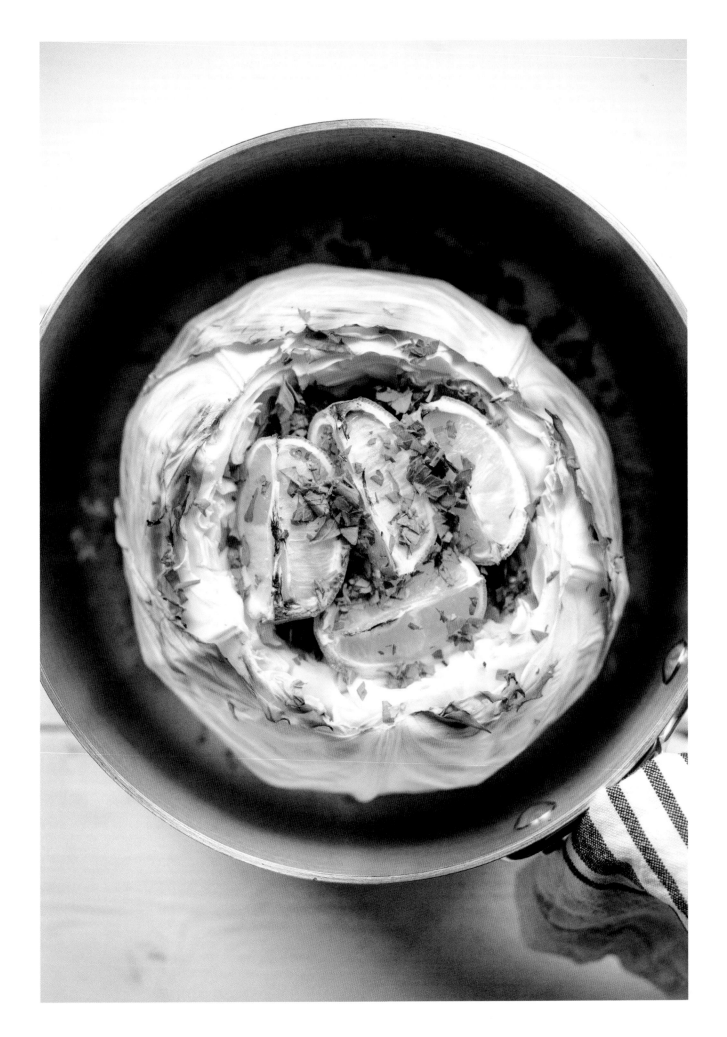

Summer Squash Casserole

I know this dish sounds simple and (potentially) not noteworthy. The first time I made it, I had the same thought! Then I gave it a whirl and was blown away by the bright flavor and freshness. I gobbled up more of this casserole than I did of the bowl of Old-Fashioned Mashed Potatoes (page 289) sitting next to it. Layering the vegetables is so worth the effort—they flavor one another, creating a truly unique and satisfying dish.

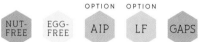

NUT-FREE · EGG-FREE · OPTION AIP · OPTION LF · GAPS

prep time: 20 minutes | *cook time: 30 minutes* | *yield: 6 servings*

2 zucchini, sliced into thin rounds

2 yellow squash, sliced into thin rounds

4 tomatoes, sliced into thin rounds (omit for AIP)

2 purple onions, sliced into thin rounds and then quarters (omit for low-FODMAP)

2 tablespoons extra-virgin olive oil

1 teaspoon Italian seasoning (omit for low-FODMAP)

½ teaspoon fine sea salt

⅛ teaspoon ground black pepper (omit for AIP)

1. Preheat the oven to 375°F.

2. Working in a 9-inch casserole dish or pie dish, create alternating layers of the zucchini, yellow squash, tomatoes, and purple onions until the dish is full. Sprinkle the tops with the olive oil, Italian seasoning, salt, and pepper. Bake for 30 minutes, or until the tops are starting to blister and bubble.

3. Remove from the oven and let rest for about 5 minutes. Serve warm.

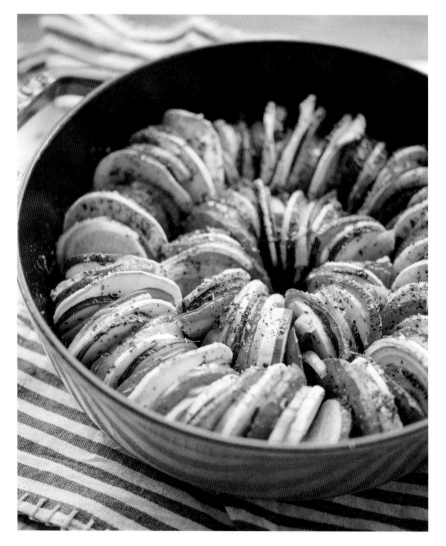

APPROXIMATE NUTRITION BREAKDOWN	
(per serving)	
CALORIES: 118	FAT: 5 g
PROTEIN: 4 g	CARBS: 16 g

Tangy New-Fashioned Coleslaw

Am I alone in this, or is there nothing better than seriously awesome coleslaw? I'm not talking about that soupy mayo-drenched raw cabbage salad with a frightening amount of sugar. I'm talking about a bright, crisp, colorful salad that has you dreaming of the meal combination possibilities. Though stand-up on its own, I like this coleslaw with grilled shrimp, pan-fried steak, or salmon.

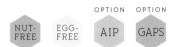

NUT-FREE | EGG-FREE | OPTION AIP | OPTION GAPS

prep time: 20 minutes | *yield: 10 servings*

½ medium head green cabbage, sliced very thin

½ medium head purple cabbage, sliced very thin

4 medium carrots, peeled and grated

1 small jicama, peeled and julienned (omit for GAPS)

½ packed cup fresh cilantro leaves and stems, coarsely chopped

1 jalapeño pepper, thinly sliced (omit for AIP)

½ cup apple cider vinegar

2 tablespoons fresh lime juice (about 1 lime)

2 tablespoons coconut aminos

½ teaspoon fine sea salt

½ teaspoon ground black pepper (omit for AIP)

¼ cup fresh cilantro leaves, for garnish

1. Toss all of the ingredients, except the cilantro, together in a large mixing bowl. Transfer to a serving bowl and top with the cilantro.

2. Enjoy right away or chill before serving.

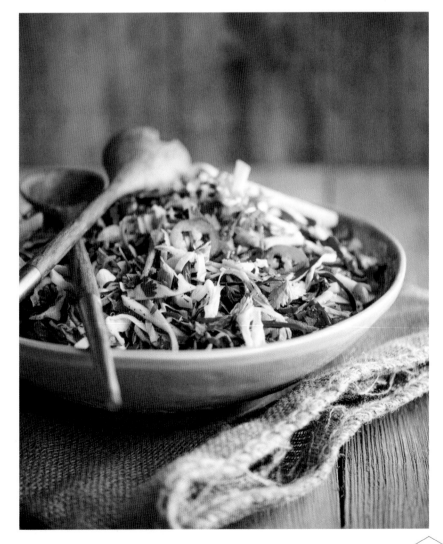

Tips

• *Seed the jalapeño or omit it altogether if you're sensitive to spice.*

• *Leftovers will keep refrigerated for up to 5 days.*

APPROXIMATE NUTRITION BREAKDOWN *(per serving)*			
CALORIES:	52	FAT:	0 g
PROTEIN:	2 g	CARBS:	11 g

Whole Brussels Bake

The first time I really nailed this recipe, I ate almost half of the entire batch while standing in the kitchen. It's that good. I created this recipe because I wanted to offer you an option for cooking up whole Brussels sprouts. This comes together much more quickly than a recipe that calls for cutting or slicing the Brussels sprouts before cooking. Wonderfully flavorful, crispy on the outside, and easy to pair with a wide variety of foods, this dish is a great candidate for your regular rotation. What's more, it freezes exceptionally well and is simple to portion out into individual servings; simply pull a serving from the freezer to add a crunchy vegetable to a meal.

NUT-FREE · **EGG-FREE** · OPTION **AIP** · **GAPS**

prep time: 5 minutes | *cook time: 45 minutes* | *yield: 5 servings*

2 pounds Brussels sprouts

2 tablespoons melted bacon fat or extra-virgin olive oil

Grated zest of 1 lemon (about 2 teaspoons)

2 tablespoons fresh lemon juice (about 1 small lemon)

1 tablespoon balsamic vinegar

½ teaspoon fine sea salt

¼ teaspoon ground black pepper (omit for AIP)

1. Preheat the oven to 375°F.

2. Toss the Brussels sprouts in the bacon fat, lemon zest, lemon juice, and vinegar. Spread out the sprouts in a single layer in a 9-inch casserole or pie dish and sprinkle the tops with the salt and pepper.

3. Bake for 45 minutes, or until the tops start to brown and the sprouts are tender enough to be pierced with a knife. Enjoy warm.

tips

• *Leftovers will keep refrigerated for up to 5 days or frozen for up to 5 months.*

• *To reheat, spread out the Brussels sprouts on a parchment paper–lined rimmed baking sheet and bake at 350°F for 10 minutes if thawed or 25 minutes if frozen, being careful to watch that they don't burn.*

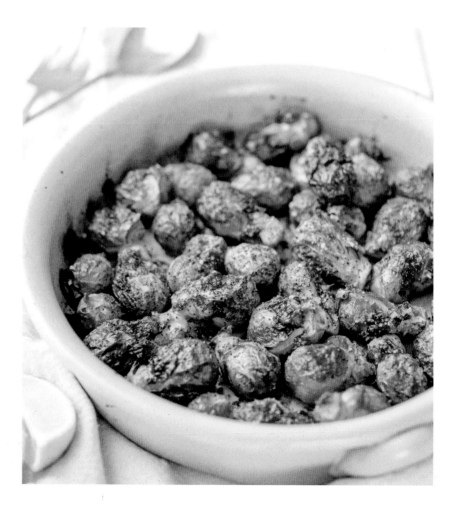

APPROXIMATE NUTRITION BREAKDOWN *(per serving)*			
CALORIES:	128	FAT:	6 g
PROTEIN:	6 g	CARBS:	18 g

Zesty Okra Fries

Okra fries are a thing. They are! At least, now they are? These guys are crispy, flavorful, and simple to whip up, and I know you're going to love them. I planted some okra in my home garden and was blown away by how easy it is to grow. Long story short, we ate okra for about three months straight and always found these fries craveable.

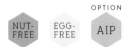

OPTION

NUT-FREE   EGG-FREE   AIP

prep time: 10 minutes | *cook time: 35 minutes* | *yield: 4 servings*

1 pound fresh okra, quartered lengthwise

2 tablespoons fresh lemon juice (about 1 small lemon)

1 tablespoon extra-virgin olive oil

1 teaspoon fine sea salt

¼ teaspoon ground black pepper (omit for AIP)

½ teaspoon garlic powder

1. Preheat the oven to 350°F. Line a rimmed baking sheet with parchment paper.

2. Toss the okra pieces in the lemon juice and olive oil. Lay them out on the prepared baking sheet so that no two pieces overlap. Sprinkle with the salt, pepper, and garlic powder. Bake for 30 to 35 minutes, until the pieces are starting to turn golden brown; be careful that the ends don't burn. Serve warm.

tips

• *Leftovers will keep refrigerated for up to 5 days or frozen for up to 5 months.*

• *Leftovers reheat best on the stovetop or in the oven. To reheat on the stovetop, place the okra in a lightly greased frying pan over medium heat for 5 minutes if thawed or 15 minutes if frozen. To reheat in the oven, spread out the okra on a parchment paper–lined rimmed baking sheet and bake in a preheated 350°F oven for 10 minutes if thawed or 25 minutes if frozen, being careful to watch that they don't burn.*

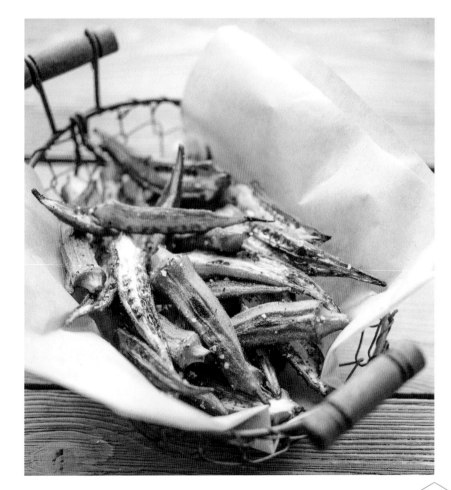

APPROXIMATE NUTRITION BREAKDOWN			
(per serving)			
CALORIES:	68	FAT:	3 g
PROTEIN:	2 g	CARBS:	9 g

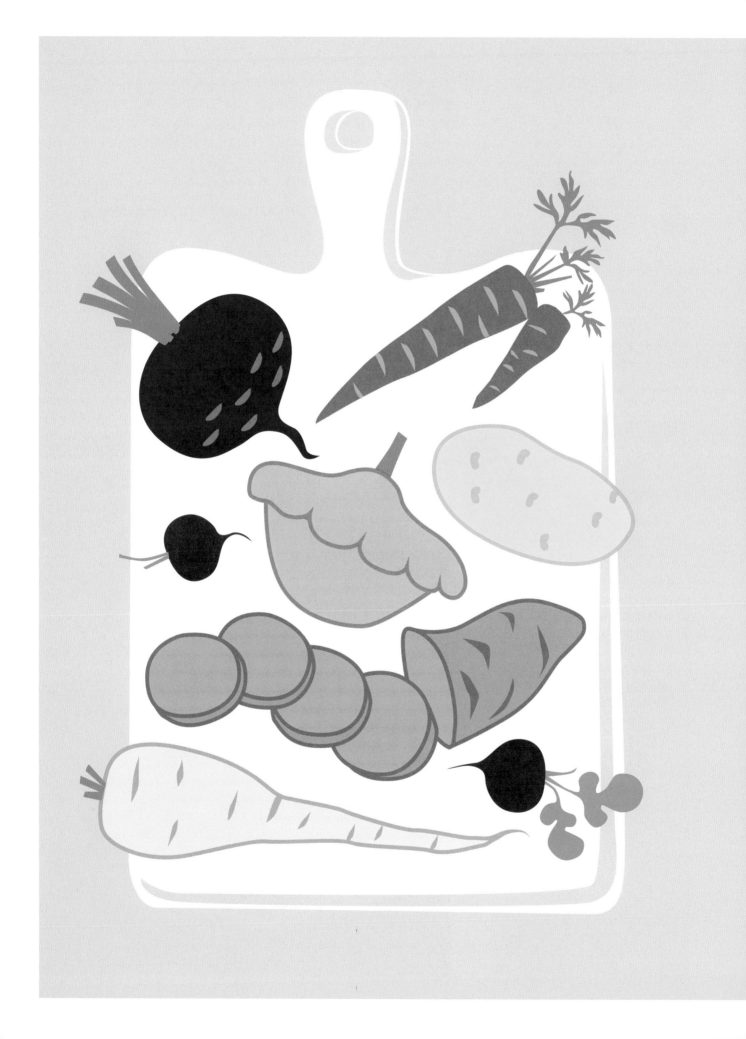

CHAPTER 9:
SATISFYING STARCHES

 Browned Butter
Butternut Mash
286

 Cowboy Potatoes
287

 Crispy Garlic Steak
Fries
288

 Old-Fashioned Mashed
Potatoes
289

 Parsnip Fries
290

Oven-Baked Tostones
291

 Roasted
Citrus Beets
292

 Root Veggie Hash
294

Download the Fed & Fit iPhone and Android app! You can scan the
above QR codes directly in the app, which will then populate a
consolidated grocery shopping list for the scanned recipes.

Browned Butter Butternut Mash

This mash is the new black. Or the new orange. I'm not exactly sure what it's replacing, but it is new and delicious and will leave other mashed orange foods in the dust! Because butternut squash is so easy to prepare in large quantities, this mash is ideal for make-ahead meal prep.

NUT-FREE · EGG-FREE · OPTION AIP · LF · GAPS

prep time: 10 minutes | *cook time: 1 hour* | *yield: 6 to 8 servings*

1 large butternut squash (4 to 5 pounds), cut in half lengthwise and seeded (if tolerated on low-FODMAP)

1 tablespoon extra-virgin olive oil

2 tablespoons salted butter (use coconut oil for AIP)

2 tablespoons fresh lemon juice (about 1 small lemon)

1 teaspoon fine sea salt

½ teaspoon ground black pepper (omit for AIP)

1. Preheat the oven to 400°F.

2. Place the squash in a baking or casserole dish with about ½ inch of water in the bottom. Rub the cut sides of the squash with the olive oil. Bake for 1 hour, or until a fork easily slides into the thickest part of the squash. Allow the squash to cool slightly until it's safe to handle.

3. While the squash is baking, brown the butter: In a small (preferably light-colored) pot or saucepan, melt the butter over medium heat. Continue to stir the butter until it has stopped foaming (indicating that all of the water has evaporated) and you start to see browned bits at the bottom, about 10 minutes. Turn off the heat and set aside.

4. Scrape the cooked squash flesh into a 12-cup or larger food processor or large mixing bowl. Add the browned butter, lemon juice, salt, and pepper and process (or hand mash with a potato masher) until smooth.

tips

- *I recommend using a light-colored pot or saucepan when making the browned butter so that it's easier to see when the milk solids have started to brown. It can be more difficult (though not impossible) to note when the solids are browned, not burned black, in dark-colored cookware.*

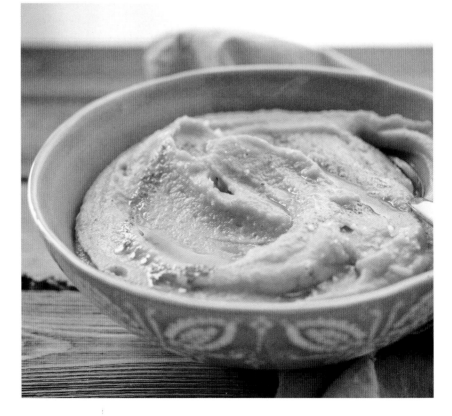

APPROXIMATE NUTRITION BREAKDOWN	
(based on 1 of 8 servings)	
CALORIES: 118	FAT: 5 g
PROTEIN: 2 g	CARBS: 20 g

Cowboy Potatoes

This is one of my default starchy side dishes. When dinner sneaks up on me, I know that I can quickly whip up this dish and have a table of happy campers! If you ever find yourself on a camp-out, this is an ideal "toss it in the fire" food, too. Wrap it in aluminum foil and set it near the coals.

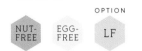

prep time: 15 minutes | *cook time: 1 hour 15 minutes* | *yield: 6 to 10 servings*

3½ pounds yellow potatoes (about 5 medium), cut into thin discs

1 pound bacon, chopped and fried to a crisp

2 tablespoons salted butter, melted

1 teaspoon garlic powder (omit for low-FODMAP)

1 teaspoon fine sea salt

¼ teaspoon ground black pepper

2 tablespoons chopped fresh chives, for garnish

1. Preheat the oven to 375°F.

2. Toss the potatoes in a large bowl with the bacon, melted butter, garlic powder, salt, and pepper. Transfer to a 9-inch square or similar-sized baking dish.

3. Cover the baking dish with aluminum foil and bake for 1 hour, then remove the foil and bake for an additional 15 minutes, or until the tops are starting to brown.

4. Garnish with the chives and serve warm.

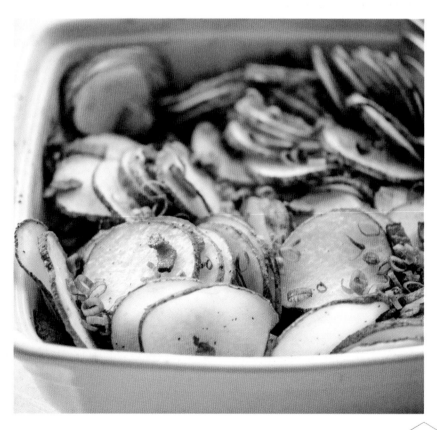

APPROXIMATE NUTRITION BREAKDOWN *(based on 1 of 10 servings)*			
CALORIES:	221	FAT:	12 g
PROTEIN:	4 g	CARBS:	24 g

Crispy Garlic Steak Fries

I can't get over these steak fries. They're so delicious and so easy! Truly, the oven does most of the work. Note that different potatoes require different cooking times, so keep an eye on them in the oven if you choose to experiment. I like to serve these up on burger nights or when I want a special "steak and fries date-night-in" with my husband!

NUT-FREE · EGG-FREE · OPTION LF

prep time: 10 minutes | cook time: 1 hour | yield: 4 to 6 servings

2 pounds russet or other white potatoes (about 6), scrubbed, dried well, and cut into 8 wedges each

3 tablespoons salted butter, melted

1 teaspoon garlic powder (omit for low-FODMAP)

1 teaspoon fine sea salt

½ teaspoon ground black pepper

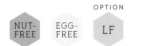

- *Leftovers will keep refrigerated for up to 4 days or frozen for up to 5 months.*

- *For the best crispy results, reheat these fries in the oven. Spread them out on a parchment paper–lined rimmed baking sheet and bake in a preheated 350°F oven for 10 minutes if thawed or 25 minutes if frozen, being careful to watch that they don't burn.*

1. Preheat the oven to 350°F. Line a rimmed baking sheet with parchment paper.

2. Toss the potatoes in the melted butter, garlic powder, salt, and pepper. Lay them out on the prepared baking sheet so that they aren't touching one another.

3. Bake for 30 minutes, then turn up the oven temperature to 425°F and bake for an additional 15 minutes, or until the tops start to look golden brown. Remove the baking sheet from the oven and flip each wedge over. Return the potatoes to the oven and bake for an additional 15 minutes, or until golden brown. Take care that they don't burn during the last couple minutes.

4. Sprinkle the tops of the fries with additional salt to taste and serve warm.

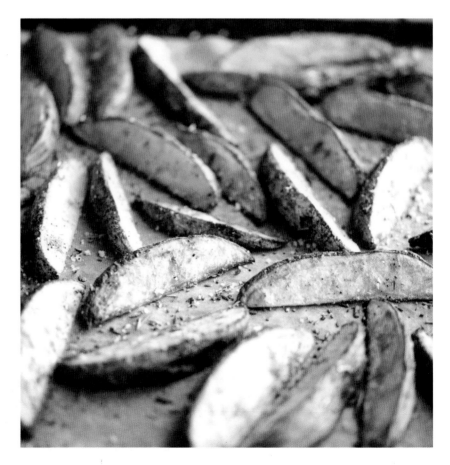

APPROXIMATE NUTRITION BREAKDOWN (based on 1 of 6 servings)			
CALORIES:	167	FAT:	6 g
PROTEIN:	3 g	CARBS:	27 g

Old-Fashioned Mashed Potatoes

I'm not kidding around with the name of this recipe. I could feel my grandmother's presence in the kitchen with me while I was pulling it together. The potato skins are left on, just the way she liked it, and I was decidedly not shy about adding butter and cream. Don't worry about the coconut milk flavoring the mashed potatoes. You can't taste it in the finished product, and the consistency is wonderfully creamy.

NUT-FREE EGG-FREE OPTION LF

| prep time: 10 minutes | cook time: 15 minutes | yield: 6 to 8 servings |

2 pounds red potatoes, rinsed and cut into ½-inch pieces

4 tablespoons salted butter

¼ cup canned, full-fat coconut milk (omit for low-FODMAP)

½ teaspoon garlic powder (omit for low-FODMAP)

1 teaspoon fine sea salt

½ teaspoon ground black pepper

2 tablespoons chopped fresh chives, for garnish

1. Place the potatoes in a large pot and cover with water. Bring to a boil, then reduce the heat and simmer for 15 minutes, or until the potatoes are easily pierced with a fork.

2. Once the potatoes are cooked, place them in a large bowl with the butter, coconut milk, garlic powder, salt, and pepper. Using a potato masher, mash until well incorporated.

3. Serve garnished with the fresh chives.

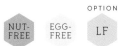

- *This recipe is easily made Autoimmune Protocol–friendly! I recommend using white-fleshed sweet potatoes, prepared the same way. Omit the pepper, use ghee instead of butter, and add 1 tablespoon lemon juice to cut the sweetness of the sweet potatoes.*

- *Leftovers will keep refrigerated for up to 5 days or frozen for up to 5 months.*

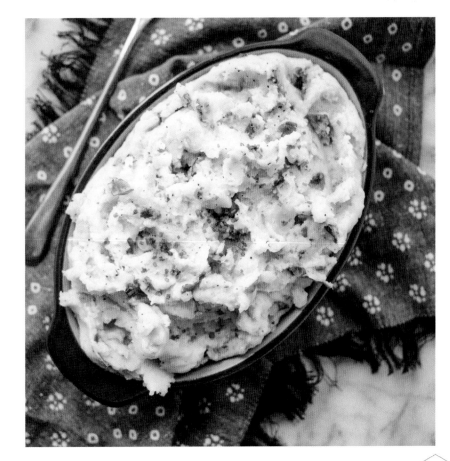

APPROXIMATE NUTRITION BREAKDOWN *(based on 1 of 8 servings)*	
CALORIES: 141	FAT: 7 g
PROTEIN: 2 g	CARBS: 18 g

Parsnip Fries

I just love parsnips. I didn't really discover them until a few years ago, but we became fast friends. Parsnips look like odd-shaped white carrots. They're slightly sweet and have a great nutty flavor. Though I love them roasted and then whipped into a buttery mash, these fries are absolutely dreamy. It's a great way to get more veggies on your plate!

NUT-FREE · EGG-FREE · **OPTION** AIP · LF

prep time: 15 minutes | *cook time: 30 minutes* | *yield: 4 to 6 servings*

2 pounds parsnips, peeled and cut into long, ¼-inch-wide matchsticks

1 tablespoon extra-virgin olive oil

½ teaspoon fine sea salt

¼ teaspoon ground black pepper (omit for AIP)

1. Preheat the oven to 350°F. Line a rimmed baking sheet with parchment paper.

2. Toss the parsnip sticks in the oil and lay them out on the prepared baking sheet so that they touch as little as possible and no two pieces overlap. If needed, line a second rimmed baking sheet with parchment paper and divide the fries between the two baking sheets. Sprinkle the tops of the parsnips with the salt and pepper.

3. Bake for 25 minutes, or until the tops start to turn golden, then turn the oven temperature up to 400°F and set the timer for an additional 5 minutes. The fries should be golden.

4. Serve warm and enjoy!

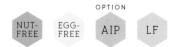

- *When parsnips are in season, I often load up my shopping cart so that I can cook and then freeze several batches of these fries. They freeze really well and can go straight from the freezer into either a preheated 350°F oven or an ungreased frying pan on the stovetop over medium heat for a quick thaw and warm-up (about 25 minutes in the oven or 10 minutes in a frying pan).*

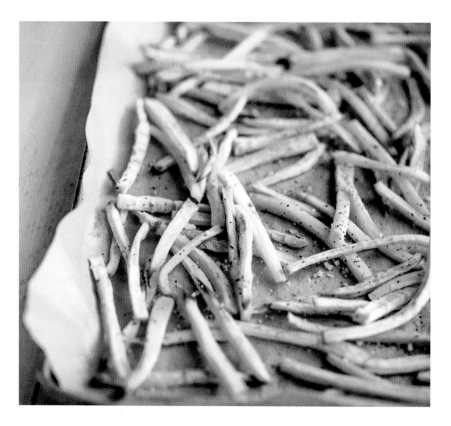

APPROXIMATE NUTRITION BREAKDOWN		
(based on 1 of 6 servings)		
CALORIES: 133		FAT: 3 g
PROTEIN: 2 g		CARBS: 27 g

Oven-Baked Tostones

Strange or not, I have a distinct food group that I think of as "vehicle starches." When I kicked flour-based tortillas to the curb, I went on the hunt for a real-food-based starch that could satisfy the same need: to add necessary carbohydrates to a meal and work as a vehicle for proteins! These oven-baked tostones fit the bill nicely. They're almost like thick, delicious, slightly crispy chalupas.

NUT-FREE · **EGG-FREE** · **AIP** · **LF**

prep time: 10 minutes | *cook time: 45 minutes* | *yield: 4 to 6 servings*

2 large green plantains

1 tablespoon extra-virgin olive oil

¼ teaspoon fine sea salt

Tips

- *The plantain peels will turn black during their first bake. This is completely normal!*

- *If the plantains break apart while you're flattening them, don't fret! Simply smash the broken pieces onto the larger portion to get them to adhere. They will bake together during their second spell in the oven.*

- *These bad boys keep well in the refrigerator for about 4 days and reheat decently, but they may lose their original crisp after the first serving. To reheat and get a nice crisp, fry them in 1 tablespoon melted butter or ghee over high heat until warmed through.*

1. Preheat the oven to 350°F.

2. Score the plantains by making one cut lengthwise down the side of each plantain, cutting through the skin so that you just touch the flesh. Place the plantains on a rimmed baking sheet and bake for 20 minutes, until the peels are black.

3. Remove the plantains from the oven and turn up the heat to 425°F. Swiftly (but carefully so as not to burn yourself) peel the hot plantains. Cut each plantain into about 1-inch-thick pieces, then flatten each piece with the back of a spoon or a stable spatula. Line the baking sheet with parchment paper and place the flattened pieces on the baking sheet.

4. Baste the plantain pieces with the oil and sprinkle the salt on top. Bake for 10 minutes, flip each piece over, and bake for an additional 10 minutes.

5. Season with more salt, if desired, and serve warm.

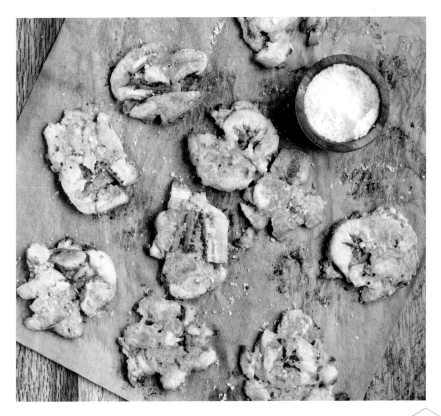

APPROXIMATE NUTRITION BREAKDOWN			
(based on 1 of 6 servings)			
CALORIES:	112	FAT:	2 g
PROTEIN:	1 g	CARBS:	24 g

Roasted Citrus Beets

I make these beets all the time. They are so simple and have such great flavor. They can stand on their own as a great starchy side dish, and they're also delicious when thrown into a salad. Get creative and have fun! If golden beets aren't in season, you can just double the quantity of red beets.

OPTION

NUT-FREE EGG-FREE AIP GAPS

prep time: 15 minutes | *cook time: 45 minutes* | *yield: 6 to 8 servings*

4 red beets, peeled and cut into ½-inch rounds or wedges

4 golden beets, peeled and cut into ½-inch rounds or wedges

1 grapefruit, peeled, seeded, and segmented (see Tips)

2 tablespoons extra-virgin olive oil

¼ teaspoon fine sea salt

⅛ teaspoon ground black pepper (omit for AIP)

1 tablespoon fresh lemon juice (about ½ small lemon)

1. Preheat the oven to 375°F. Line a rimmed baking sheet with parchment paper.

2. Toss the beets and grapefruit sections in the olive oil. Spread them out on the prepared baking sheet and sprinkle the tops with the salt and pepper. Bake for 45 minutes, or until the tops of the beets are starting to look crispy.

3. Drizzle the cooked beets with the lemon juice, lightly toss, and then serve either warm or chilled.

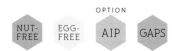

tips

- *To segment citrus fruits, cut off the outer skin (the peel and pith). Slide a sharp paring knife inward toward the center of the fruit, as close to the membrane as possible. Repeat on the adjoining side of the membrane until a wedge of fruit is set free. Continue with the rest of the fruit.*

- *Leftovers will keep refrigerated for up to 5 days.*

APPROXIMATE NUTRITION BREAKDOWN *(based on 1 of 8 servings)*			
CALORIES:	79	FAT:	4g
PROTEIN:	1g	CARBS:	11g

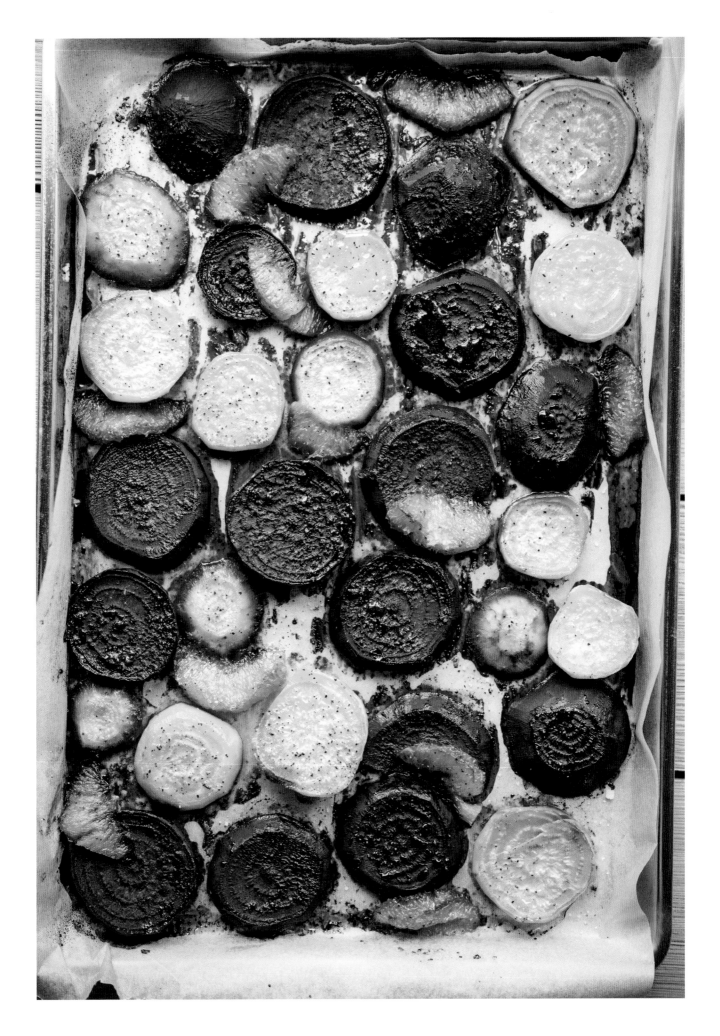

Root Veggie Hash

Consider this list of ingredients a guideline, not a rule. The possibilities are endless! I often whip up this hash at the end of the week when I have several root veggies on their last legs. A quick shred, a toss in some oil and seasonings, and then a spell in the oven can transform forgotten vegetables into the most delicious starchy side dish.

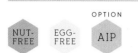

NUT-FREE   EGG-FREE   OPTION AIP

prep time: 20 minutes | *cook time: 40 minutes* | *yield: 6 to 10 servings*

4 carrots, scrubbed and shredded

3 parsnips, peeled and shredded

2 large sweet potatoes, peeled and shredded

2 red beets, peeled and shredded

2 golden beets, peeled and shredded

1 bunch radishes, scrubbed and shredded

¼ cup extra-virgin olive oil

2 tablespoons fresh lemon juice (about 1 small lemon)

2 tablespoons dried thyme leaves

1 teaspoon fine sea salt

½ teaspoon ground black pepper (omit for AIP)

6 to 10 lemon wedges (1 to 2 lemons), for garnish

1. Preheat the oven to 325°F. Line two rimmed baking sheets with parchment paper.

2. Toss the shredded vegetables together in a large mixing bowl. Add the olive oil, lemon juice, thyme, salt, and pepper and toss to mix well.

3. Spread out the veggie mixture on the prepared baking sheets. Bake for 20 minutes, flip the position of the two pans in the oven, and then return to the oven for an additional 20 minutes. The hash is finished when the top is starting to look crispy.

4. Serve warm with lemon wedges.

tips

• *Leftovers will keep refrigerated for up to 5 days or frozen for up to 5 months.*

• *To reheat the hash on the stovetop, toss it in 1 tablespoon melted butter or ghee, place it in a large frying pan over medium heat, and then cover and let steam (if frozen) for 5 to 10 minutes, until warmed through. To reheat it in the oven, spread it out on a parchment paper–lined rimmed baking sheet and bake in a preheated 350°F oven for 10 minutes if thawed or 20 minutes if frozen.*

APPROXIMATE NUTRITION BREAKDOWN *(based on 1 of 10 servings)*	
CALORIES: 110	FAT: 6 g
PROTEIN: 2 g	CARBS: 15 g

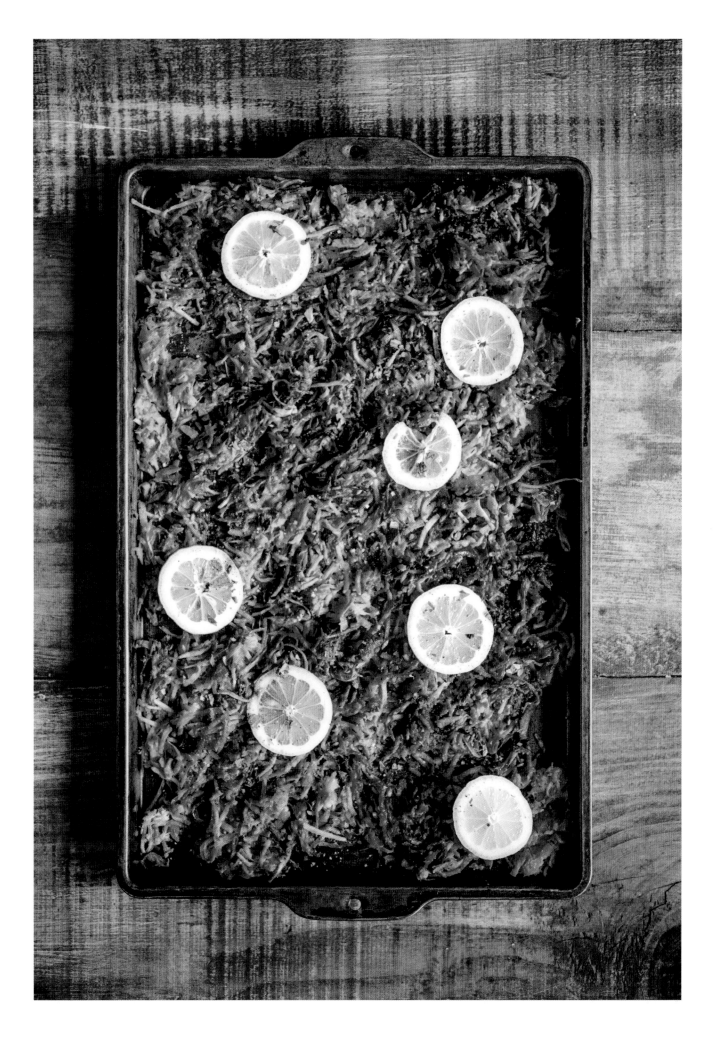

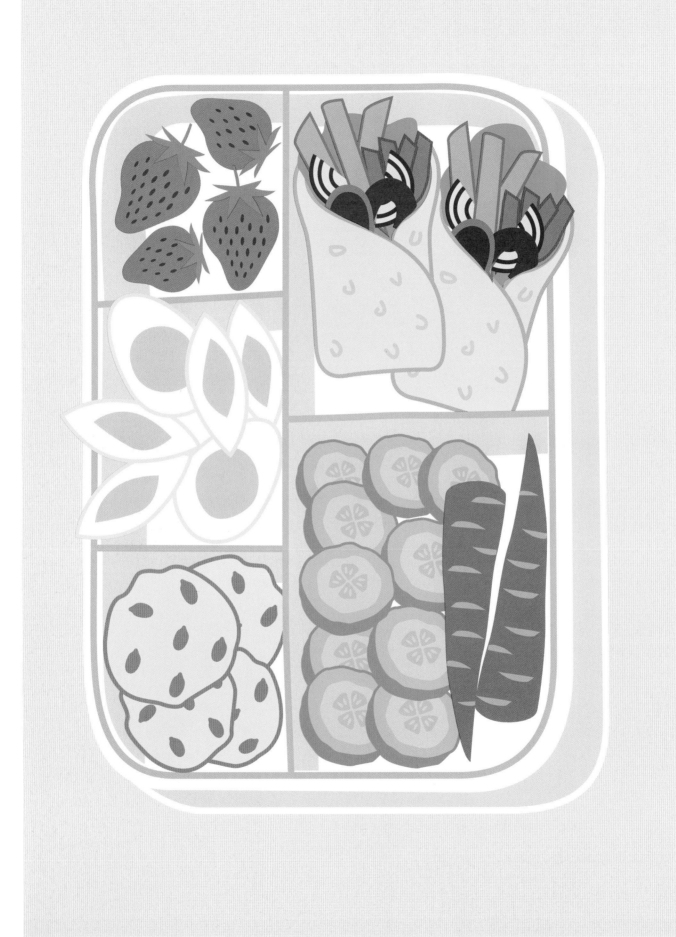

CHAPTER 10:
TAKE IT WITH YOU

 Cold Cut
Roll-Ups
298

 Pesto Chicken Salad
Wraps
299

 Sonoma
Chicken Salad
300

 Curried Sardine
& Tuna Salad
301

 Flax Crackers
302

 Cheddar
Kale Chips
304

 Perfect
Hard-Boiled Eggs
305

 Blueberry Protein Bar
306

 Dark Chocolate Sea
Salt Protein Bar
306

 Sour Cherry
Protein Bar
306

 Teriyaki Beef Jerky
308

 Trail Mix:
Salt & Pepper Cashews
310

 Trail Mix:
Curried Pecans
310

 Trail Mix:
Cinnamon Vanilla Almonds
310

Download the Fed & Fit iPhone and Android app! You can scan the
above QR codes directly in the app, which will then populate a
consolidated grocery shopping list for the scanned recipes.

Cold Cut Roll-Ups

Cold cut roll-ups are a grain-free girl's best friend. When I hit the road for a long trip, I like to pack plenty of supplies to make several meals. Make these roll-ups to your liking! Experiment with different cuts of meat, crunchy vegetables, and sauces (like mayo, pesto, or even ranch).

NUT-FREE | OPTION EGG-FREE | OPTION AIP | OPTION LF | GAPS

prep time: 10 minutes | *yield: 1 serving*

2 ounces deli turkey (about 2 slices)

2 ounces deli roast beef (about 2 slices)

1 tablespoon mustard

1 teaspoon mayo, store-bought or homemade (page 349) (omit for egg-free and AIP)

¼ teaspoon fine sea salt

⅛ teaspoon ground black pepper (omit for AIP)

3 kale, collard, or chard leaves

1 red bell pepper, seeded and cut into long strips (omit for AIP)

¼ purple onion, cut into long strips (omit for low-FODMAP)

1. Lay the turkey slices on a cutting board and layer the roast beef slices on top. Spread the mustard and mayo on the roast beef. Sprinkle with the salt and pepper.

2. Tear or fold the kale leaves so that they fit in the center of the meat. Add an even amount of bell pepper and onion to each pile.

3. Roll the meat over the vegetable filling and secure with a toothpick, kitchen twine, or even a sheet of parchment paper. Enjoy right away or store for later.

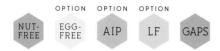

tips

• *The roll-ups can be made ahead and stored in the fridge for up to 4 days.*

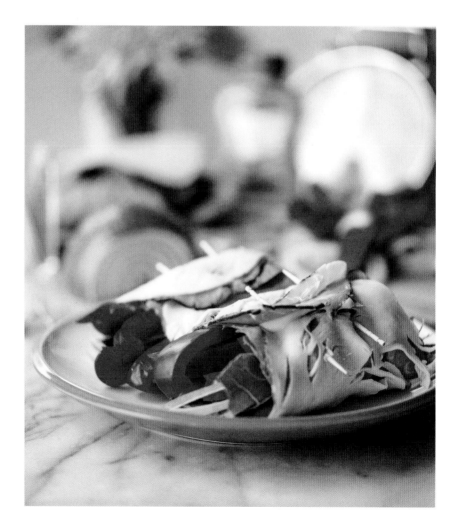

APPROXIMATE NUTRITION BREAKDOWN *(based on 1 serving)*	
CALORIES: 266	FAT: 9 g
PROTEIN: 29 g	CARBS: 20 g

Pesto Chicken Salad Wraps

Pesto chicken salad is a staple in my house. Once it's spooned inside a couple collard green leaves, it is one of the tastiest on-the-go lunches you can imagine! And with veggies provided by the collards, fat by the pesto, and protein by the chicken, this is a near-complete meal. Just find a convenient starch and you're set!

EGG-FREE | GAPS

prep time: 10 minutes (not including pesto) | *cook time: 20 minutes* | *yield: 2 to 4 servings*

2 boneless, skinless chicken breast halves (about 1 pound), rinsed and patted dry

½ teaspoon fine sea salt

¼ teaspoon ground black pepper

¼ cup Roasted Garlic Pesto 2.0 (page 348)

8 large collard leaves, bottom stems removed (see Tips)

1. Preheat the oven to 450°F. Sprinkle the chicken with the salt and pepper. Place the chicken on a rimmed baking sheet and bake for 15 to 18 minutes, until the juices run clear. Set aside to cool for about 10 minutes.

2. When it's cool enough to handle, cut the chicken into ½-inch dice. In a small bowl, toss the chicken with the pesto.

3. Stack two collard leaves on top of each other, creating four stacks total. Spoon an equal amount of pesto chicken salad along the stem of each stack. Roll the edges of the leaves over the salad and secure with toothpicks or kitchen twine. Enjoy right away or store in the refrigerator for up to 4 days.

Tips

- *If you prefer less-tough collard greens, I suggest using smaller leaves and creating more wraps. The larger, more mature leaves will hold more filling but tend to be tougher.*

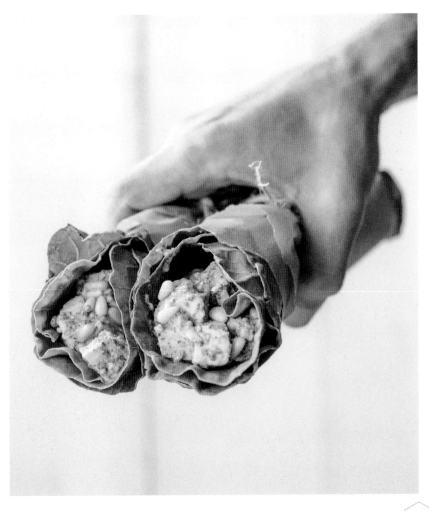

APPROXIMATE NUTRITION BREAKDOWN *(based on 1 of 4 servings)*	
CALORIES: 268	FAT: 10 g
PROTEIN: 40 g	CARBS: 3 g

Sonoma Chicken Salad

When I hop down the hall to the office break room to retrieve my lunch from the refrigerator, I really feel like I've got my life together when I pull out this salad. It's incredibly delicious, satisfying, and energizing! I'm able to keep hopping into the afternoon at full speed. Enjoy it as is or wrap it up in a couple collard green leaves.

OPTION | OPTION | OPTION
NUT-FREE | EGG-FREE | AIP | GAPS

prep time: 20 minutes (not including the baked chicken breast)

yield: 6 to 8 servings

1 batch Perfect Baked Chicken Breast (page 122), coarsely chopped, or meat from 1 whole store-bought rotisserie chicken, coarsely chopped (skin and bones discarded)

3 stalks celery, chopped (about 1 cup)

½ cup halved purple grapes

½ cup raw pecans (omit for nut-free and AIP)

½ cup mayo, store-bought or homemade (page 349) (omit for egg-free and AIP)

1 tablespoon apple cider vinegar

2 teaspoons poppy seeds (omit for nut-free and AIP)

½ teaspoon fine sea salt

¼ teaspoon ground black pepper (omit for AIP)

1. Place the chicken, celery, grapes, and pecans in a large bowl.

2. In a separate small bowl, whisk the mayo, vinegar, poppy seeds, salt, and pepper until the mixture has a smooth, even consistency. Pour the dressing over the salad ingredients and toss to combine.

tips

- *Leftover salad will keep in the refrigerator for up to 4 days.*

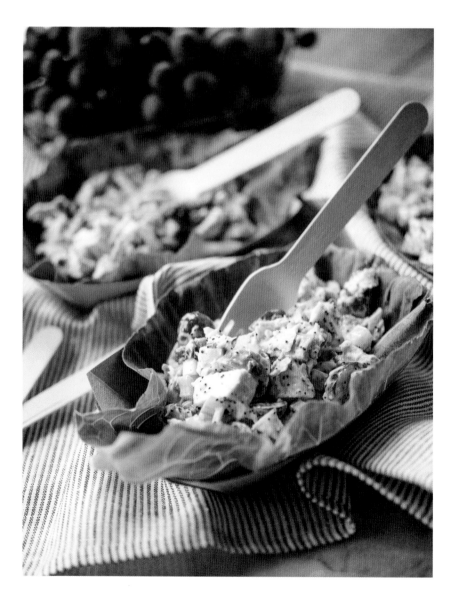

APPROXIMATE NUTRITION BREAKDOWN *(based on 1 of 8 servings)*	
CALORIES: 607	FAT: 45 g
PROTEIN: 41 g	CARBS: 5 g

Curried Sardine & Tuna Salad

Thanks to the sardines, spices, fresh cilantro, and jalapeño pepper, this is a more nutrient-dense version of my childhood lunchtime favorite, tuna salad. If you're trying to find a way to incorporate sardines into your routine, this recipe is a great option! The tuna and curry powder help mask the sardine flavor, resulting in a truly craveable, packable lunch.

OPTION · OPTION · OPTION

NUT-FREE · EGG-FREE · LF · GAPS

prep time: 10 minutes | *yield: 2 to 4 servings*

2 (5-ounce) cans tuna packed in water, drained

1 (4.375-ounce) tin sardines packed in water, drained

1 jicama, peeled and cut into ¼-inch dice (omit for GAPS)

¼ cup mayo, store-bought or homemade (page 349) (omit for egg-free and low-FODMAP)

2 tablespoons fresh lime juice (about 1 lime)

2 heaping tablespoons curry powder

1 tablespoon garlic powder (omit for low-FODMAP)

1 tablespoon turmeric powder

½ teaspoon fine sea salt

¼ teaspoon ground black pepper

¼ cup chopped fresh cilantro, for garnish

1 jalapeño pepper, cut into rounds, for garnish

1. Place all of the ingredients, except the cilantro and jalapeño, in a large mixing bowl. Using a fork, break up the chunks of tuna and sardines into the rest of the ingredients. Stir until well combined and showing an even color.

2. Garnish with the chopped cilantro and jalapeño slices and serve.

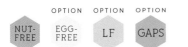

tips

- *Leftover salad will keep in the refrigerator for up to 3 days.*

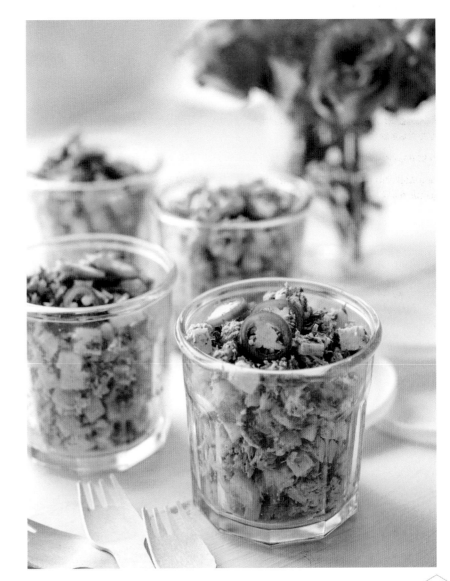

APPROXIMATE NUTRITION BREAKDOWN	
(based on 1 of 4 servings)	
CALORIES: 334	FAT: 17 g
PROTEIN: 24 g	CARBS: 20 g

Flax Crackers

These crackers are the bomb! They're a breeze to whip up, and they pack some great healthy fats. I like them on their own, served with roll-ups (page 298), or even with Curried Sardine & Tuna Salad (page 301). If you like spicy foods, try adding ¼ teaspoon cayenne pepper to the dough!

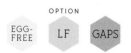

OPTION

EGG-FREE   LF   GAPS

| prep time: 10 minutes | cook time: 18 minutes | yield: 4 dozen crackers (6 crackers per serving) |

1 cup very finely ground hulled, raw sunflower seeds (see Tips)

½ cup flax seeds

½ teaspoon garlic powder (omit for low-FODMAP)

½ teaspoon onion powder (omit for low-FODMAP)

1 teaspoon fine sea salt

1 tablespoon melted coconut oil

2 tablespoons lemon juice (about 1 small lemon)

2 tablespoons water

1. Preheat the oven to 350ºF. Line a baking sheet with parchment paper.

2. In a medium-sized bowl, whisk the ground sunflower seeds, flax seeds, garlic powder, onion powder, and salt until thoroughly combined.

3. Pour the melted coconut oil, lemon juice, and water over the dry ingredients and stir until an even paste forms.

4. Scoop a 1 teaspoon–sized ball of the dough and drop it onto the prepared baking sheet. Repeat with the rest of the dough, spacing the balls at least 2 inches apart.

5. Using a coaster or flat-bottomed glass and a square of parchment paper set on top of the dough, press each ball of dough into a flat disc. The crackers will not spread as they bake, so it's okay if they get a little close together.

6. Bake for 15 minutes, then rotate the baking sheet 180 degrees and bake for another 3 minutes. Remove the crackers from the oven when they are slightly golden brown.

tips

• To make the ground sunflower seeds, measure out at least 1 cup of hulled, raw sunflower seeds and place them in a food processor. Pulse about 10 times, until the seeds become a fine powder and no clumps are visible.

• If you want to save time the day of, you can pre-grind the sunflower seeds. Store the ground seeds in an airtight container in the refrigerator for up to 1 month or in the freezer for up to 5 months.

• Leftover crackers will keep refrigerated or on the shelf for up to 1 week.

APPROXIMATE NUTRITION BREAKDOWN		
(per serving)		
CALORIES: 199		FAT: 17 g
PROTEIN: 7 g		CARBS: 8 g

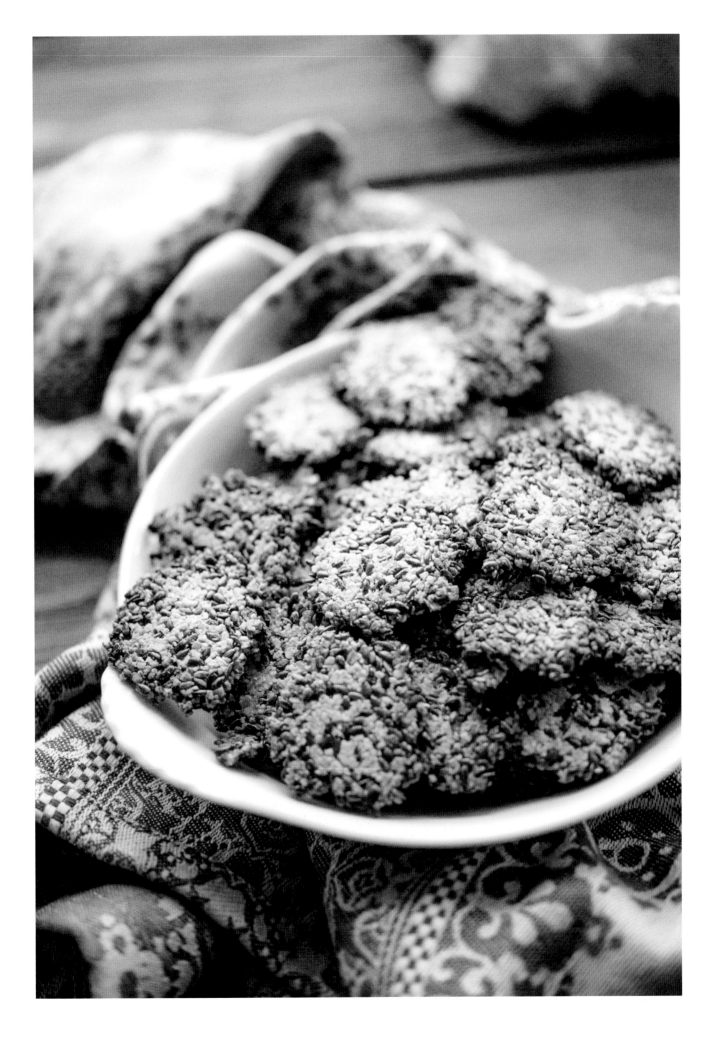

Cheddar Kale Chips

This recipe goes out to everyone who grew up on cheesy nacho chips. I used to so look forward to my after-school snack of cheesy chips that I would practically sprint from the school bus directly to the pantry. Though the days of highly processed, artificial ingredient–loaded chips are behind me, these cheddar kale chips hit the same satisfying spot. They're crunchy and cheesy (thanks to the nutritional yeast) and make a great grab-and-go green snack.

NUT-FREE · EGG-FREE · AIP · LF · GAPS

prep time: 15 minutes | *cook time: 1 hour or 3 to 4 hours, depending on method* | *yield: 6 servings*

¼ cup nutritional yeast

¼ cup fresh lemon juice (about 2 small lemons)

2 tablespoons melted coconut oil

2 bunches kale, destemmed and cut into large pieces

½ teaspoon fine sea salt

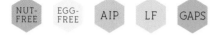

- *Leftover chips will keep in a sealed container at room temperature for up to 5 days.*

1. In a small bowl, whisk the nutritional yeast, lemon juice, and coconut oil until well combined. Note that the yeast isn't expected to dissolve, just incorporate evenly.

2. Place the kale in a large mixing bowl and pour the nutritional yeast mixture over the top. Using your hands, toss the kale, making sure that each piece is evenly coated.

3. Dehydrate the chips using one of these two methods:

   Oven method: Preheat the oven to 210°F. Line two rimmed baking sheets with parchment paper. Spread out the kale in a single layer on the baking sheets, then sprinkle the tops with the salt. Bake for 1 hour, or until the chips are crispy to the touch.

   Dehydrator method: Spread out the kale on the racks of a dehydrator, then sprinkle the tops with the salt. Set the temperature to 135°F and dehydrate for 3 to 4 hours, until the chips are crispy to the touch.

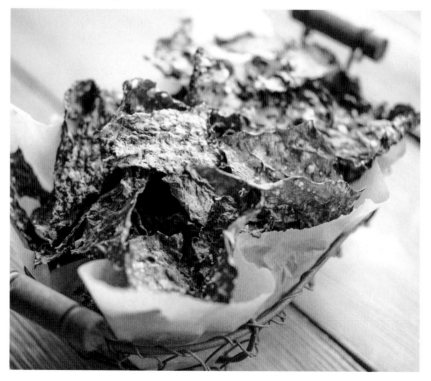

APPROXIMATE NUTRITION BREAKDOWN			
(per serving)			
CALORIES:	71	FAT:	5 g
PROTEIN:	3 g	CARBS:	5 g

Perfect Hard-Boiled Eggs

If I were to craft a list of the on-the-go foods that I turn to most often, hard-boiled eggs would be at the tippy top. They are an incredibly convenient protein, are a cinch to make in bulk, and can serve as a base for so many fun flavors. Creating an easy-to-peel hard-boiled egg is actually really simple once you understand a single principle: drastic temperature variations between really hot and really cold. I've steamed, baked, and boiled countless eggs so that I could provide you with the most direct route to an eggshell that comes right off and leaves your eggs looking beautiful!

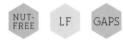

prep time: 15 minutes | *cook time: 10 minutes* | *yield: 12 eggs (2 per serving)*

12 large eggs, chilled

TOPPING SUGGESTIONS

3-Ingredient Paleo Ranch (page 338)

Capers, smoked salmon, and fresh dill

Mustard, mayo [store-bought or homemade (page 349)], and chives

Buffalo Sauce (page 337) and diced purple onion

1. Bring about 3 inches of water to a boil in a large pot. Once boiling, pull the eggs from the refrigerator. Using a slotted spoon or fitted strainer basket, carefully place or submerge the eggs in the boiling water. Boil the eggs for exactly 10 minutes.

2. While the eggs are boiling, prepare an ice bath by filling a large bowl with at least 5 cups of ice cubes. Add enough water to cover the ice cubes.

3. Use a slotted spoon (or the strainer basket) to pull the eggs from the boiling water. Immediately place them in the ice bath, making sure that each egg is submerged. Let them sit in the bath for at least 15 minutes.

4. Once completely chilled, either peel the eggs and enjoy right away or transfer to the refrigerator for up to 7 days.

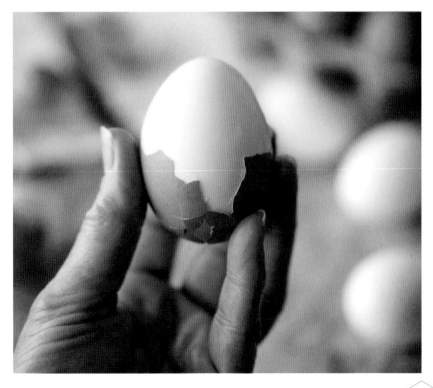

APPROXIMATE NUTRITION BREAKDOWN *(per serving)*			
CALORIES:	140	FAT:	8 g
PROTEIN:	12 g	CARBS:	0 g

Blueberry, Dark Chocolate Sea Salt, Sour Cherry

Of all the recipes I've ever created—around 500 of them now—I don't think I worked as hard for any of them as I did for these protein bars. You see, I don't actually like normal protein bars. They're chalky, usually dipped in chocolate, and don't make me feel very energized. However, I do love the idea of one. A convenient package of protein, fat, and carbohydrate to supplement a meal? I'm in. After (I'm not kidding) about thirty attempts, I finally landed on a bar that I'm exceptionally proud to include in this book. I hope you love it as much as I do!

EGG-FREE   OPTION GAPS

prep time: 15 minutes, plus 1 hour to chill | *yield: 4 bars each (1 bar per serving)*

BLUEBERRY

8 pitted Medjool dates

8 tablespoons collagen peptides

½ cup freeze-dried blueberries

¼ cup raw almonds

¼ teaspoon fine sea salt

2 teaspoons water

DARK CHOCOLATE SEA SALT (not GAPS compliant)

8 pitted Medjool dates

8 tablespoons collagen peptides

¼ cup raw almonds

2 tablespoons unsweetened cocoa powder

½ teaspoon fine sea salt

2 teaspoons water

SOUR CHERRY

8 pitted Medjool dates

8 tablespoons collagen peptides

½ cup freeze-dried cherries

¼ cup raw almonds

¼ teaspoon fine sea salt

2 teaspoons water

tips

• *These bars are sticky at room temperature, so I recommend keeping them chilled.*

1. Place all of the dry ingredients in a food processor and chop until the mixture has a fine, even texture. Add the water and pulse 3 to 5 times, until the dough comes together and forms a ball.

2. Place the dough ball in the middle of a 12-inch square piece of parchment paper, folding the paper over the top of the dough. Working over the top of the parchment paper, shape the dough into a rectangle that's approximately 4 by 8 inches. Transfer the slab to the refrigerator to chill for at least 1 hour. Use a sharp knife to score or divide into 4 bars.

3. Enjoy right away or wrap in parchment paper so that the bars don't stick together. They'll keep refrigerated for up to 2 weeks or frozen for up to 6 months.

BLUEBERRY

APPROXIMATE NUTRITION BREAKDOWN *(per bar)*	
CALORIES: 285	FAT: 5 g
PROTEIN: 21 g	CARBS: 44 g

DARK CHOCOLATE SEA SALT

APPROXIMATE NUTRITION BREAKDOWN *(per bar)*	
CALORIES: 269	FAT: 5 g
PROTEIN: 21 g	CARBS: 39 g

SOUR CHERRY

APPROXIMATE NUTRITION BREAKDOWN *(per bar)*	
CALORIES: 282	FAT: 5 g
PROTEIN: 21 g	CARBS: 43 g

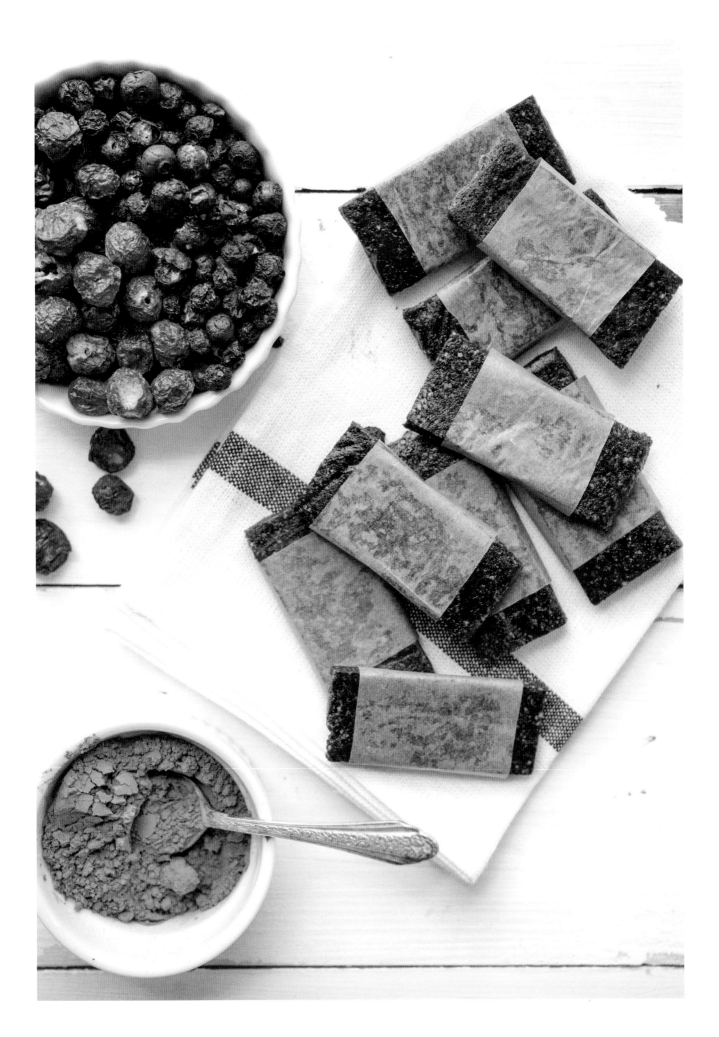

Teriyaki Beef Jerky

This jerky is a hot commodity in my house. I make it in huge batches, and if I don't keep a stash hidden in the freezer, Austin will claim every last strip. I like to bring beef jerky with me on long hikes and road trips and when I travel for work. It's such a convenient, travel-friendly protein with amazing flavor. You're going to love this jerky!

OPTION **NUT-FREE** · OPTION **EGG-FREE** · OPTION **AIP** · **LF** · **GAPS**

prep time: 10 minutes, plus at least 8 hours to marinate | *cook time: 20 minutes plus 4 to 6 hours, depending on method* | *yield: 10 to 15 servings*

2 pounds beef skirt steak or rump roast, sliced wafer-thin

2 teaspoons sesame oil (untoasted) (use EVOO for nut-free, AIP, and low-FODMAP)

3 cloves garlic, grated (omit for low-FODMAP)

2 teaspoons peeled and grated fresh ginger

2 teaspoons red pepper flakes (omit for AIP)

1 cup coconut aminos

½ cup apple cider vinegar

¼ cup fresh lime juice (about 2 limes)

½ teaspoon fine sea salt

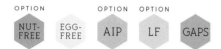

tips

• *The jerky will keep in the refrigerator for up to 2 weeks or in the freezer for up to 6 months.*

1. Place the beef strips in a large glass bowl.

2. Heat the sesame oil in a small saucepan over high heat. Add the garlic and ginger, stir to coat, and sauté for 4 minutes, or until fragrant. Add the red pepper flakes and sauté for an additional 3 minutes, or just until fragrant. Add the coconut aminos, whisk to combine, and bring to a simmer. Continue to simmer and reduce for at least 20 minutes, until it coats the back of a spoon.

3. Move the pan off the heat, then add the vinegar, lime juice, and salt. Stir until the salt has dissolved. Set the marinade aside and let cool to room temperature.

4. Pour the cooled marinade over the beef and stir to combine. Cover the bowl with plastic wrap and place in the refrigerator to marinate for at least 8 hours.

5. Dehydrate the marinated beef using one these two methods:

   Dehydrator method: Lay the beef strips on the grates of the dehydrator. Dehydrate at 185°F for 5 to 6 hours, until shriveled and reduced in size but still bendable.

   Oven method: Preheat the oven to 225°F. Line two rimmed baking sheets with parchment paper. Lay the beef strips on the prepared baking sheets. Bake for 4 hours, or until shriveled and reduced in size but still bendable.

APPROXIMATE NUTRITION BREAKDOWN *(based on 1 of 15 servings)*	
CALORIES: 134	FAT: 5g
PROTEIN: 17g	CARBS: 4g

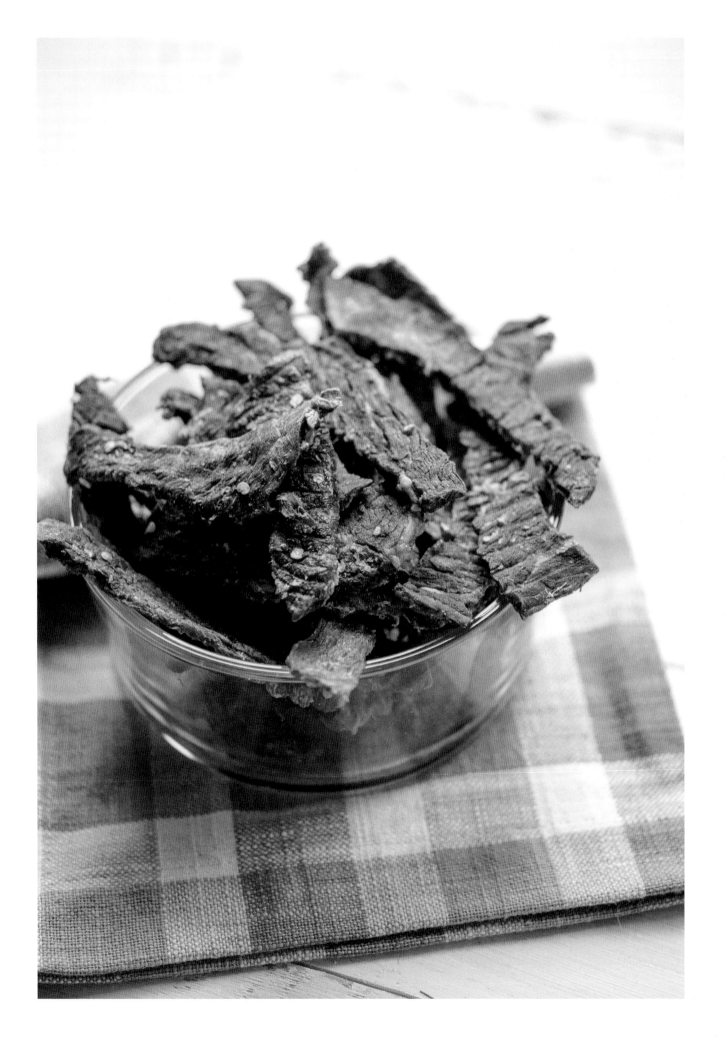

Trail Mix

3 Ways

I was a proud Girl Scout for a little over a decade, and as such, I considered myself an authority on trail mix. My favorite variety included one part peanuts, one part chocolate chips, one part M&Ms, and one part dried fruit—though, truth be told, I would pick out the candy and leave the rest. Now that I'm an adult on a mission to fuel my body with the best available nutrients, I still think that my Girl Scout self would've loved these new, more fun, more flavorful varieties.

OPTION NUT-FREE · EGG-FREE · OPTION AIP · OPTION LF · OPTION GAPS

prep time: 5 minutes | *cook time: 15 minutes* | *yield: 8 servings*

SALT & PEPPER CASHEWS
(not AIP friendly)

1 cup raw cashews (omit for nut-free and low-FODMAP)

1 teaspoon melted coconut oil

½ teaspoon fine sea salt

¼ teaspoon ground black pepper

1 cup dehydrated tomato slices

1 cup salted plantain chips (omit for GAPS)

CURRIED PECANS
(not low-FODMAP friendly)

1 cup raw pecans (omit for nut-free and AIP)

1 teaspoon melted coconut oil

½ teaspoon fine sea salt

1 tablespoon curry powder (omit for AIP)

Pinch of cayenne pepper (omit for AIP)

1 cup salted beet chips

1 cup freeze-dried cherries

CINNAMON VANILLA ALMONDS

1 cup raw almonds (omit for nut-free, AIP, and low-FODMAP)

1 teaspoon melted coconut oil

1 teaspoon ground cinnamon

½ teaspoon vanilla extract

1 cup unsweetened toasted coconut flakes

1 cup salted plantain chips (omit for GAPS)

1. Preheat the oven to 325°F. Toss the nuts in the coconut oil, salt (if included), spices, and vanilla extract (if included). Spread out the nuts on a rimmed baking sheet. Bake for 15 minutes, or until slightly fragrant. Let cool on the counter for at least 5 minutes.

2. Toss the nuts with the rest of the ingredients and enjoy!

3. Trail mix will keep on the shelf for up to 2 weeks or in the freezer for up to 6 months.

SALT & PEPPER CASHEWS

APPROXIMATE NUTRITION BREAKDOWN *(per serving)*	
CALORIES: 174	FAT: 10 g
PROTEIN: 5 g	CARBS: 16 g

CURRIED PECANS

APPROXIMATE NUTRITION BREAKDOWN *(per serving)*	
CALORIES: 187	FAT: 15 g
PROTEIN: 4 g	CARBS: 12 g

CINNAMON VANILLA ALMONDS

APPROXIMATE NUTRITION BREAKDOWN *(per serving)*	
CALORIES: 241	FAT: 19 g
PROTEIN: 5 g	CARBS: 13 g

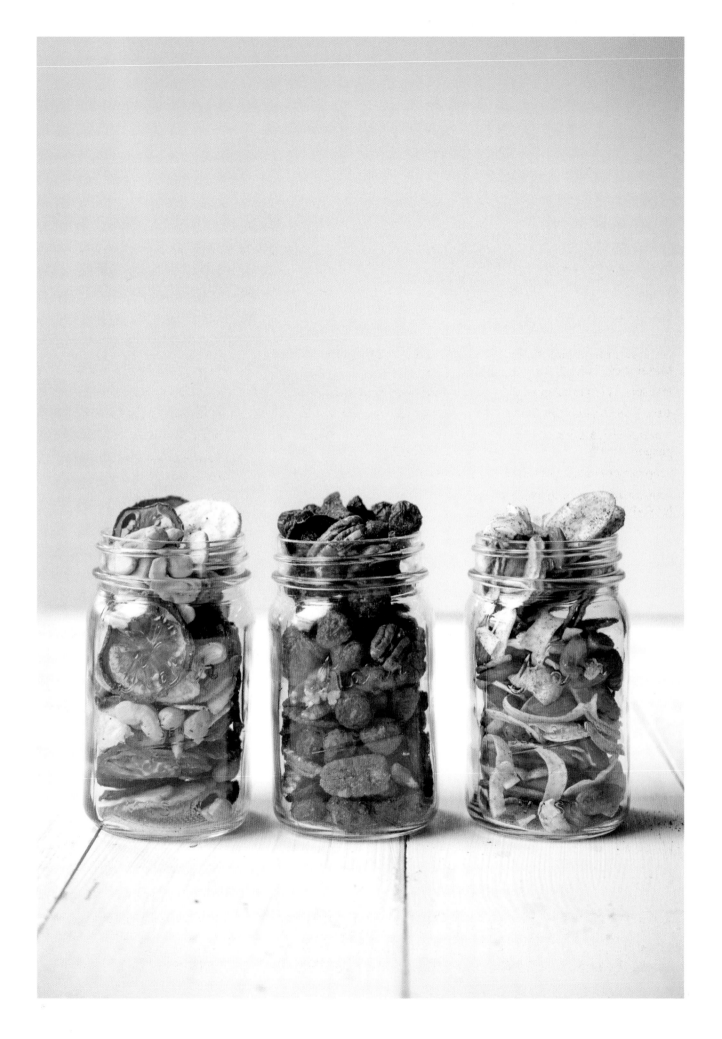

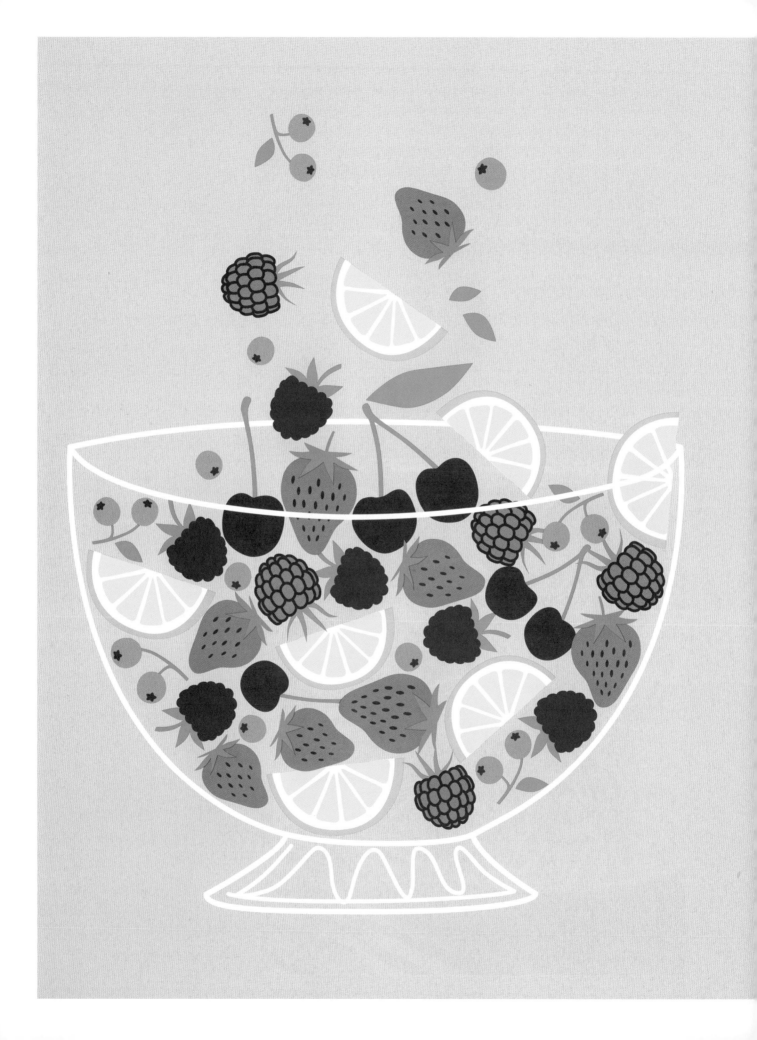

CHAPTER 11:
NATURALLY SWEET

 Vanilla Bean Pudding
314

 Chocolate Pudding
314

 Toasted Coconut Pudding
314

 Blueberry Cherry Gummies
316

 Strawberry Raspberry Gummies
316

 Carrot Orange Gummies
316

 Lemon Lime Gummies
316

 Ginger Kale Gummies
316

 Roasted Blueberry Pops
318

 Roasted Cherry Pops
318

 Roasted Grapefruit Pops
318

 Roasted Strawberry Pops
318

 Roasted Raspberry Pops
318

 Fudgesicles
320

 Berries and Cream
321

Download the Fed & Fit iPhone and Android app! You can scan the
above QR codes directly in the app, which will then populate a
consolidated grocery shopping list for the scanned recipes.

Puddings

3 Ways

Oh, how I adore these little puddings. They're perfectly portioned for when you want a sweet treat, and they freeze exceptionally well (so you don't feel like you have to devour them all at once). Because they're delicious, healthy, and great to make ahead, they're also an excellent dessert option for a dinner party!

NUT-FREE · EGG-FREE · OPTION AIP · OPTION GAPS

prep time: 5 minutes, plus 3 to 4 hours to set | cook time: 10 minutes | yield: 5 servings each

TOASTED COCONUT PUDDING

1 (13½-ounce) can full-fat coconut milk

½ cup unsweetened shredded coconut, toasted (see Tips), plus extra for garnish

2 pitted Medjool dates

2 teaspoons unflavored gelatin

1 teaspoon vanilla extract (omit if sensitive on AIP)

CHOCOLATE PUDDING (not AIP or GAPS-friendly)

1 (13½-ounce) can full-fat coconut milk

2 tablespoons unsweetened cocoa powder, plus extra for garnish

2 pitted Medjool dates

2 teaspoons unflavored gelatin

1 teaspoon vanilla extract

VANILLA BEAN PUDDING

1 (13½-ounce) can full-fat coconut milk

2 pitted Medjool dates

2 teaspoons unflavored gelatin

Vanilla bean seeds scraped from 2 pods (omit if sensitive on AIP)

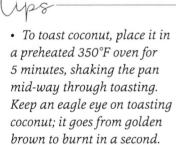

tips

• *To toast coconut, place it in a preheated 350°F oven for 5 minutes, shaking the pan mid-way through toasting. Keep an eagle eye on toasting coconut; it goes from golden brown to burnt in a second.*

• *Leftovers will keep refrigerated for up to 5 days or frozen for up to 4 months.*

• *To defrost, transfer a container to the refrigerator and let it soften for at least 24 hours.*

1. In a heavy-bottomed saucepan, warm the coconut milk over medium heat until it simmers. Pour it into a blender and add the rest of the ingredients. Blend until smooth, transfer to five 4-ounce jars or small ramekins, and refrigerate for 3 to 4 hours, until set. Be sure to use freezer-safe jars if you plan to freeze the leftovers.

2. Garnish the Toasted Coconut or Chocolate Puddings with additional toasted coconut or cocoa powder before serving.

TOASTED COCONUT

APPROXIMATE NUTRITION BREAKDOWN *(per serving)*	
CALORIES: 231	FAT: 20 g
PROTEIN: 2 g	CARBS: 11 g

CHOCOLATE

APPROXIMATE NUTRITION BREAKDOWN *(per serving)*	
CALORIES: 182	FAT: 15 g
PROTEIN: 2 g	CARBS: 11 g

VANILLA BEAN

APPROXIMATE NUTRITION BREAKDOWN *(per serving)*	
CALORIES: 177	FAT: 15 g
PROTEIN: 2 g	CARBS: 10 g

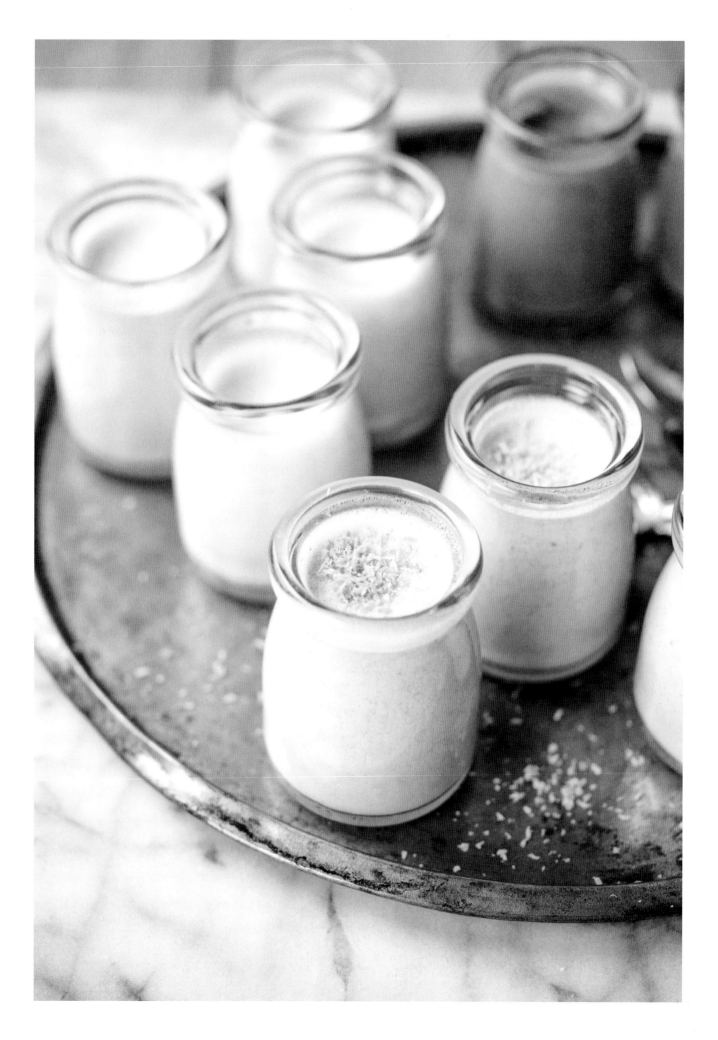

Gummies

5 Ways

The first time I made healthy gummies at home, I almost cried. I took them to work and insisted that everyone try a bite. These gummies are delicious, wonderfully healthy, and really versatile! Because of their small size and negligible caloric impact, they are an exception to the no-snacking rule. They are essentially Fed & Fit Project–approved candy!

NUT-FREE · EGG-FREE · AIP · LF OPTION · GAPS

prep time: 10 minutes, plus at least 3 hours to set | *yield: 1 dozen each (3 gummies per serving)*

BLUEBERRY CHERRY JAM GUMMIES
(not low-FODMAP friendly)

1½ cups fresh blueberries

1½ cups pitted fresh cherries

2 tablespoons fresh lemon juice (about 1 small lemon)

¼ cup unflavored gelatin

CARROT ORANGE JUICE GUMMIES

Store-bought juice option:

1 cup orange carrot juice

Homemade juice option:

3 carrots

2 oranges, peeled, seeded, and segmented (see Tips, page 292)

¼ cup unflavored gelatin

STRAWBERRY RASPBERRY JAM GUMMIES

2 cups fresh strawberries, hulled

2 cups fresh raspberries

2 tablespoons fresh lemon juice (about 1 small lemon)

¼ cup unflavored gelatin

LEMON LIME JUICE GUMMIES

½ cup fresh lemon juice (about 4 small lemons)

½ cup fresh lime juice (about 4 limes)

¼ cup unflavored gelatin

GINGER KALE JUICE GUMMIES

Store-bought juice option:

1 cup green juice

Homemade juice option:

2 packed cups kale leaves (with stems)

½ packed cup fresh cilantro leaves and stems

2 lemons, peeled, seeded, and segmented (see Tips, page 292)

1 (1-inch) piece fresh ginger, peeled and grated

¾ cup water

¼ cup unflavored gelatin

SPECIAL EQUIPMENT

Juicer (for homemade juice gummies)

Silicone gummy mold (optional)

BLUEBERRY CHERRY JAM

APPROXIMATE NUTRITION BREAKDOWN *(per serving)*			
CALORIES:	136	FAT:	0 g
PROTEIN:	16 g	CARBS:	23 g

CARROT ORANGE JUICE

APPROXIMATE NUTRITION BREAKDOWN *(per serving)*			
CALORIES:	92	FAT:	0 g
PROTEIN:	15 g	CARBS:	9 g

1. Prepare the jam or homemade juice base for the gummies:

    For the jam gummies: Place the fruit and lemon juice in a small saucepot over medium heat. Cover and bring to a simmer. Remove the lid, stir, and let simmer for an additional 20 minutes, or until all of the fruit has softened and the jam has a deep color. Transfer the hot fruit to a blender and blend for 1 minute, or until smooth. Set aside.

    For the homemade juice gummies: Process the juice ingredients in a juicer and set the juice aside.

2. Dissolve the gelatin in ½ cup boiling water. If any clumps remain, scoop them out and discard them.

3. Whisk the jam or juice into the gelatin water until smooth. Pour the mixture into a silicone mold or an 8-inch square ceramic or glass baking dish.

4. Refrigerate the gummies for at least 3 hours. If using a silicone mold, I recommend freezing the tray so that the gummies are easier to extract. If using a baking dish, use a butter knife to cut the gummies into squares or other shapes. Store in an airtight container in the refrigerator for up to 5 days.

STRAWBERRY RASPBERRY JAM

APPROXIMATE NUTRITION BREAKDOWN *(per serving)*	
CALORIES: 136	FAT: 0 g
PROTEIN: 16 g	CARBS: 19 g

LEMON LIME JUICE

APPROXIMATE NUTRITION BREAKDOWN *(per serving)*	
CALORIES: 104	FAT: 0 g
PROTEIN: 16 g	CARBS: 13 g

GINGER KALE JUICE

APPROXIMATE NUTRITION BREAKDOWN *(per serving)*	
CALORIES: 84	FAT: 0 g
PROTEIN: 15 g	CARBS: 8 g

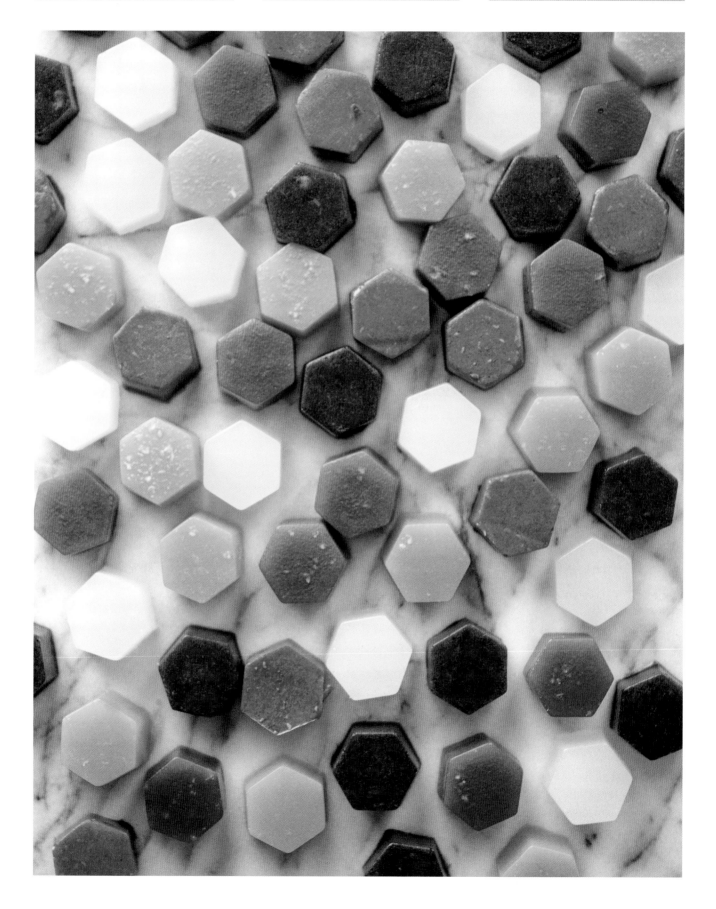

Roasted Fruit Pops

5 Ways

I lean on these ice pops BIG TIME when I'm overcoming a sugar withdrawal (like after a holiday or girls' weekend). The portions work out so that each pop, no matter the flavor, contains the equivalent of one serving of fruit. Roasting the fruit really deepens the flavor and brings out the natural sugars. I recommend that you make a few batches and keep these on hand for when you need a frozen sweet treat!

NUT-FREE · EGG-FREE · AIP · LF OPTION · GAPS

prep time: 10 minutes, plus at least 4 hours to set | cook time: 40 minutes | yield: 4 pops each (1 pop per serving)

ROASTED BLUEBERRY POPS

1 cup fresh blueberries

1 tablespoon extra-virgin olive oil

1 cup water

2 tablespoons fresh lemon juice (about 1 small lemon)

¼ teaspoon fine sea salt

ROASTED CHERRY POPS (not low-FODMAP friendly)

1 cup pitted fresh cherries

1 tablespoon extra-virgin olive oil

1 cup water

2 tablespoons fresh lemon juice (about 1 small lemon)

¼ teaspoon fine sea salt

ROASTED RASPBERRY POPS

2 cups fresh raspberries

1 tablespoon extra-virgin olive oil

1 cup water

2 tablespoons fresh lemon juice (about 1 small lemon)

¼ teaspoon fine sea salt

ROASTED STRAWBERRY POPS

2 cups fresh strawberries, hulled and cut in half

1 tablespoon extra-virgin olive oil

1 cup water

2 tablespoons fresh lemon juice (about 1 small lemon)

¼ teaspoon fine sea salt

ROASTED GRAPEFRUIT POPS

2 grapefruits, peeled, seeded, and segmented (see Tips, page 292)

1 tablespoon extra-virgin olive oil

1 cup water

2 tablespoons fresh lemon juice (about 1 small lemon)

¼ teaspoon fine sea salt

SPECIAL EQUIPMENT

4 Popsicle molds and sticks

BLUEBERRY

APPROXIMATE NUTRITION BREAKDOWN (per serving)	
CALORIES: 52	FAT: 4g
PROTEIN: 0g	CARBS: 6g

CHERRY

APPROXIMATE NUTRITION BREAKDOWN (per serving)	
CALORIES: 51	FAT: 4g
PROTEIN: 0g	CARBS: 5g

STRAWBERRY

APPROXIMATE NUTRITION BREAKDOWN (per serving)	
CALORIES: 59	FAT: 4g
PROTEIN: 1g	CARBS: 6g

GRAPEFRUIT

APPROXIMATE NUTRITION BREAKDOWN (per serving)	
CALORIES: 85	FAT: 3g
PROTEIN: 1g	CARBS: 14g

RASPBERRY

APPROXIMATE NUTRITION BREAKDOWN (per serving)	
CALORIES: 64	FAT: 4g
PROTEIN: 1g	CARBS: 8g

1. Preheat the oven to 350°F and line a rimmed baking sheet with parchment paper. Toss the fruit in the olive oil and spread it out on the prepared baking sheet. Bake for 40 minutes, or until the fruit has released its juices but is not burning.

2. Transfer the roasted fruit to a blender and add the remaining ingredients. Blend on high speed for 3 minutes, or until smooth.

3. Pour the puree into 4 Popsicle molds. Add a stick and freeze for 4 hours or overnight.

4. To loosen the pops, place the bottoms of the molds in warm water, then remove the pops from the molds. Store in a sealed container in the freezer for up to 1 month.

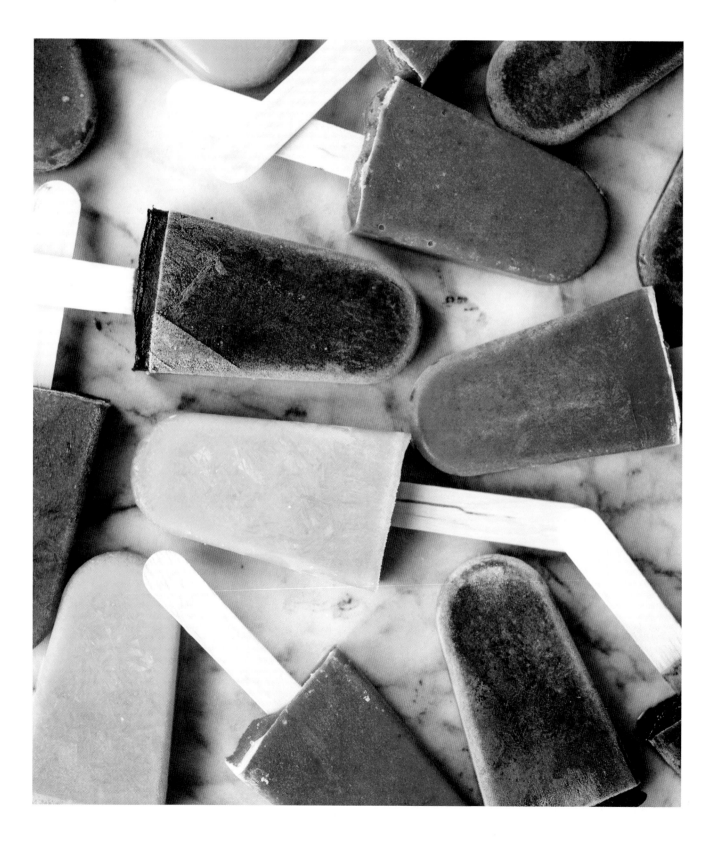

Fudgesicles

All I can say is, you're welcome. If you're on the Fed & Fit Project and frantically looking for a recipe that contains chocolate, I promise that these will hit the spot. I like to make a big batch so that I've got a fudgesicle at the ready when an ice cream or chocolate craving strikes!

NUT-FREE   EGG-FREE

prep time: 5 minutes, plus time to set overnight | *cook time: 10 minutes* | *yield: 8 fudgesicles (1 per serving)*

½ cup water

3 tablespoons unflavored gelatin

2½ cups full-fat coconut milk [about 1½ (13½-ounce) cans]

4 pitted Medjool dates

¼ cup unsweetened cocoa powder

SPECIAL EQUIPMENT

8 Popsicle molds and sticks

1. Bring the water to a boil. Whisk the gelatin into the boiling water and continue to stir until it is completely dissolved. Remove from the heat.

2. Place the coconut milk, dates, and cocoa powder in a blender. Blend on high speed for 3 minutes, or until the dates are completely liquefied. Pour the hot gelatin water into the coconut milk mixture and blend for about 20 seconds to combine.

3. Pour the mixture into 8 Popsicle molds. Place in the freezer for 1 hour to firm slightly. After 1 hour, push a Popsicle stick into each mold and place back in the freezer to set overnight.

4. To loosen the fudgesicles, place the bottoms of the molds in warm water, then pull the fudgesicles from the molds.

5. Enjoy right away or store in a large plastic bag in the freezer. To soften the fudgesicles before serving, let them sit out at room temperature for 3 to 5 minutes.

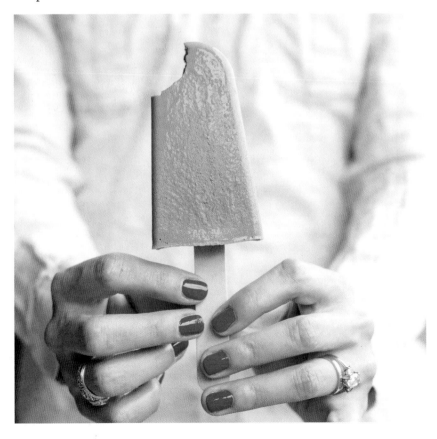

APPROXIMATE NUTRITION BREAKDOWN *(per serving)*			
CALORIES:	186	FAT:	14 g
PROTEIN:	4 g	CARBS:	13 g

Berries & Cream

This is one of my most favorite desserts of all time! In fact, it's even pictured on the cover of this book. It is delicious, is a breeze to pull together, and, if you're looking for a healthy dessert to serve a large group, can wow a crowd. I serve this simple whipped cream over any type of berry that's fresh and in season. Note that this whipped cream doesn't contain any added sweetener, which you'll find you don't need after completing the 28-Day Fed & Fit Project!

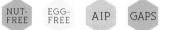

prep time: 5 minutes | *yield: 4 servings*

1 (13½-ounce) can full-fat coconut milk, chilled overnight

½ teaspoon vanilla extract

2 cups fresh berries of choice

1. Scoop the cream from the top of the can of coconut milk, leaving the water behind, and place the cream in a mixing bowl. Add the vanilla extract and, using either a stand mixer or a hand mixer, mix on high speed until the cream is smooth, forms soft peaks, and is slightly increased in volume.

2. To serve, divide the berries among four serving bowls. Add a dollop of whipped cream (about 2 tablespoons) to each dish.

3. The whipped cream will keep in the refrigerator for up to 4 days. If it's difficult to scoop when chilled, let it sit out at room temperature until softened.

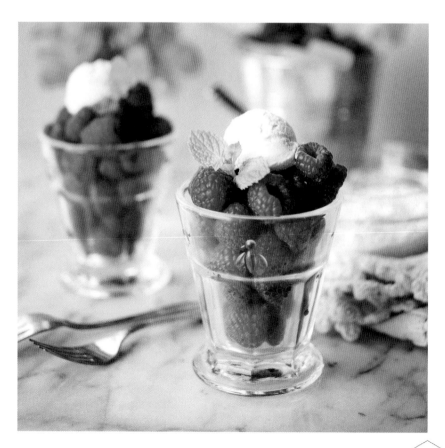

APPROXIMATE NUTRITION BREAKDOWN *(per serving)*			
CALORIES:	207	FAT:	19 g
PROTEIN:	1 g	CARBS:	9 g

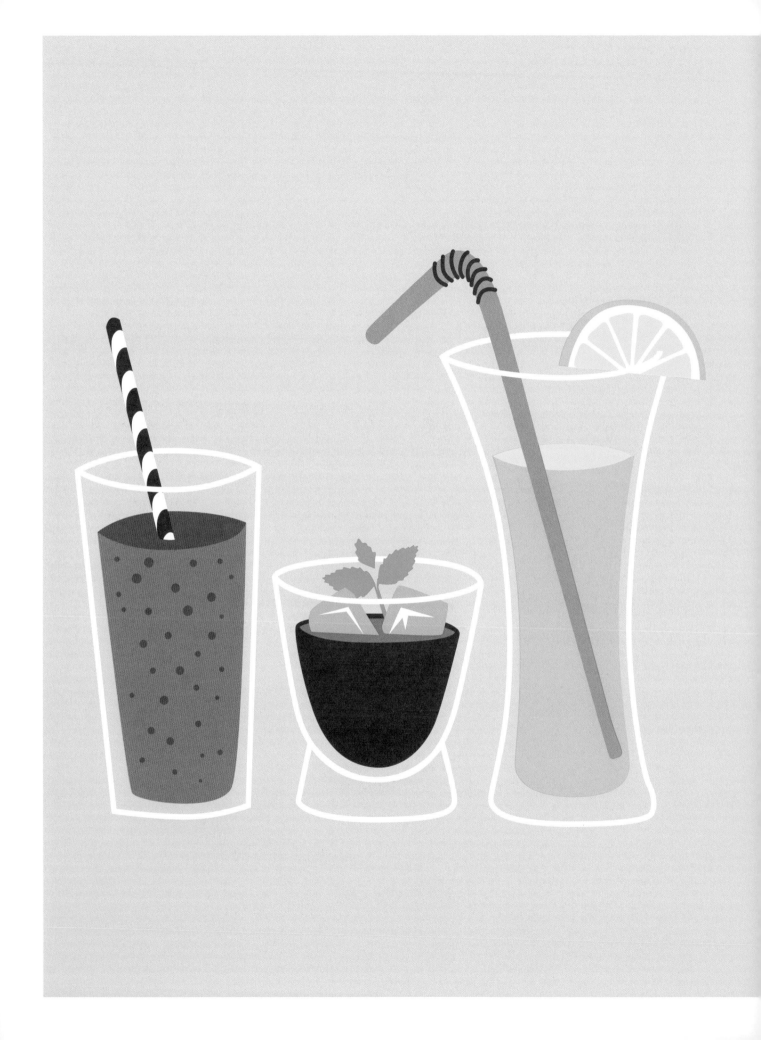

CHAPTER 12

I'M THIRSTY FOR MORE!

 Blackberry Rosemary
Agua Fresca
324

 Lavender Grapefruit
Agua Fresca
324

 Lemon Thyme
Agua Fresca
324

 Cucumber Mint
Agua Fresca
324

 Strawberry Lime
Agua Fresca
324

 Pumpkin Pie Spice
Coffee Creamer
326

 French Vanilla
Coffee Creamer
326

 Peppermint Mocha
Coffee Creamer
326

 Salted Caramel
Macchiato Coffee
Creamer
326

 Cold-Brew Coffee
Concentrate
328

 Hibiscus Mint Sparkler
329

 Almond Milk
330

 Cashew Milk
330

 Sunflower Seed Milk
330

 Soothing Lemon Ginger
Tea
331

 Bone Broth—Chicken
332

 Bone Broth—
Roasted Beef
332

Download the Fed & Fit iPhone and Android app! You can scan the
above QR codes directly in the app, which will then populate a
consolidated grocery shopping list for the scanned recipes.

Agua Fresca

5 Ways

I completely understand that not indulging in a Friday happy hour cocktail, Sunday evening glass of wine, or pitcher of margaritas at the neighborhood BBQ can make you feel like you're missing out. While I recommend that the majority of our daily hydration comes from water, sparkling water, or herbal tea, these agua frescas are a totally Fed & Fit Project–compliant treat. They're great to make when you're ready for something new or something special. An ice-cold glass of your favorite flavor will erase any feelings of missing out.

NUT-FREE · EGG-FREE · AIP · LF OPTION **· GAPS**

prep time: 5 to 15 minutes

yield: 6 servings each

LAVENDER GRAPEFRUIT AGUA FRESCA

4 grapefruits, peeled and broken into large pieces

2 tablespoons chopped fresh lavender leaves

3 cups water, divided

3 sprigs fresh lavender, for garnish

BLACKBERRY ROSEMARY AGUA FRESCA
(not low-FODMAP friendly)

1 pound fresh blackberries

2 tablespoons chopped fresh rosemary

6 cups water, divided

6 fresh rosemary sprigs, for garnish

CUCUMBER MINT AGUA FRESCA

3 cucumbers, cut into large pieces

2 tablespoons chopped fresh mint

3 cups water, divided

3 sprigs fresh mint, for garnish

LEMON THYME AGUA FRESCA

6 lemons, peeled and seeded

2 tablespoons chopped fresh thyme

6 cups water, divided

3 sprigs fresh thyme, for garnish

STRAWBERRY LIME AGUA FRESCA

1 pound fresh strawberries, hulled

¼ cup fresh lime juice (about 2 limes)

6 cups water, divided

6 lime wedges, for garnish

1. Place the fruit and any non-garnish herbs or lime juice in a blender with 3 cups of the water. Blend on high speed for 3 minutes, or until completely smooth. Pour the mix through a nut milk bag, cheesecloth, or fine-mesh strainer into a large pitcher.

2. Stir the rest of the water into the mix, add ice, and pour into glasses. Garnish and enjoy!

3. Agua fresca will keep refrigerated for 3 days. Even though the mixture was strained, small fruit particles left behind may settle to the bottom of the pitcher; just give it a stir and serve.

LAVENDER GRAPEFRUIT

APPROXIMATE NUTRITION BREAKDOWN *(per serving)*	
CALORIES: 71	FAT: 0 g
PROTEIN: 1 g	CARBS: 18 g

LEMON THYME

APPROXIMATE NUTRITION BREAKDOWN *(per serving)*	
CALORIES: 18	FAT: 0 g
PROTEIN: 1 g	CARBS: 6 g

BLACKBERRY ROSEMARY

APPROXIMATE NUTRITION BREAKDOWN *(per serving)*	
CALORIES: 33	FAT: 0 g
PROTEIN: 1 g	CARBS: 7 g

STRAWBERRY LIME

APPROXIMATE NUTRITION BREAKDOWN *(per serving)*	
CALORIES: 27	FAT: 0 g
PROTEIN: 1 g	CARBS: 7 g

CUCUMBER MINT

APPROXIMATE NUTRITION BREAKDOWN *(per serving)*	
CALORIES: 23	FAT: 0 g
PROTEIN: 2 g	CARBS: 6 g

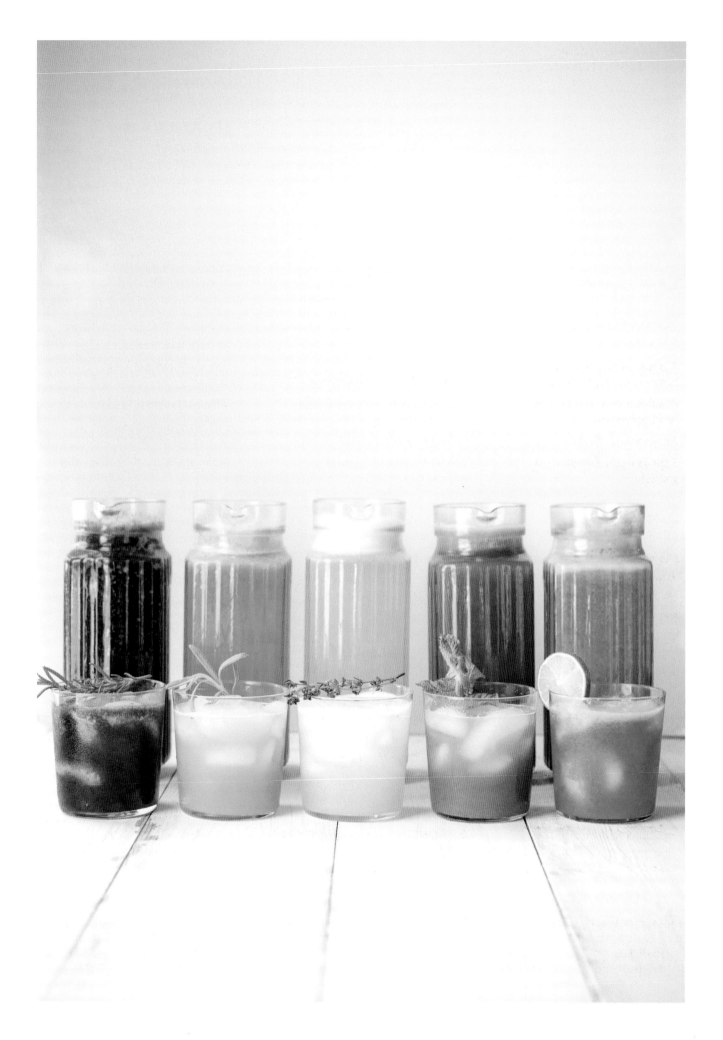

Coffee Creamer

4 Ways

I've lost count of the number of people who've told me that they're happy to "go Paleo" but can't possibly fathom giving up their sugary, artificial ingredient–filled, poor-quality-dairy–laden coffee creamer. Well, by golly, I can't let that fly anymore. Here are four different varieties for you to choose from! I prefer to freeze my creamer into small cubes so that they cool and flavor my coffee.

NUT-FREE · EGG-FREE · OPTION AIP · OPTION GAPS

prep time: 5 minutes | *yield: 2 scant cups (30 servings)*

PUMPKIN PIE SPICE COFFEE CREAMER

1 (13½-ounce) can full-fat coconut milk

2 tablespoons water

2 pitted Medjool dates

1 teaspoon vanilla extract (omit if sensitive on AIP)

½ teaspoon ground cinnamon

½ teaspoon ginger powder

½ teaspoon ground nutmeg

⅛ teaspoon ground allspice

⅛ teaspoon ground cloves

PEPPERMINT MOCHA COFFEE CREAMER
(not AIP or GAPS-friendly)

1 (13½-ounce) can full-fat coconut milk

2 tablespoons water

2 pitted Medjool dates

1 tablespoon unsweetened cocoa powder

½ teaspoon peppermint extract

⅛ teaspoon fine sea salt

SALTED CARAMEL MACCHIATO COFFEE CREAMER

1 (13½-ounce) can full-fat coconut milk

2 tablespoons water

2 pitted Medjool dates

½ teaspoon vanilla extract (omit if sensitive on AIP)

¼ teaspoon fine sea salt

FRENCH VANILLA COFFEE CREAMER

1 (13½-ounce) can full-fat coconut milk

2 tablespoons water

2 pitted Medjool dates

1 teaspoon vanilla extract (omit if sensitive on AIP)

In a blender, puree all of the ingredients for 3 to 5 minutes, until completely smooth. Use right away or store in a jar in the refrigerator for up to 7 days.

tips

- *If your canned coconut milk is extra thick and/or the creamer is too thick after being chilled, add 1 to 2 tablespoons water to thin it.*

- *If you prefer not to include any sweetener, skip the dates!*

- *Freeze the creamer in silicone molds to have convenient portions available anytime! Individual portions of creamer will keep in the freezer for up to 5 months.*

PUMPKIN PIE

APPROXIMATE NUTRITION BREAKDOWN *(per serving)*		
CALORIES: 29	FAT:	3 g
PROTEIN: 0 g	CARBS:	2 g

FRENCH VANILLA

APPROXIMATE NUTRITION BREAKDOWN *(per serving)*		
CALORIES: 28	FAT:	3 g
PROTEIN: 0 g	CARBS:	2 g

PEPPERMINT MOCHA

APPROXIMATE NUTRITION BREAKDOWN *(per serving)*		
CALORIES: 29	FAT:	3 g
PROTEIN: 0 g	CARBS:	2 g

SALTED CARAMEL

APPROXIMATE NUTRITION BREAKDOWN *(per serving)*		
CALORIES: 28	FAT:	3 g
PROTEIN: 0 g	CARBS:	2 g

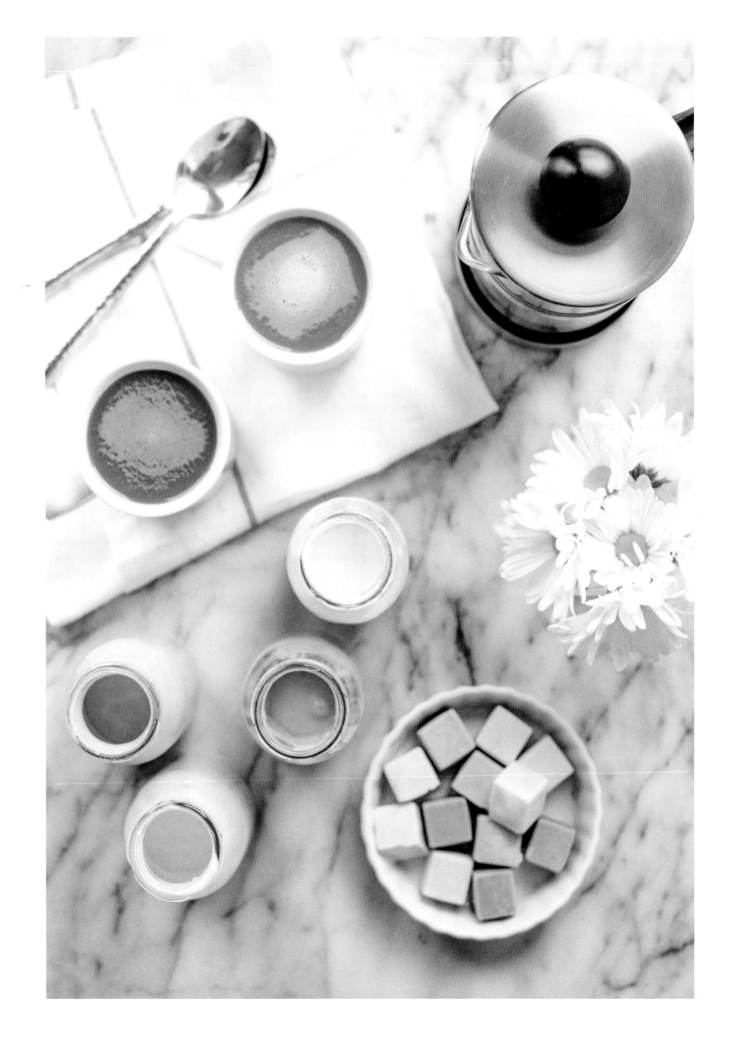

Cold-Brew Coffee Concentrate

I did the math and discovered that, for the same amount of money I've spent on store-bought cold-brew coffee over the past two years, I could be the proud owner of the coveted Manolo Blahnik 'Hangisi' Jeweled Pumps in two colors. While quality coffee grounds aren't free, they stretch a lot further and, thanks to this incredibly delicious home cold-brew method, get me much closer to my first pair. (Hot pink, in case you're wondering.) I adore cold-brew coffee because it tends to be less bitter and slightly stronger than its hot-brewed counterpart. I enjoy it over ice, but you can heat it up if you prefer!

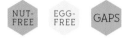

NUT-FREE **EGG-FREE** **GAPS**

prep time: 5 minutes, plus at least 12 hours to brew

yield: eight 8-ounce servings

2 cups coarsely ground coffee

4 cups water

FOR SERVING

Coffee creamer of choice [page 326] (optional)

SPECIAL EQUIPMENT

8-cup French coffee press (optional)

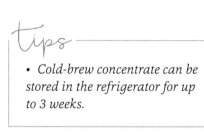

tips

- Cold-brew concentrate can be stored in the refrigerator for up to 3 weeks.

1. Place the coffee grounds in an 8-cup French press (ideal), a 2-quart glass mason jar, or a medium-sized glass bowl. Pour the water over the coffee grounds, cover, and refrigerate for at least 12 hours but no more than 2 days.

2. Press the French press stopper down to separate the grounds from the coffee, or strain the grounds through a fine-mesh strainer. Pour the coffee into a mason jar or pitcher for storage.

3. To serve, mix 1 part cold-brew concentrate (about ½ cup) with 1 part cool water (about ½ cup). Serve over ice with your favorite coffee creamer!

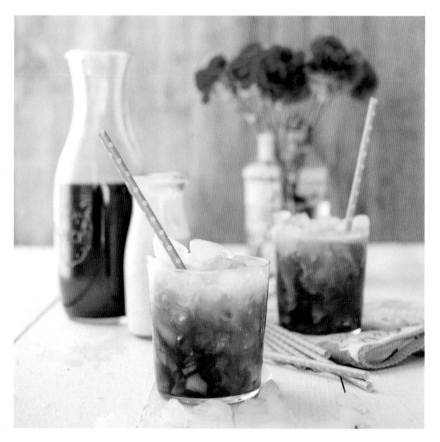

APPROXIMATE NUTRITION BREAKDOWN *(per serving)*			
CALORIES:	5	FAT:	0 g
PROTEIN:	1 g	CARBS:	0 g

Hibiscus Mint Sparkler

Homemade herbal tea inspired by the famous passion tea from Starbucks! If I'm out and about and want a non-water drink in the afternoon (I try not to drink caffeine after noon), I'll swing through a Starbucks for an "unsweetened iced venti passion." It's tart and so refreshing—but it needed something more. I found myself cutting the passion tea with my own bottles of sparkling water to make it more of an herbal tea–infused flavored soda. The added mint makes it an even more delicious treat.

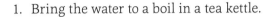

NUT-FREE · EGG-FREE · AIP · LF · GAPS

prep time: 10 minutes | *cook time: 10 minutes* | *yield: ten 12-ounce servings*

HIBISCUS MINT TEA

7 cups water

1 cup dried hibiscus flowers

½ packed cup fresh mint leaves

FOR SERVING

2 quarts unflavored sparkling mineral water

Fresh mint sprigs (optional)

1. Bring the water to a boil in a tea kettle.

2. Place the hibiscus flowers in a colander or strainer and run cold water over them for about 1 minute. Transfer the rinsed, dried flowers to a heatproof 2-quart (or larger) pitcher or pot and add the mint. Pour the boiling water over the flowers and mint and let steep for 5 minutes.

3. Strain out the hibiscus and mint by pouring the tea through fine-mesh strainer into a clean pitcher. Let the tea cool completely before drinking.

4. To serve, fill glasses with ice and pour in 1 part cooled, strained tea and 1 part sparkling water. Garnish with fresh mint, if desired.

tips

• *Dried hibiscus flowers are pretty easy to find. If your local grocer doesn't carry them, check out any nearby Spanish market. Otherwise, you can order them online.*

• *Once the package is opened, dried hibiscus flowers will keep in the pantry for about 2 months. For longer storage, store the flowers in a freezer-safe bag or container in the freezer for up to 5 months. This will ensure their freshness.*

• *The strained tea will keep refrigerated for up to 10 days.*

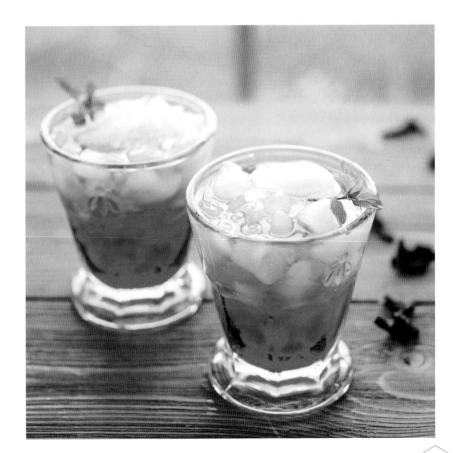

APPROXIMATE NUTRITION BREAKDOWN *(per serving)*			
CALORIES:	8	FAT:	0 g
PROTEIN:	0 g	CARBS:	1 g

Almond, Cashew, or Sunflower Seed Milk

Finding store-bought nut or seed milk made with healthy ingredients is more difficult than it sounds. Sweeteners, emulsifiers, and various preservatives are found in most national brands. The good news is that making your own milks at home is actually much easier than it sounds! It's almost as simple as making a pot of coffee. If you don't already have one, I highly recommend that you purchase a nut milk bag. It will make this process even easier!

 EGG-FREE   GAPS

prep time: 5 minutes, plus at least 4 hours to soak the nuts or seeds

yield: 1 quart (four 1-cup servings)

1 cup raw almonds, cashews, or sunflower seeds

4 cups cool water

½ teaspoon vanilla extract

¼ teaspoon fine sea salt

SPECIAL EQUIPMENT

High-powered blender or food processor

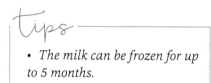

- *The milk can be frozen for up to 5 months.*

1. Place the nuts or seeds in a small bowl. Cover with water and set in the refrigerator to soak for 4 to 8 hours.

2. Discard the soaking liquid, rinse the nuts or seeds, and then place them in a high-powered blender or food processor. Add 4 cups of fresh cool water and blend on high speed for 3 minutes, or until all of the clumps are gone.

3. Pour the nut milk through a nut milk bag or cheesecloth, discarding the pulp or saving it for later use (you could, for example, dehydrate the pulp for grain-free baking).

4. Transfer the filtered milk to a large mason jar or pitcher with a lid. Season with the vanilla extract and salt. Enjoy right away or store in the refrigerator for up to 7 days. Note that the milk will separate as it sits in the refrigerator. This is completely normal; just give it a stir before serving.

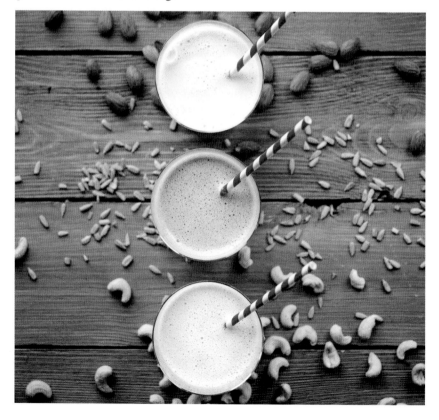

ALMOND

APPROXIMATE NUTRITION BREAKDOWN *(per serving)*			
CALORIES:	9	FAT:	1 g
PROTEIN:	0 g	CARBS:	3 g

SUNFLOWER SEED

APPROXIMATE NUTRITION BREAKDOWN *(per serving)*			
CALORIES:	9	FAT:	1 g
PROTEIN:	0 g	CARBS:	3 g

CASHEW

APPROXIMATE NUTRITION BREAKDOWN *(per serving)*			
CALORIES:	11	FAT:	1 g
PROTEIN:	0 g	CARBS:	3 g

Soothing Lemon Ginger Tea

I drink lemon ginger tea almost every single day. While I adore the flavor, I really love this tea because of its healing, anti-inflammatory properties. A warm glass first thing in the morning or even on ice at the end of a long day always soothes my stomach and staves off emotional eating.

NUT-FREE · EGG-FREE · AIP · LF · GAPS

prep time: 5 minutes | *cook time: 10 minutes* | *yield: six 8-ounce servings*

4 ounces fresh ginger (about 4 inches), sliced thin

4 lemons, halved

6 cups water

1. Bring 6 cups of water to a boil.

2. Place the lemons and ginger in a heatproof 2-quart pitcher. Once the water is boiling, pour it over the top. Stir and let steep for at least 5 minutes.

3. To store, you can either strain out the lemon and ginger if you prefer a milder tea, or leave them in if (like me) you prefer a stronger tea.

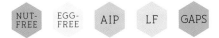

- *Leftover tea will keep in the refrigerator for up to 2 weeks.*

- *If you opt to keep the lemon and ginger in the tea, it will continue to deepen in flavor.*

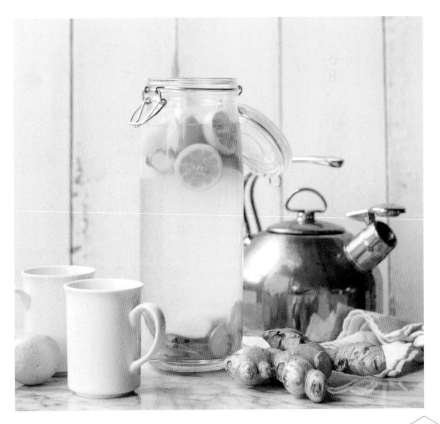

APPROXIMATE NUTRITION BREAKDOWN			
(per serving)			
CALORIES:	8	FAT:	0 g
PROTEIN:	0 g	CARBS:	2 g

Bone Broth— Chicken & Roasted Beef

With its seemingly magical healing properties, bone broth is a deserving staple in every healthy kitchen. While its obvious uses are geared toward soups and stews, the less-obvious uses make it a daily indulgence in my house. I'll sip on a mug of seasoned broth in the morning, especially if my stomach is unsettled, and toss a frozen broth cube in a bowl for our Great Pyrenees, Gus, to enjoy as an afternoon treat. For the beef bone broth, I suggest roasting the beef bones before making the broth; this extra step really helps bring out a wonderful flavor.

NUT-FREE · EGG-FREE · AIP (OPTION) · LF · GAPS

prep time: 10 minutes | *cook time: 1½ or 10 to 12 hours, depending on method, plus 35 minutes for beef broth* | *yield: 6 quarts each (twelve 2-cup servings)*

BEEF BONE BROTH

2 tablespoons extra-virgin olive oil

3 pounds beef stock bones with marrow (see Tips)

CHICKEN BONE BROTH

3 pounds chicken feet, wings, or necks

2 onions, unpeeled and quartered (omit for low-FODMAP)

2 carrots, unpeeled and cut into large chunks

2 cloves garlic, peeled and smashed with the side of knife (omit for low-FODMAP)

2 tablespoons apple cider vinegar

2 bay leaves

6 quarts water

1. If making chicken bone broth, jump ahead to Step 2. If making beef bone broth, preheat the oven to 400°F. Rub the olive oil over the beef bones. Spread them out on a rimmed baking sheet and bake for 35 minutes, or until they develop a deep brown color. Remove the bones from the pan and set aside. Pour a small amount of hot water (about ½ cup) into the pan and work to scrape up any remaining bits of meat or fat stuck to the bottom of a pan; set the pan aside.

2. Cook the broth using one of these two methods:

   Pressure cooker method: Place the chicken or roasted beef bones and the rest of the broth ingredients in a pressure cooker. If making beef bone broth, pour the water and scraped-up meat and fat pieces in the roasting pan into the pressure cooker. Seal and, following the manufacturer's instructions for your pressure cooker, bring it up to temperature. Let cook for 1 hour, then slowly release the pressure. Let the pot sit for 30 minutes after the pressure dissipates.

   Slow cooker method: Place the chicken or roasted beef bones and the rest of the broth ingredients in a 10-quart slow cooker. If making beef bone broth, pour the water and scraped-up meat and fat pieces in the roasting pan into the slow cooker. Cover and cook on low for 10 to 12 hours.

3. Skim off and discard any scum that may have collected on the top of the broth. Strain the broth through a nut milk bag, cheesecloth-lined colander, or fine-mesh strainer.

CHICKEN

APPROXIMATE NUTRITION BREAKDOWN *(per serving)*			
CALORIES:	20	FAT:	0 g
PROTEIN:	4 g	CARBS:	2 g

BEEF

APPROXIMATE NUTRITION BREAKDOWN *(per serving)*			
CALORIES:	30	FAT:	0 g
PROTEIN:	6 g	CARBS:	2 g

- Knuckle bones are great for making broth, especially if cut in half. Ask your butcher to do this for you.

- Store the broth in the refrigerator for up to 7 days or freeze for up to 5 months.

- To freeze small amounts of broth, pour it into a plastic ice cube tray. Freeze the cubes, then transfer them to a large bag for long-term storage.

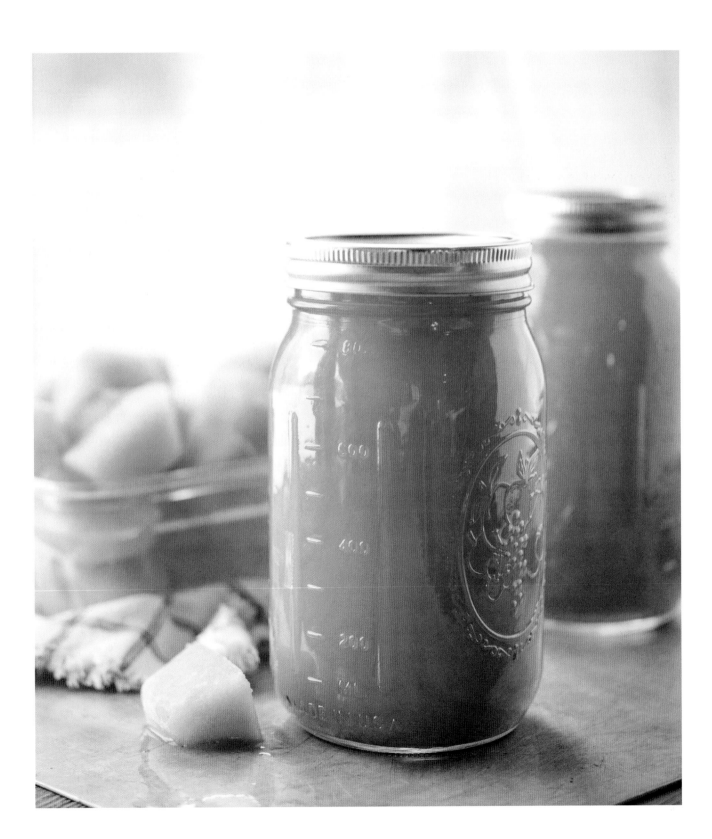

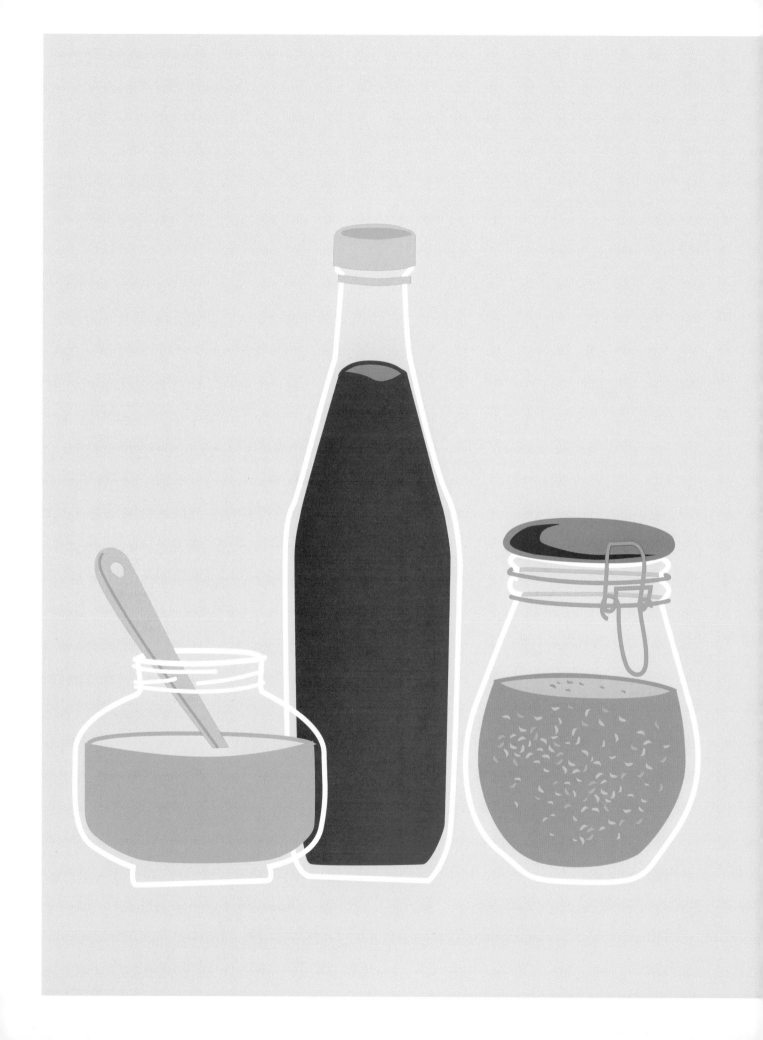

CHAPTER 13

MORE FLAVOR, PLEASE!

 BBQ Sauce 2.0
336

 Buffalo Sauce
337

3-Ingredient
Paleo Ranch
338

 Creamy
Jalapeño Ranch
339

 Ketchup: Classic
340

 Ketchup: Spicy
340

 Paleo
Sour Cream
341

 Pico de Gallo
342

Guacamole
343

 Salsa Verde
344

 Salsa Rojo
345

Roasted Garlic
346

 Roasted Garlic Pesto
2.0
348

 Super Simple Paleo
Mayo
349

Download the Fed & Fit iPhone and Android app! You can scan the
above QR codes directly in the app, which will then populate a
consolidated grocery shopping list for the scanned recipes.

BBQ Sauce 2.0

I don't think I could rightly call myself a proud Texan if I didn't have a killer BBQ sauce recipe up my sleeve. Here's my mission with this sauce: when you plop it down next to all of the off-the-shelf BBQ sauces at your next family gathering, folks won't just rave about how it's their new favorite, but they'll have no clue that it's made with healthy, wholesome ingredients. As a bonus, this sauce freezes really well!

NUT-FREE   EGG-FREE   OPTION GAPS

prep time: 5 minutes | *cook time: 6 minutes* | *yield: 3½ cups (2 tablespoons per serving)*

1 (15-ounce) can strained tomatoes or tomato sauce*

1 (6-ounce) can tomato paste*

½ cup apple cider vinegar

½ cup coconut aminos

1 tablespoon chili powder

1 tablespoon garlic powder

1 tablespoon onion powder

1 teaspoon fine sea salt

½ teaspoon ground black pepper

*If following a GAPS protocol, check the labels of the strained tomatoes and tomato paste carefully to make sure that they are free of additives.

1. In a medium-sized saucepan over medium heat, whisk together all of the ingredients until well combined. Bring to a simmer and continue to whisk for an additional 5 minutes.

2. Remove from the heat and let cool for at least 5 minutes.

3. Use right away or transfer to a jar for storage in the refrigerator for up to 2 weeks.

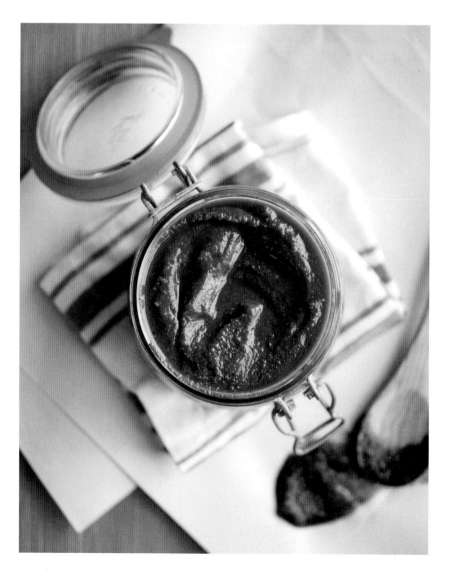

tips

• *This sauce will keep in the freezer for up to 5 months. You can either freeze it in freezer-safe jars or pour it into an ice cube tray to have convenient portions for later use.*

APPROXIMATE NUTRITION BREAKDOWN *(per serving)*			
CALORIES:	27	FAT:	0 g
PROTEIN:	1 g	CARBS:	6 g

Buffalo Sauce

This truly magical sauce keeps my recipe inspiration brimming with flavorful family favorites. It's entirely customizable, depending on whether you prefer more or less heat, and it adds mega flavor to casseroles, baked or grilled chicken, roasted vegetables, and salads. Experiment and keep this winner on hand for when you need more variety in your routine!

NUT-FREE   EGG-FREE   OPTION LF   GAPS

prep time: 5 minutes | *cook time: 6 minutes* | *yield: 1 cup (1 tablespoon per serving)*

⅓ cup avocado oil (use EVOO for low-FODMAP)

⅓ cup apple cider vinegar

⅓ cup fresh lemon juice (2 to 3 lemons)

2 teaspoons garlic powder (omit for low-FODMAP)

2 teaspoons onion powder (omit for low-FODMAP)

2 teaspoons fine sea salt

1 teaspoon cayenne pepper

1 teaspoon paprika

½ teaspoon ground black pepper

1. In a medium saucepan over medium heat, whisk all of the ingredients until well combined. Bring to a simmer and continue to whisk for an additional 5 minutes.

2. Remove from the heat. Either use right away or transfer to a jar and store in the refrigerator for up to 2 weeks.

tips

• *When chilled, the olive oil in the sauce may separate and rise to the top of the jar. This is normal! Just let it come to room temperature before using and stir to combine or heat it either in a microwave for 30 seconds or on the stovetop and stir until the oil is incorporated.*

• *This sauce can be stored in the freezer for up to 5 months. You can either freeze it in freezer-safe jars or pour it into an ice cube tray to have convenient portions for later use.*

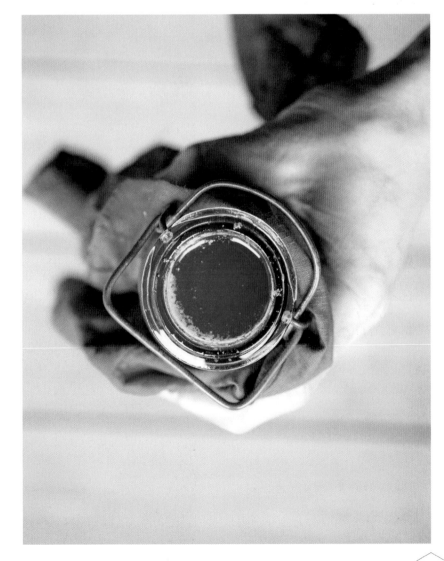

APPROXIMATE NUTRITION BREAKDOWN *(per serving)*			
CALORIES:	47	FAT:	5 g
PROTEIN:	0 g	CARBS:	1 g

3-Ingredient

Paleo Ranch

This ranch dressing is probably the single most consistently popular recipe on my blog. Why? Because it is so easy to make and is really flavorful. I'm updating this Fed & Fit classic by substituting avocado oil for the "light-tasting" olive oil in the mayo of the original recipe. I've found that avocado oil yields a much milder and more consistent flavor.

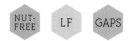

prep time: 5 minutes | *yield: about 2 cups (2 tablespoons per serving)*

2 cups mayo, store-bought or homemade (page 349)

¼ cup fresh lemon juice (about 2 small lemons)

1 tablespoon dried dill weed

1. Whisk the lemon juice and dill into the mayo until well combined.

2. Enjoy right away or transfer to a jar and store in the refrigerator. It will keep for about 1 month.

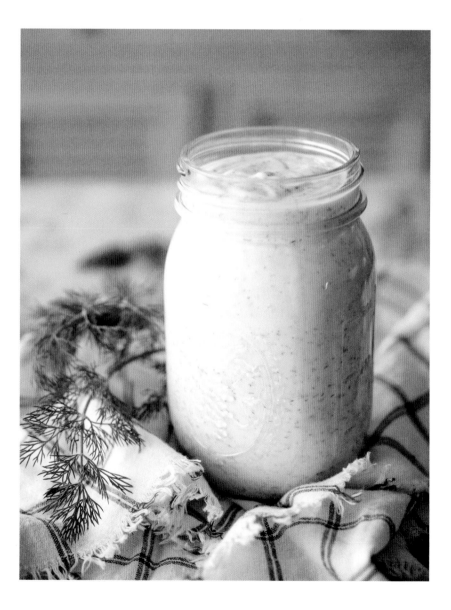

APPROXIMATE NUTRITION BREAKDOWN *(per serving)*			
CALORIES:	201	FAT:	21g
PROTEIN:	0g	CARBS:	1g

Creamy Jalapeño Ranch

Let's be honest. This recipe came to be because if a restaurant has a "creamy jalapeño ranch" on the menu, then I'm going to order it. Though I was first introduced to this spicy version of ranch as a dipping sauce for tortilla chips, I've also come to love it as a sauce for Pan-Fried Plantains (page 145), as a salad dressing, and as a finishing sauce for a simple protein (pages 122 to 127).

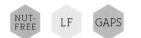

prep time: 5 minutes | *yield: 2 cups (2 tablespoons per serving)*

2 cups mayo, store-bought or homemade (page 349)

½ cup fresh lime juice (about 4 limes)

2 jalapeño peppers, seeded and coarsely chopped

1. In a blender, puree the mayo, lime juice, and jalapeños for at least 1 minute, until the mixture is smooth and has an even consistency. Season to taste.

2. Enjoy right away or transfer to a jar and store in the refrigerator. It will keep covered in the refrigerator for about 1 week.

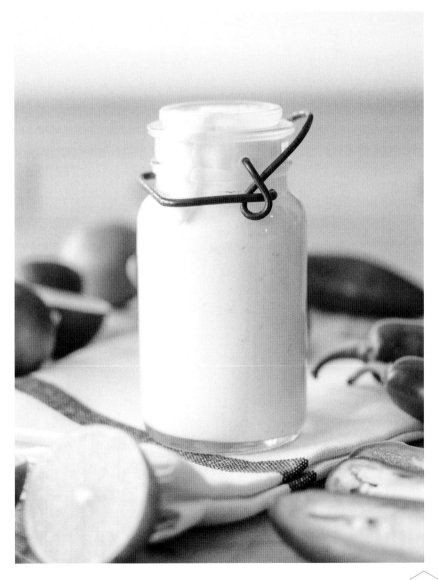

APPROXIMATE NUTRITION BREAKDOWN	
(per serving)	
CALORIES: 201	FAT: 21 g
PROTEIN: 0 g	CARBS: 1 g

Ketchup: Classic & Spicy

After going Paleo, I thought I wouldn't miss ketchup. I thought that all of the other vibrant and flavorful foods would keep my attention elsewhere. Then, years later, when I dipped a steak fry into a jar of my spicy ketchup for the first time, I almost cried. Yes, all of the other foods in my Paleo template were vibrant and delicious, but good grief, I love ketchup, too.

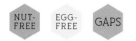

NUT-FREE · EGG-FREE · GAPS

prep time: 5 minutes, plus at least 4 hours to soak the dates

yield: 1¼ cups (2 tablespoons per serving)

6 ounces tomato paste

2 Medjool dates, pitted and soaked in warm water for 4 hours or overnight

1 teaspoon date water (reserved from soaking dates)

1 tablespoon apple cider vinegar

1 tablespoon plus 1 teaspoon fresh lemon juice (about ½ small lemon)

3 tablespoons water

½ teaspoon fine sea salt

¼ teaspoon garlic powder

FOR SPICY KETCHUP

½ teaspoon fresh lemon juice

⅛ to ¼ teaspoon cayenne pepper

1. Place all of the ingredients for the ketchup in a bowl, adding an additional ½ teaspoon lemon juice and cayenne pepper if making spicy ketchup (⅛ teaspoon cayenne will create a medium-spiced ketchup with just a hint of heat, and ¼ teaspoon will create a truly spicy ketchup). Whisk together until the ketchup has a smooth consistency.

2. Use right away or transfer to a jar and store in the refrigerator.

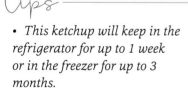

tips

- *This ketchup will keep in the refrigerator for up to 1 week or in the freezer for up to 3 months.*

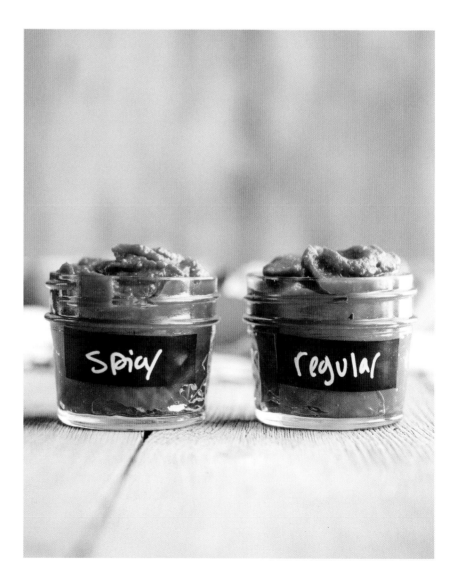

REGULAR

APPROXIMATE NUTRITION BREAKDOWN *(per serving)*			
CALORIES:	23	FAT:	0 g
PROTEIN:	0 g	CARBS:	6 g

SPICY

APPROXIMATE NUTRITION BREAKDOWN *(per serving)*			
CALORIES:	23	FAT:	0 g
PROTEIN:	0 g	CARBS:	6 g

Paleo
Sour Cream

Leave it to a Garcia to invent a Paleo sour cream recipe that comes together in under 5 minutes. Sometimes a girl just needs sour cream on her stuffed potato, salad, or chili relleno casserole that won't make her break out from exposure to dairy! I make a bowl of this sour cream about once every two weeks—it's that good and that easy.

NUT-FREE   EGG-FREE   AIP   GAPS

prep time: 5 minutes, plus at least 8 hours to chill the cans of coconut milk

yield: 1 cup (2 tablespoons per serving)

2 (13½-ounce) cans full-fat coconut milk, refrigerated overnight

2 tablespoons fresh lemon juice (about 1 small lemon)

½ teaspoon fine sea salt

1. Open the cans of chilled coconut milk. Scoop off the cream that has risen to the top and place it in a food processor or blender. Save the coconut water for shakes or other uses.

2. Add the lemon juice and salt to the food processor or blender and blend for about 1 minute, until it has a smooth, even consistency.

3. Use right away or transfer to a jar and store in the refrigerator.

tips

- *This sour cream will keep in the refrigerator for about 1 week.*

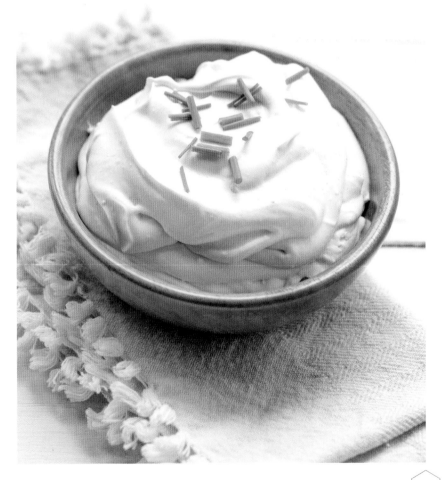

APPROXIMATE NUTRITION BREAKDOWN	
(per serving)	
CALORIES: 40	FAT: 4 g
PROTEIN: 0 g	CARBS: 1 g

Pico de Gallo

Finding food substitutions is always easier (and more sustainable) than eliminating foods entirely. Am I right? A trick that I've kept up my sleeve for years is using (or asking for) extra pico in place of cheese. Think of the flavorful possibilities! This trick works on casseroles, salads, nachos, and so on. Get creative!

NUT-FREE   EGG-FREE   OPTION LF   GAPS

prep time: 10 minutes | *yield: 2 cups (¼ cup per serving)*

3 medium tomatoes, diced small

½ medium-sized purple onion, diced small (omit for low-FODMAP)

¼ cup fresh cilantro leaves and stems, chopped

1 jalapeño pepper, seeded and finely chopped

1 clove garlic, minced (omit for low-FODMAP)

2 tablespoons fresh lime juice (about 1 lime)

½ teaspoon fine sea salt

1. Place all of the ingredients in a small mixing bowl and stir until well combined.

2. Use right away or cover and store in the refrigerator for up to 1 week.

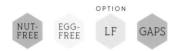

- *Like more heat? Leave the jalapeño seeds in or add an extra chopped jalapeño!*

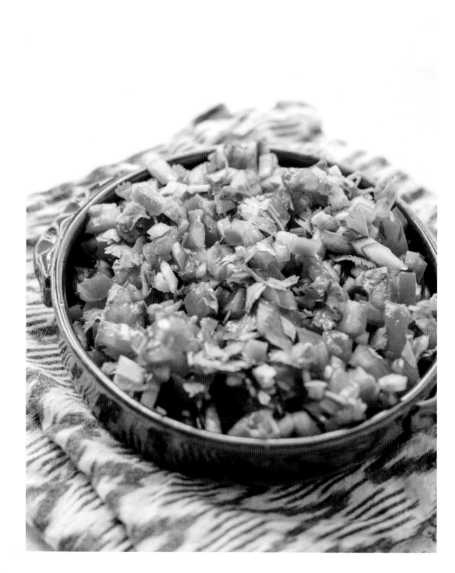

APPROXIMATE NUTRITION BREAKDOWN			
(per serving)			
CALORIES:	14	FAT:	0 g
PROTEIN:	0 g	CARBS:	3 g

Guacamole

Born and raised in the capital of Tex-Mex (San Antonio, that is), I've tasted thousands of guacamole variations. Yes, thousands. As such, I've decided that the best guacamole 1) is simple to pull together; 2) is not overly fancy; and 3) allows the star of the show (the avocado) to remain the star of the show. This guacamole recipe is just that! It is a cinch to pull together, calls for straightforward ingredients, and really highlights the luscious avocado.

NUT-FREE   EGG-FREE   GAPS

prep time: 5 minutes | *yield: 4¼ cups (¼ cup per serving)*

3 avocados, peeled and pitted

½ cup pico de gallo, store-bought or homemade (page 342)

2 tablespoons fresh lime juice (about 1 lime)

1 teaspoon fine sea salt

1. Place the avocados in a large mixing bowl and roughly mash them with a fork. Add the rest of the ingredients and mix everything together with a fork until the pico is evenly mixed into the avocado.

2. Use right away or cover and store in the refrigerator for up to 5 days.

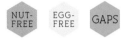

tips

• *If you don't have any pico de gallo on hand, you can substitute an equal amount of fresh salsa.*

• *To keep leftover guacamole from browning too quickly, I recommend pressing a sheet of wax paper directly on top. This will help keep the air off and, therefore, will reduce oxidative browning.*

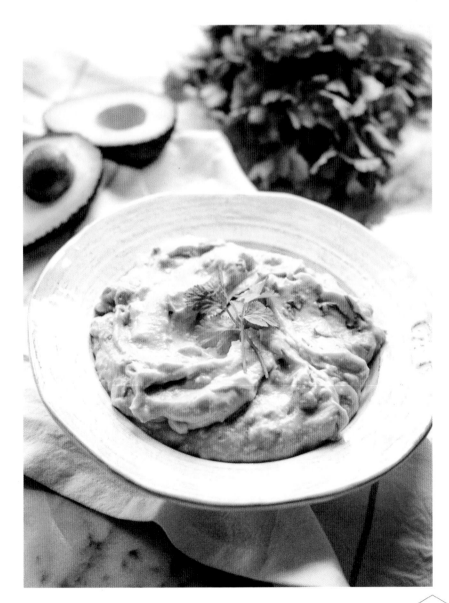

APPROXIMATE NUTRITION BREAKDOWN *(per serving)*			
CALORIES:	112	FAT:	10 g
PROTEIN:	2 g	CARBS:	7 g

Salsa Verde

I lived in Austin, Texas, for a hot minute after I graduated from Texas A&M University, and two of my favorite things about the city were the bustling walking trail around Lake Austin (where I used to train for my long-distance runs) and the salsa verde at Guero's Taco Bar, a Mexican restaurant on South Congress. I used to go to Guero's just for the salsa. In true food love affair fashion, I fashioned my own salsa verde recipe worthy of adoration.

 NUT-FREE   EGG-FREE GAPS

prep time: 15 minutes | *yield: 3 cups (¼ cup per serving)*

1 pound tomatillos (about 14), husked and quartered

1 yellow onion, coarsely chopped

8 cloves garlic, smashed with the side of a knife

4 jalapeño peppers, seeded and coarsely chopped

1 cup fresh cilantro leaves and stems, coarsely chopped

½ cup fresh lime juice (about 4 limes)

½ teaspoon fine sea salt

1. Place all of the ingredients in a blender or food processor. Blend for 2 minutes, or until the salsa has an even consistency and there aren't any chunks.

2. Use immediately or transfer to a jar and store in the refrigerator. It will keep refrigerated for up to 1 week.

tips

- *This salsa actually freezes well! You can either freeze it in one large freezer-safe jar for a single use or pour it into an ice cube tray for convenient portions. It will keep in the freezer for up to 5 months.*

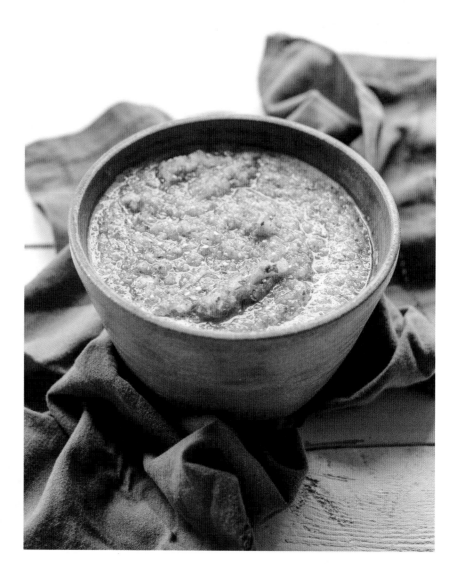

APPROXIMATE NUTRITION BREAKDOWN *(per serving)*			
CALORIES:	18	FAT:	0 g
PROTEIN:	0 g	CARBS:	3 g

Salsa Rojo

Because I can't take you to my favorite Mexican restaurant in San Antonio, I'll have to settle for sharing my restaurant-style salsa recipe. I love using salsa as a dressing on salads and as a simple dip when folks come over! I suggest serving it with plantain chips or other crunchy vegetables.

NUT-FREE   EGG-FREE   **OPTION** LF   GAPS

prep time: 10 minutes | *yield: 4 cups (¼ cup per serving)*

1 (28-ounce) can diced tomatoes, drained

½ medium-sized purple onion, coarsely chopped (about ½ cup) (omit for low-FODMAP)

¼ cup fresh cilantro leaves and stems

¼ cup fresh lime juice (about 2 limes)

2 cloves garlic, smashed with the side of a knife (omit for low-FODMAP)

1 jalapeño pepper, seeded and coarsely chopped

1 teaspoon fine sea salt

1. Place all of the ingredients in a blender or food processor. Pulse about 15 times, or until the mixture has an even, slightly textured consistency and no large chunks remain.

2. Use immediately or transfer to a jar and store in the refrigerator. The salsa will keep refrigerated for up to 1 week.

tips

• *This salsa actually freezes well! You can either freeze it in one large freezer-safe jar for a single use or pour it into an ice cube tray for convenient portions. It will keep frozen for up to 5 months.*

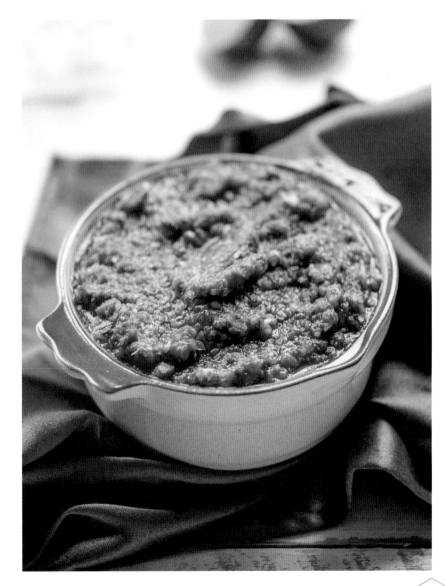

APPROXIMATE NUTRITION BREAKDOWN *(per serving)*			
CALORIES:	17	FAT:	0 g
PROTEIN:	0 g	CARBS:	3 g

Roasted Garlic

If you want to add instant, life-changing flavor to a sauce, protein, or side, look no further than good old-fashioned roasted garlic. While it's true that raw garlic has a strong, bright flavor, roasted garlic is much milder and sweeter.

NUT-FREE · EGG-FREE · AIP · GAPS

prep time: 5 minutes | *cook time: 45 minutes* | *yield: ¼ cup cloves (1 tablespoon roasted garlic paste per serving)*

2 garlic bulbs

tips

- *To extend the life of your roasted garlic, after squeezing the roasted garlic out of the cloves, mash it into a paste. Drop 1-tablespoon amounts of the roasted garlic paste onto a baking sheet, freeze until firm, and transfer to a freezer-safe bag for up to 4 months.*

1. Preheat the oven to 375°F.

2. Cut off the very top of each garlic bulb to expose the tips of the individual cloves. Peel away the outer papery skin, but make sure that all of the cloves stay attached to the main bulb. For cloves that don't reach the top, use a paring knife to cut off their tops so that every clove is exposed.

3. Wrap each prepared bulb in a square piece of aluminum foil. Place the wrapped bulbs, evenly spaced, in two wells of a metal muffin tin. (This keeps them upright.) Bake for 45 minutes.

4. Remove from the oven and let cool completely in the foil, about 1 hour.

5. To extract the roasted garlic, squeeze the bulbs or individual cloves until all of the roasted garlic is pushed out of the cloves.

6. Use right away or store in the refrigerator for up to 1 week.

APPROXIMATE NUTRITION BREAKDOWN *(per serving)*			
CALORIES:	26	FAT:	0g
PROTEIN:	1g	CARBS:	6g

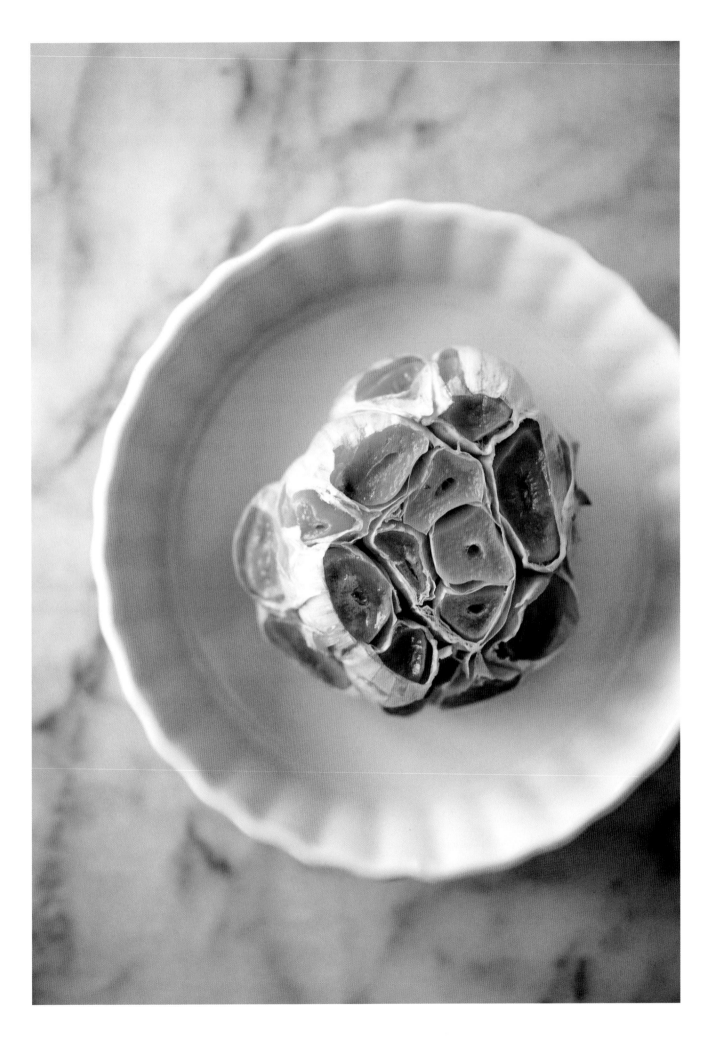

Roasted Garlic Pesto 2.0

This is one of the most popular recipes on my blog. I originally posted it with an accompanying recipe for chicken salad, but readers quickly decided that it could be used in other ways. They published photos of their creations, showing it used in other salads, mixed with zucchini noodles, and used as a rub for slow-cooked roasts! The possibilities are endless, and the flavor is through the roof.

EGG-FREE   GAPS

prep time: 5 minutes (not including the roasted garlic)

yield: 1 cup (2 tablespoons per serving)

1 packed cup fresh basil leaves (about 2 ounces)

1 bulb Roasted Garlic (page 346)

¼ cup pine nuts (see Tips)

¼ cup fresh lemon juice (about 2 small lemons)

¼ cup extra-virgin olive oil

¼ teaspoon fine sea salt

⅛ teaspoon ground black pepper

1. Place all of the ingredients in a food processor or blender. Blend for about 1 minute, until the pesto is smooth, without any chunks.

2. Use right away or transfer to a jar and store in the refrigerator. The pesto will keep covered in the refrigerator for about 1 week.

tips

• *For extra flavor, toast the pine nuts in a small dry frying pan over medium-low heat. Shake or stir often because they burn easily. They will brown in 4 to 5 minutes. You will start to smell pine nuts when they are close to finished.*

• *I always double this recipe because it freezes so well! To freeze, spoon the pesto into an ice cube tray and freeze until solid. Transfer the pesto cubes to a freezer-safe bag and use as you need them. They will keep frozen for up to 5 months.*

• *The pine nuts can be swapped out for walnuts, almonds, or even pecans. The flavor will change slightly, but if you tolerate one nut better than others, feel free to experiment.*

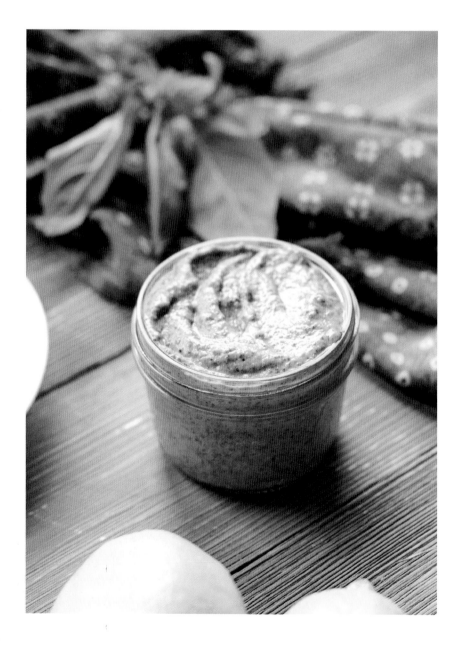

APPROXIMATE NUTRITION BREAKDOWN *(per serving)*			
CALORIES:	98	FAT:	10 g
PROTEIN:	1 g	CARBS:	3 g

Super Simple Paleo Mayo

You need to know three things about Paleo-friendly mayo: 1) it tastes just like the real thing, 2) it's easier to make than you might think, and 3) once you've got it made, the possibilities for its use are limitless. If you need a large quantity of mayo, you can easily double this recipe.

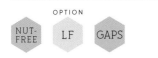

OPTION

NUT-FREE · LF · GAPS

prep time: 5 minutes | *yield: 2 cups (2 tablespoons per serving)*

1 large egg, room temperature

2 tablespoons fresh lemon juice (about 1 small lemon)

½ teaspoon fine sea salt

1½ cups avocado oil (use olive oil for low-FODMAP)

1. Place the egg, lemon juice, and salt in a food processor or blender. Blend for about 30 seconds, until smooth and frothy.

2. With the machine running, drizzle in the avocado oil as slowly as possible. This should take at least 2 minutes. After all of the oil has been added, stop the machine to check that the mayo has formed. It should be thick enough to form a peak on your finger.

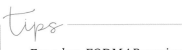

- *For a low-FODMAP version, use "light-tasting" olive oil instead of avocado oil.*

- *Mayo will keep in the fridge for up to 1 month.*

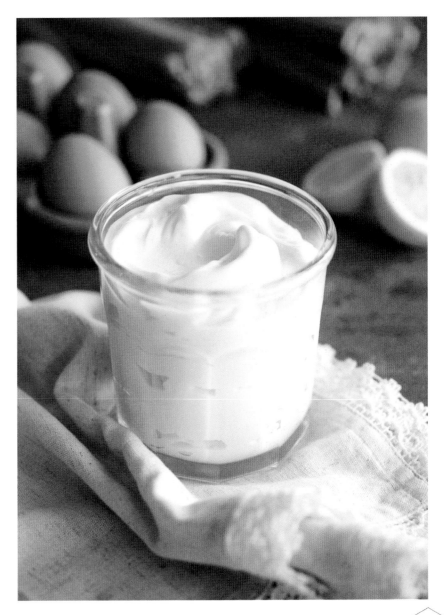

APPROXIMATE NUTRITION BREAKDOWN *(per serving)*			
CALORIES:	200	FAT:	21g
PROTEIN:	0g	CARBS:	0g

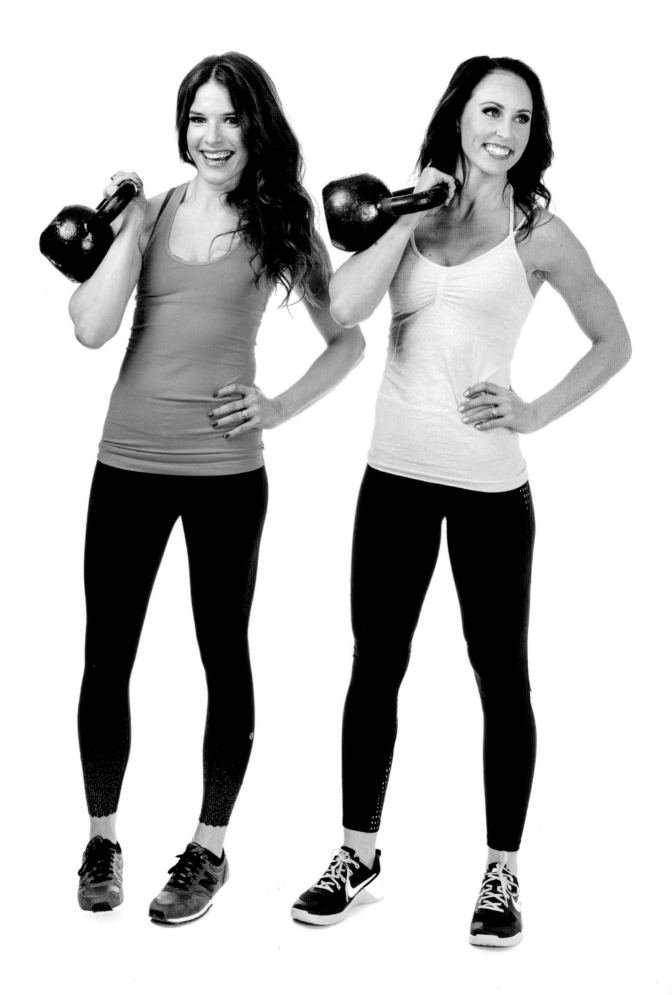

THE FITNESS INDEX

abs: ab leg lifts

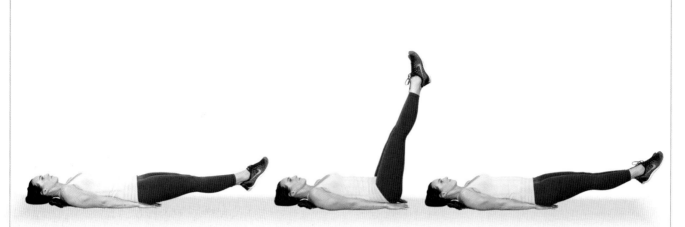

1) Lie flat on your back and place your hands under your butt. Tighten your glutes and abs to prepare for the movement, keeping your head resting on the ground.

2) Squeeze your abs, raising your legs off the mat in a controlled manner until they are pointing straight up.

3) Slowly lower your legs back toward the ground. Keep your abs engaged throughout the movement to prevent your feet from touching the floor. When your heels are about 6 inches from the floor, fully contract your hip flexors and reverse the movement for another repetition.

abs: flutter kicks

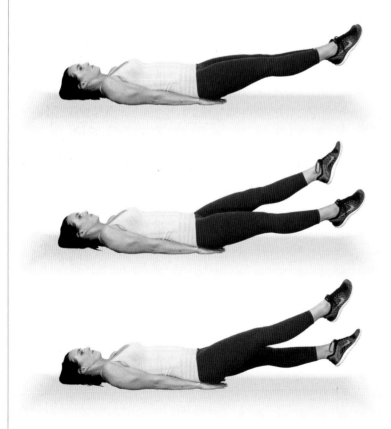

1) Lie flat on your back and place your hands under your butt. Engage your hip flexors and raise your legs about 6 inches off the ground.

2) Engage one set of hip flexors to slowly raise one leg while simultaneously relaxing the other side of your body and allowing the other leg to drop slightly.

3) Once your feet are about 6 to 10 inches apart, reverse the movement, relaxing your top leg and allowing it to drop while flexing your bottom leg and forcing it to move upward. Repeat the desired number of times.

abs: russian twists

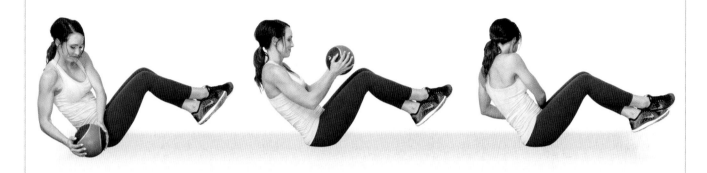

1) Place a medicine ball on the floor and sit next to it. Elevate and cross your feet while leaning back slightly. Engage your abs to balance on your butt. Then grab the ball with both hands.

2) Lift the ball off the ground while keeping your torso locked in place. As the weight rises, keep your trunk locked in place and your spine stable. The goals here are to resist the rotational force of the weight and to keep your belly button facing forward throughout the movement.

3) Gently touch the ball to the floor by your opposite hip, then slowly reverse the movement for another repetition.

abs: abmat sit-ups

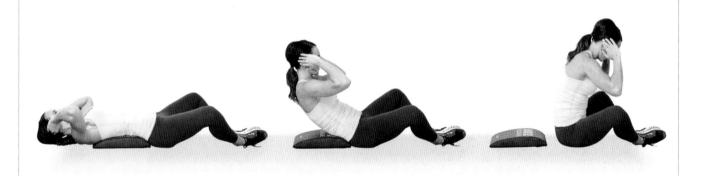

1) Lie on the AbMat with the gently tapered end facing your head. Your butt should be pressed against the bottom end of the mat and supporting your lower back. Assume the sit-up position with your knees bent, your feet on the floor, and your hands behind your head.

2) Contract your abs until your shoulders begin to rise off the floor. Although you should try to maintain a tight arch, if your abs are too weak or your muscles are exhausted, the AbMat will support your lumbar spine if you fail to maintain your forward curvature, making the ascent portion of the exercise safer than a traditional sit-up.

3) Continue to rise until your lower back loses contact with the mat. At this point you should have sufficient leverage to pull your torso into a forward arch without the support of the mat. Once your torso is completely vertical, slowly reverse the movement by slightly relaxing your ab muscles and dropping back toward the mat. Be sure to maintain the tight curvature of your back until your spine is supported by the mat again.

abs: bicycle crunches

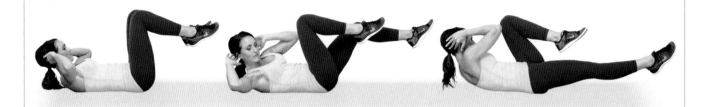

1) Lie on your back and come into the crunch position by raising your knees until your thighs are perpendicular to the floor, hanging your feet. Raise your head off the ground and place your hands behind your head.

2) Activate your abs and oblique muscles, rotating your torso and bringing one elbow forward toward the opposite knee. At the same time, activate the hip flexor of the opposite leg, bringing your opposite-side elbow and knee close enough to touch.

3) Once your elbow and knee touch, reverse the movement, twisting your torso in the opposite direction, lowering your knee, and raising the opposite knee. It's important not to twist your neck in order to gain extra reach. Keep your neck rigid and initiate the twist at your waist. For an added challenge, try straightening your bottom leg as it moves downward.

abs: sit-ups

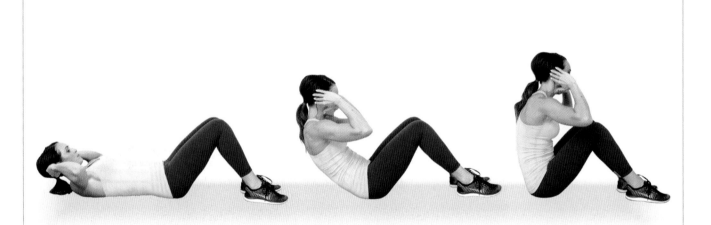

1) Lie on your back with your knees bent, your feet flat on the ground, your head slightly lifted, and your hands behind your head.

2) Flex your abdominal muscles, raising your shoulders off the floor and pulling your torso toward your knees. Make sure to keep your spine rounded forward as you sit up. If you let your back hyperextend, it can damage the discs in your back.

3) Continue to rise until your elbows touch your knees or your torso is pointing straight up. Then reverse the movement, keeping your abs tight to retain the forward curvature of your spine and maintaining a controlled descent until your shoulders touch the mat. Repeat the desired number of times.

abs: v-ups

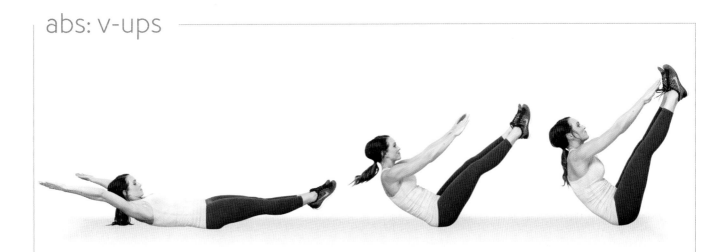

1) Lie flat on your back with your legs and arms extended, your heels about 6 inches off the ground, and your arms and head lifted.

2) Simultaneously flex your abs and hip flexor muscles to raise your legs and torso toward one another at the same speed. Reach your arms forward as your torso rises, pointing your fingers toward your toes.

3) Continue flexing until your fingers touch your toes. Then relax your abs and hips, lowering your torso and legs back to the floor. Stop the movement before your feet or head touch the ground, then do another repetition, coming completely to the ground at the end of your set.

arms: bench dips

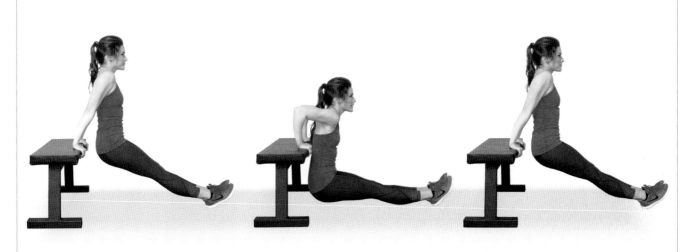

1) Begin with your hands on a bench and your legs extended in front of your body. The bench should be a few inches behind your butt.

2) Lower your butt toward the floor until your elbows are bent 90 degrees. Notice that Cassy's butt is just barely above the ground. It's important not to hit the floor in order to maintain tension throughout the movement.

3) Squeeze your triceps and force your torso upward. Keep your abs engaged and shoulders back throughout the movement.

arms: weighted bench dips

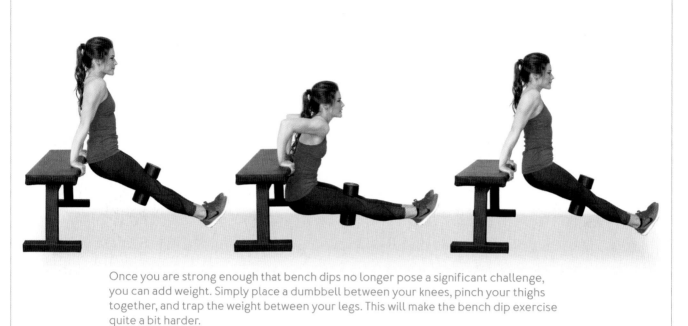

Once you are strong enough that bench dips no longer pose a significant challenge, you can add weight. Simply place a dumbbell between your knees, pinch your thighs together, and trap the weight between your legs. This will make the bench dip exercise quite a bit harder.

box jumps

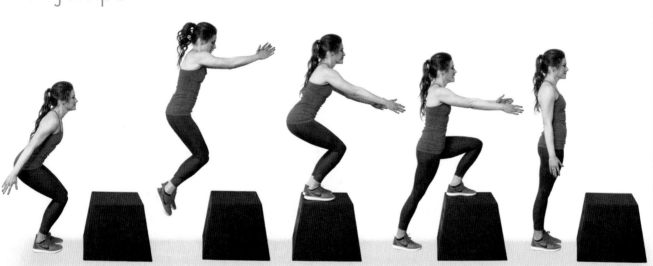

1) Begin a step away from a plyometric box. Bend your knees slightly and point your hands toward the floor.

2) Extend your legs while driving your hands upward in the direction you are jumping.

3) Land on top of the box mid-foot first, with your knees bent.

4) After settling on top of the box, step down one leg at a time. Extend your arms in front of your body for counterbalance and keep one foot flat on the box until the other foot touches the floor.

5) Step the other foot off the box, tighten your core, and prepare for another repetition.

lateral box jumps

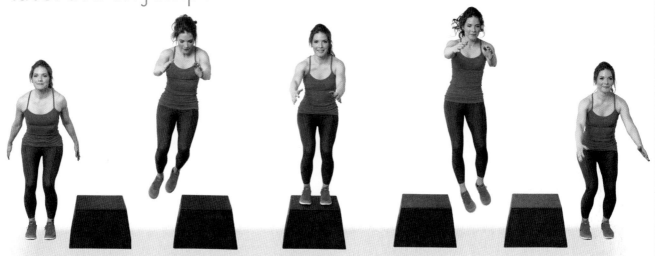

1) Begin standing to the side of a box, about a foot away from the box. Bend your knees, point your arms downward, and prepare to jump.

2) Extend your knees, drive with your outside hip, and thrust your arms upward. This will cause you to jump laterally, toward the box.

3) Land on top of the box mid-foot first, with your knees bent.

4) Jump again in the same lateral direction, this time jumping off the other side of the box. This will be a lower-elevation jump, but you still need to drive with your hip to move to the side.

5) Land on the floor on the far side of the box with your knees bent and your arms out in front of you for balance. From here, repeat the sequence in the opposite direction.

step-ups

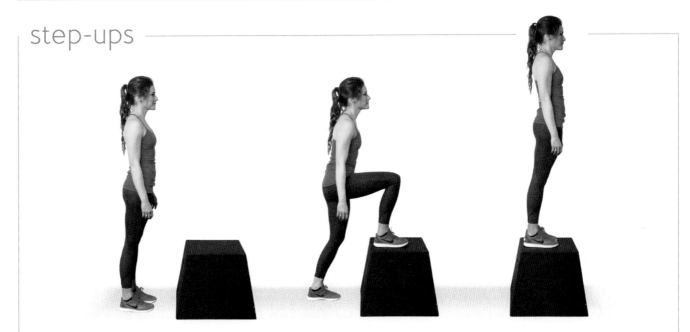

1) Begin facing a box with your feet flat on the ground and your hands at your sides.

2) Lean slightly forward while raising one foot off the floor. Plant your raised foot on top of the box, making sure that the shin of your raised leg is vertical.

3) Still leaning forward, flex the quad of your raised leg and lift your bottom foot off the floor. Keep tension in your planted leg as your torso rises, then place your feet together on top of the box. Step down one foot at a time, then repeat the movement, planting the other leg on top of the box.

burpees

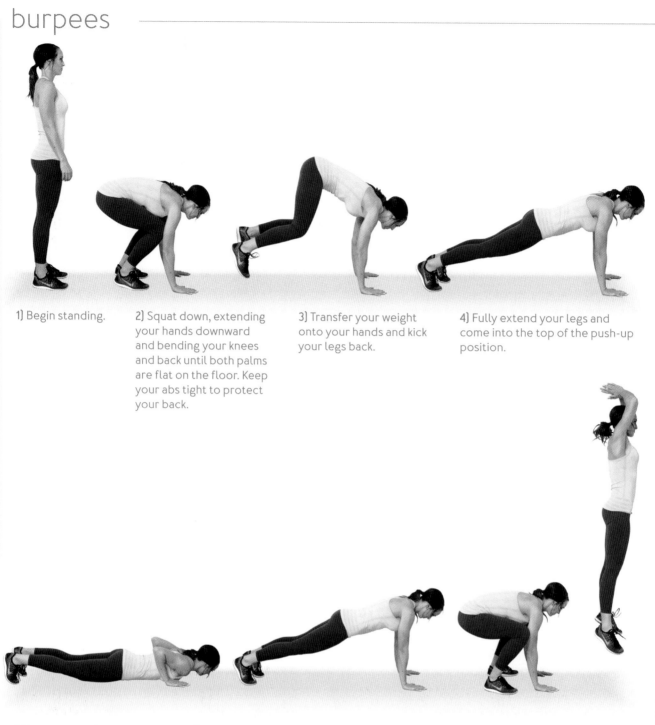

1) Begin standing.

2) Squat down, extending your hands downward and bending your knees and back until both palms are flat on the floor. Keep your abs tight to protect your back.

3) Transfer your weight onto your hands and kick your legs back.

4) Fully extend your legs and come into the top of the push-up position.

5) Lower your chest to the mat, keeping your back straight as you descend.

6) Flex your triceps and rise to the top of the push-up position.

7) From the top of the push-up, immediately jump your legs forward into the squat position.

8) Remove your hands from the floor and rapidly extend your legs. At the top of the motion, flex your toes as you come off the floor, raise your arms overhead, and touch your hands together. Land with slightly bent knees and immediately drop back down into the squat position. Repeat this sequence the desired number of times.

butt kicks

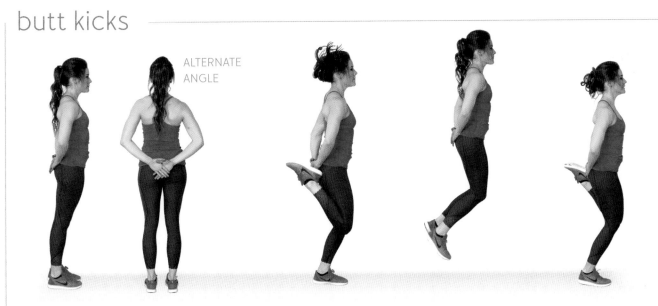

ALTERNATE ANGLE

1] Begin standing with your feet together and your hands on your butt with the palms facing outward.

2] Powerfully flex one hamstring, pulling your foot up toward your butt. Continue flexing your leg until your heel strikes your hands. Be sure to keep your thigh vertical. If your knee drifts forward, it will limit your hamstring activation.

3] Drop your foot, simultaneously flexing your opposite hamstring to raise the opposite foot.

4] Rapidly alternate legs with a hopping motion to ensure continuous hamstring flexion on one leg or the other.

handstand hold

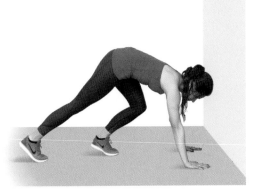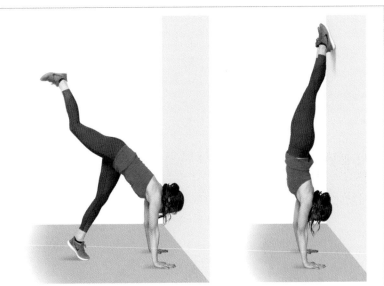

1] Begin in a sprinter's position, with both hands flat on the floor, your feet in a split stance, and your hips slightly elevated above your shoulders.

2] Raise your rear leg by flexing your hamstring and glute.

3] Take a small hop with your leg that is still on the ground and kick both legs up, tilting up into the vertical position. Holding this position is great for developing shoulder and arm strength. If your balance isn't good enough to hold the position, you can rest your heels against a wall or have a partner hold you upright.

high knees

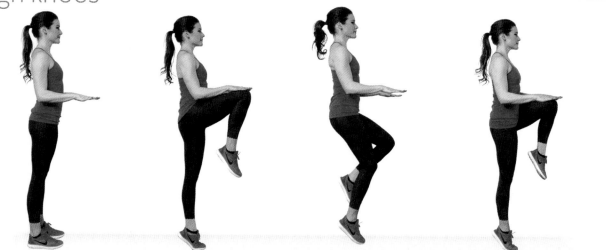

1) Begin standing with your elbows bent 90 degrees and your palms facing downward. The position of your palms will help you determine the correct height for your knees.

2) Take a quick jump and raise one knee until it touches your palms. Your knee should be bent roughly 90 degrees.

3) Quickly lower your high knee while jumping your planted leg into the air.

4) As your legs switch positions, land on your foot with your ankle slightly flexed, and raise the other knee into the high position until it touches your palms. Rapidly alternate legs, each time taking a quick hop to initiate the movement, for a set amount of time or number of repetitions.

single unders

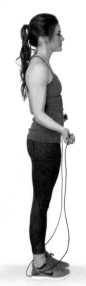 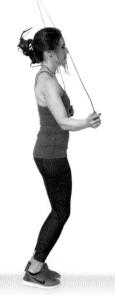

1) Start holding the jump rope handles in either hand and the rope behind your body.

2) Swing the rope forward, over your head.

3) Bend your knees and time your jump as the rope passes just in front of your legs. Continue this circular movement, timing each jump, for a set length of time. Jump rope is not only an excellent cardio exercise, but can build strength in your legs and lower arms as well.

double unders

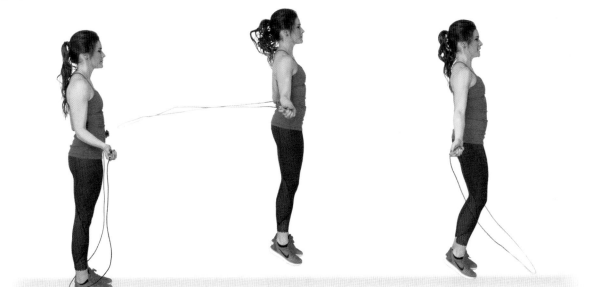

1) Start with the jump rope handles in either hand and the rope behind your body.

2) Swing the rope forward rapidly and jump over it.

3) While still in the air, continue the momentum of the rope swing and bring it back under your feet a second time. Repeat this pattern of two rope passes under your feet for every jump for a set amount of time.

jumping jacks

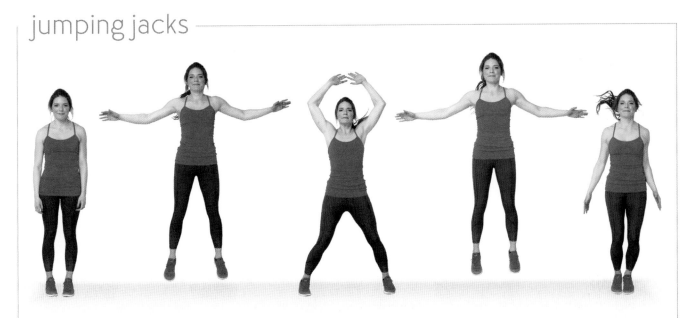

1) Begin standing with your hands at your sides.

2) Take a small jump and, while your feet are in the air, force both legs outward while simultaneously raising both arms overhead. Time your arm and leg movements so that your feet touch down in a wide stance at the same time your hands meet above your head.

3) Reverse the motion, taking a small hop and pulling your legs inward while simultaneously lowering your hands to your sides. Time the movement so that your feet land in a narrow stance at the same time your hands reach your hips. Repeat the motion for a set amount of time to get a great full-body cardio workout.

in-and-out jumps

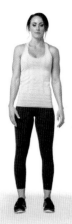
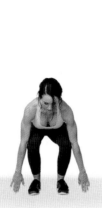
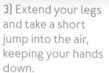
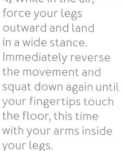
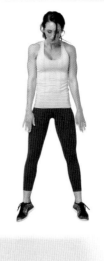

1) Begin standing with your feet in a narrow stance and your hands at your sides.

2) Hinge at the waist, bend your knees, and bend down until your fingertips touch the floor outside of your legs. Keep your abs tight to protect your back.

3) Extend your legs and take a short jump into the air, keeping your hands down.

4) While in the air, force your legs outward and land in a wide stance. Immediately reverse the movement and squat down again until your fingertips touch the floor, this time with your arms inside your legs.

5) Extend your legs and leap into the air again, this time drawing your legs into a narrow stance. Repeat this sequence the desired number of times.

jump-overs

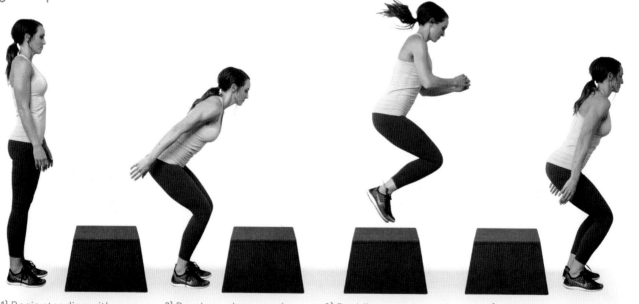

1) Begin standing with your feet shoulder width apart, facing a plyometric box.

2) Bend your knees and hinge forward at the hips, keeping your arms in line with your torso.

3) Rapidly extend your legs, push your hips forward, pull your arms in the direction of the box, and jump over the box.

4) Land on the other side of the box with your knees slightly bent, your feet shoulder width apart, and your hands at your sides.

skater jumps

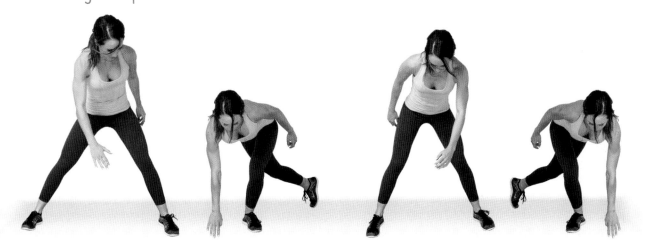

1) Begin standing with your feet in a wide stance. Reach one arm across your body toward the opposite toes.

2) Pull your other foot off the floor as you reach toward the ground, touching your fingers down next to your grounded foot. Pull your opposite leg behind your body, extending it as you touch the toes to the ground.

3) Quickly move your back leg forward and jump back to a standing position with your legs in a wide stance. Immediately reach your other hand across your body toward the opposite toes.

4) Repeat the sequence on the other side. Here Juli is touching her left fingers to the floor while her right leg is planted on the ground and her left leg is extended behind her body with the toes touching the floor. Quickly alternating sides in this fashion emulates a speed skater's motion and strengthens the hips and core muscles.

tuck jumps

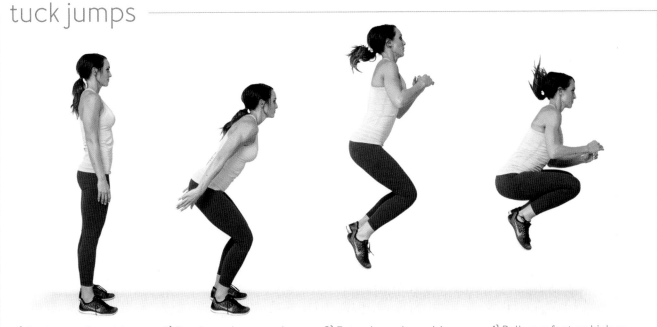

1) Begin standing with your feet shoulder width apart and your hands at your sides.

2) Bend your knees and hinge forward at the hips, keeping your arms in line with your torso.

3) Extend your legs, drive your hips forward, and raise your arms. As your body rises, extend your toes, giving you extra momentum as your body leaves the ground.

4) Pull your feet up high as your body moves through the air. Keep your hands in a neutral position for balance and prepare to land mid-foot with your knees slightly bent.

american kettlebell swings

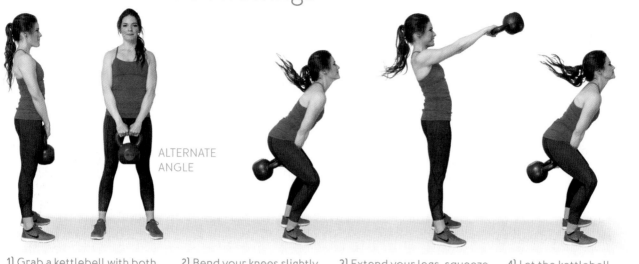

ALTERNATE ANGLE

1) Grab a kettlebell with both hands and rise to standing with your feet shoulder width apart and your palms facing your body.

2) Bend your knees slightly and hinge forward at the hips. Make sure that your legs are far enough apart that the kettlebell can swing between them.

3) Extend your legs, squeeze your butt, and drive your hips forward, which will accelerate the kettlebell forward. Keep a tight grip on the handle, forcing the weight to travel upward in an arc. Use your shoulders to control the weight and prevent it from rising higher than head level.

4) Let the kettlebell drop. As it nears your hips, bend your knees, hinge at the hips, and allow your hips to catch your arms. Once the weight stops moving, immediately reverse the motion to begin another repetition.

walking lunges

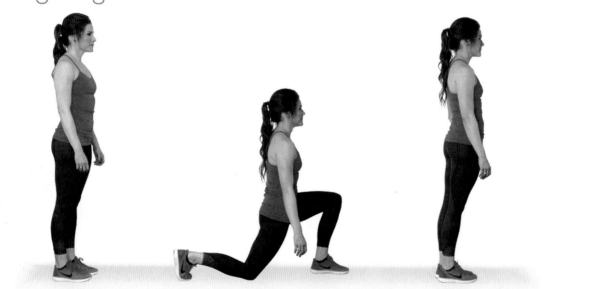

1) Begin standing with your feet shoulder width apart and your hands at your sides.

2) Take a big step forward, bend your knee as your foot contacts the ground, and then lower your rear knee until it's nearly touching the floor. Keep your torso vertical and your abs tight.

3) Shift your weight onto your lead foot, extend your lead leg, drive your torso upward, and pull your rear leg even with your front leg until you're standing again. Switch legs and repeat.

alternating walking lunges

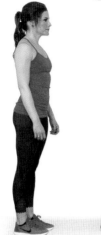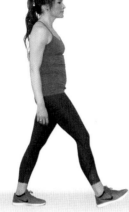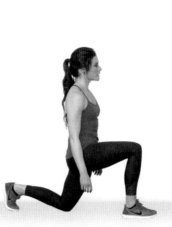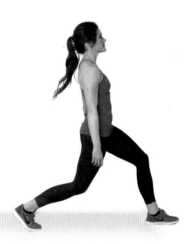

1) Begin standing with your feet together, your hands at your sides, and your abs tight.

2) Take a big step forward and plant your foot on the floor in front of you.

3) Lower your trailing knee until it touches the ground and your lead leg is bent 90 degrees.

4) Flex the quad of your lead leg, driving your torso upward. As your weight shifts onto your lead leg, bring your trailing leg forward, take a big step, and repeat the sequence with the opposite leg.

jumping lunges

1) Begin in the lunge position. Your lead leg should be bent 90 degrees with your foot flat on the floor and your rear leg bent 90 degrees with your knee and toes touching the floor. Your torso should be vertical and your hands slightly in front of your body for balance.

2) Engage the quad of your lead leg and drive yourself upward. When your legs are fully extended, flex your toes to add momentum as you jump into the air with your legs in a split stance.

3) Shift your legs into the opposite split stance, moving the front leg backward and the rear leg forward.

4) Land with your front foot flat on the floor and on the ball of your rear foot. Immediately descend into a lunge until your rear knee touches down. Drive upward again and repeat the sequence.

calf stretch

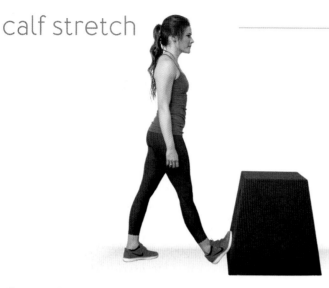

1] Stand a few feet away from a box and place the ball of one foot against the side of the box. Drive your weight forward into that leg, stretching your calf muscle and flexing your ankle joint.

2] To deepen the stretch, lean your torso toward the box, placing more of your weight on your lead leg. Place your hands on top of the box to regulate the pressure and control the tension of the stretch.

pigeon hold

ALTERNATE ANGLE

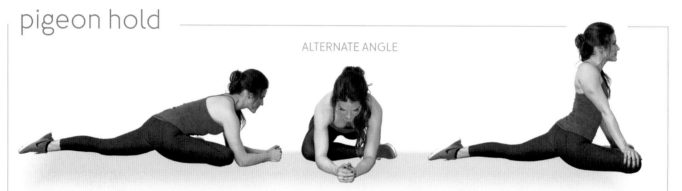

1] Begin on your knees. Extend one leg behind you and bring the other leg forward, rotating your front leg so that your foot comes in and moves toward the opposite side of your body. Position your front foot so that your lower leg is perpendicular to your body and the outside of your foot, calf, and knee are resting firmly on the ground. Keep your torso low to get comfortably into position before initiating the stretch.

2] Once you're in position, place one hand on your knee and the other on your foot and begin driving your torso upward into the vertical position. Having your hands down prevents your knee from raising off the floor, which would reduce the effectiveness of the stretch.

modification

Place the outside edge of your foot on top of a box and drive your knee outward until it is resting on the box as well. Keep your rear leg outstretched with the ball of your foot pressed into the ground for control. Once your leg is stable on top of the box, raise your torso into the vertical position. This stretch opens up the hips and loosens up tight glute muscles.

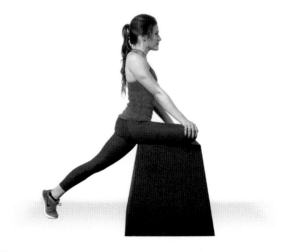

squat hold

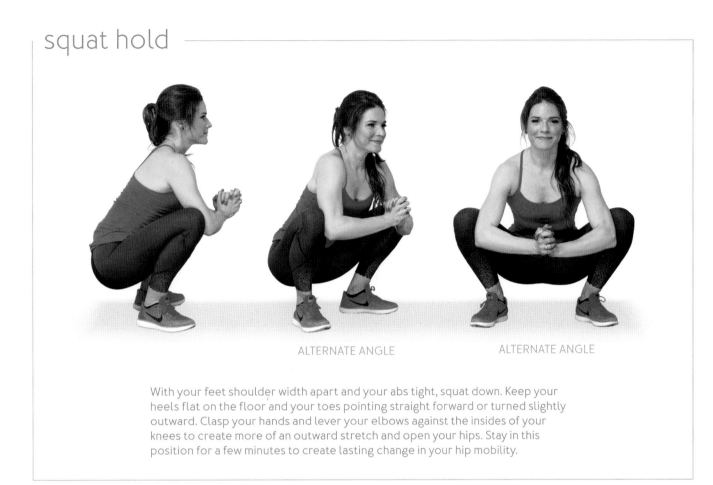

ALTERNATE ANGLE   ALTERNATE ANGLE

With your feet shoulder width apart and your abs tight, squat down. Keep your heels flat on the floor and your toes pointing straight forward or turned slightly outward. Clasp your hands and lever your elbows against the insides of your knees to create more of an outward stretch and open your hips. Stay in this position for a few minutes to create lasting change in your hip mobility.

kneeling quad stretch

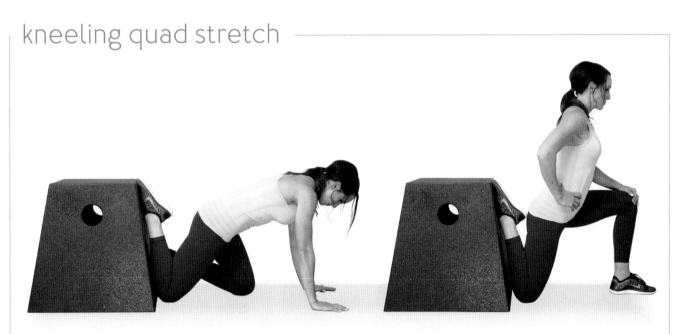

1) Back up to a box and place your knee on the floor directly in front of the box, with your shin resting against the edge of the box. Place your hands flat on the floor and your butt a fair distance away from your foot to give yourself space to maneuver your leg into position without initiating the stretch.

2) Lift your other knee off the ground and plant that foot on the floor with your knee bent 90 degrees. Use that foot as a post to raise your torso to vertical. The closer your butt comes to your foot, the deeper the stretch on your quad will be. Keep your abs tight and stretch only to a comfortable position.

runner's stretch

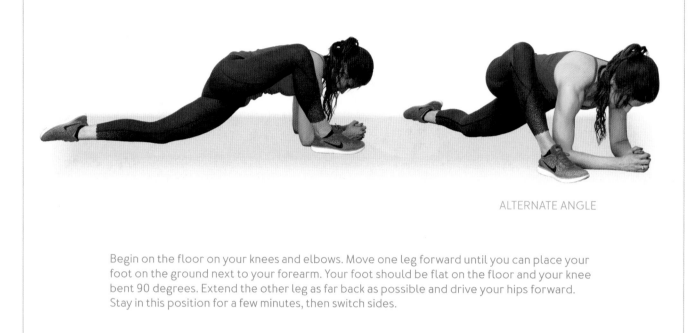

ALTERNATE ANGLE

Begin on the floor on your knees and elbows. Move one leg forward until you can place your foot on the ground next to your forearm. Your foot should be flat on the floor and your knee bent 90 degrees. Extend the other leg as far back as possible and drive your hips forward. Stay in this position for a few minutes, then switch sides.

standing forward fold

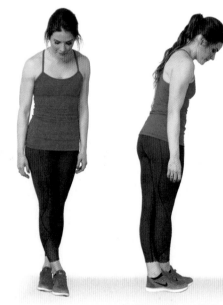

ALTERNATE ANGLE

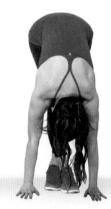 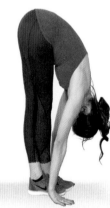

ALTERNATE ANGLE

1) From the standing position, cross one foot over the other.

2) Hinge forward at the waist, slowly bending toward the ground until your hands touch the floor. This stretches the hamstring of your back leg as well as mobilizes the joints of your back. After holding for a moment, slowly rise to standing, switch the positions of your feet, and repeat the stretch for the opposite leg.

standing shoulder stretch

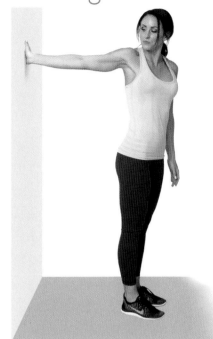
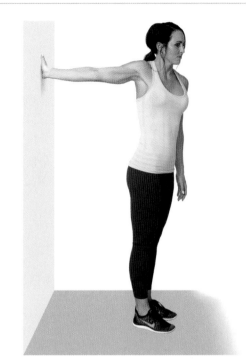

1) From the standing position, extend your hand out to your side and place your palm on a sturdy surface, such as a wall.

2) Slowly step your feet in a circle to rotate your torso away from your hand, stretching your arm behind your back. Keep your palm firmly anchored while rotating your trunk to create a stretch on the pectoral muscle. Hold the stretch, then repeat on the other side.

floor shoulder stretch

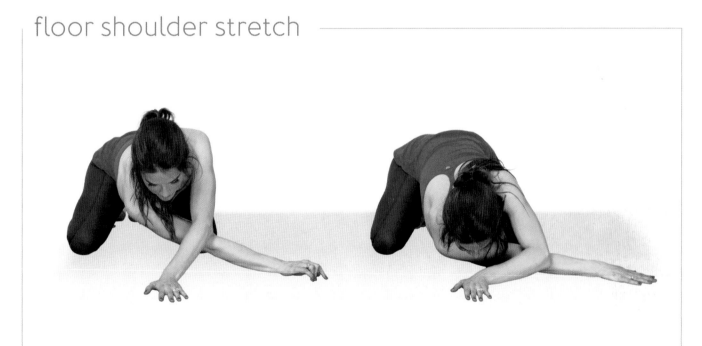

1) Begin on your hands and knees. Take one hand off the floor and slide it across your chest, under your other arm and to the opposite side of your body. Stretch this hand as far to the other side of your body as it will reach.

2) Relax your arm that's posted on the ground and allow gravity to pull your torso toward the floor to stretch your shoulder and back muscles. Keep your chest square to the ground and lower slowly to deepen the stretch. Hold for a few minutes, then raise yourself back up with your posted hand, switch arms, and repeat on the other side.

PVC shoulder stretch

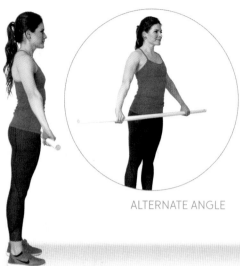

ALTERNATE ANGLE

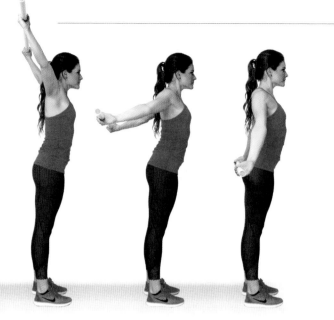

1) While standing, grab hold of a piece of PVC pipe with both hands, with your palms facing you.

2) Raise your arms overhead, then slowly rotate them behind your back. Keep a firm grip on the pipe and monitor the stretch in your back.

3) Continue rotating your arms, slowly stretching the muscles of your upper back.

4) If you have the flexibility to do it, rotate your arms until the pipe touches your butt. Then reverse the movement, slowly bringing the pipe back in front of your body.

L-sit forward fold

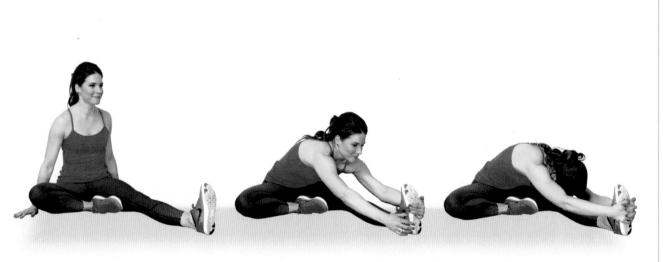

1) Sit on the floor with your torso upright and your legs extended. Bend one knee and bring your heel toward your groin, with the outside of your foot resting flat on the floor. Your knee should be facing out at a right angle from the opposite leg.

2) Reach forward one hand at a time and clasp your hands around your foot. You can interlace your fingers for a stronger grip.

3) Flex your arms and drop your head toward your knee. This will pull the hamstring tight and deepen the stretch. Hold this position for the desired amount of time, then switch legs and repeat on the other side.

sitting twists

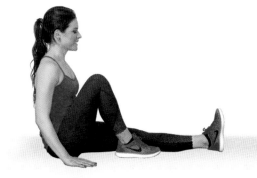
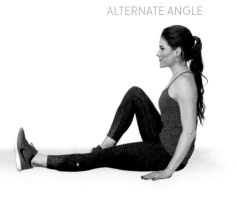

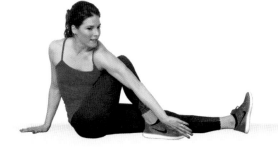
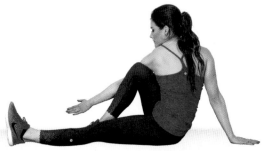

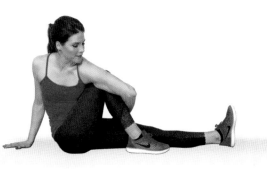
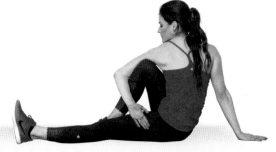

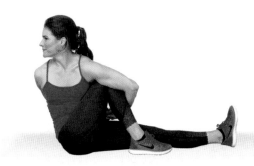

1] Begin seated on the floor with one leg straight out in front of you and the other leg bent with your foot on the floor. The knee of your bent leg should come up roughly to chest height.

2] Reach across your body with your arm opposite your bent leg, around the far side of your knee, and extend that arm fully.

3] Bend your elbow, reaching around your knee and toward your other hip. Your elbow should be hooked at your knee, keeping your knee locked in place.

4] Reach your other arm around your back and clasp hands next to your hip. Then turn your head so that you're looking over your rear shoulder. Hold the stretch for a few minutes, then release your grip, slowly coming back to the seated position. Switch sides and repeat.

downward dog

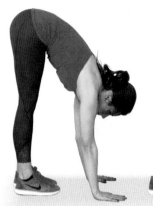 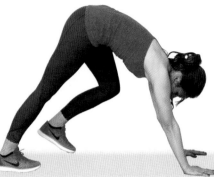 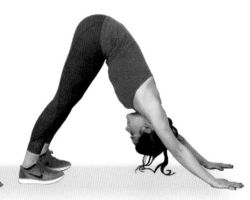

1) Begin standing, then bend forward until both hands are flat on the floor.

2) Step both feet back, one foot at a time, until you're in a comfortable position with your hands and feet flat on the floor and your hips higher than your head.

3) Extend your arms and legs and pull your shoulder blades together until your head pulls under your arms. Hold this position for the desired amount of time.

upward dog

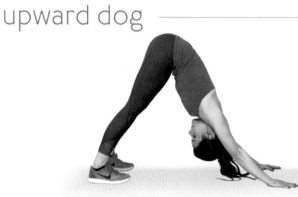 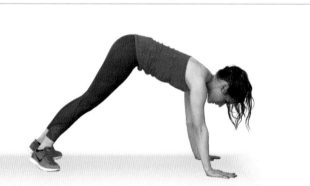

1) Begin in the downward dog position with your hands and feet flat on the floor and your body in an upside-down V position with your hips higher than your shoulders. Your weight should be equally distributed across all four points of contact with the ground.

2) Shift your weight forward onto your hands by driving with your legs and/or pulling with your shoulders. This will lower your hips and raise your shoulders.

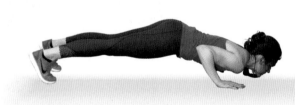 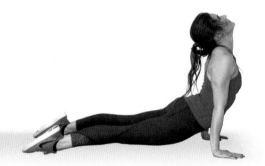

3) Once your weight is over your hands, move into a modified push-up by bending your elbows and lowering your chest to the floor.

4) Once your chest is on the floor, drive your hips downward and slowly extend your arms to raise your chest and extend your legs and toes to drop your hips toward the ground. Continue this full-body extension in a slow and controlled manner until your chest is forward and your head is high, with your gaze facing the sky. You can hold the stretch here or immediately reverse the movement to come back to the starting position.

dead bugs

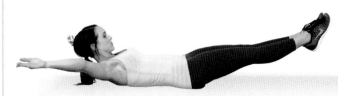

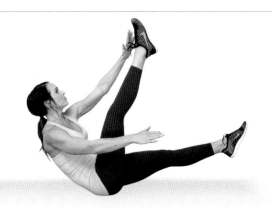

1) Lie flat on your back and flex your abs and hip flexors, raising your legs and arms a few inches off the ground. Pull your head forward and come in a full-body arch.

2) Simultaneously contract your ab muscles and one side of your hip flexors to raise one leg and your torso toward one another. At the same time, reach for your rising foot with your opposite-side hand.

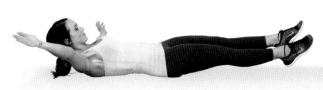

3) Relax your abs and hip flexors and come back to the arch position, making sure that neither your legs nor your arms touch the ground.

4) Repeat the movement on the other side, flexing your abs and opposite-side hip flexor and raising your other leg and arm for a fingers-to-toes touch.

hand plank to forearm plank

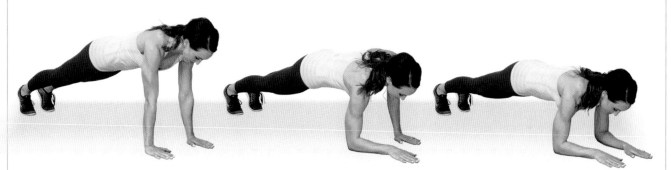

1) Begin in the top of the push-up position, with your body in a straight line from your head to your feet.

2) Slowly shift your weight onto one hand, remove the other hand from the floor, and drop your elbow to the ground. Keep your abs as tight as possible to prevent your torso from rotating as you lower your body.

3) Once your weight is on your elbow and hand, shift your weight onto that arm and lower the other arm down until both elbows and hands are flat on the ground, carrying your weight equally. Now reverse the movement, slowly raising yourself back to the push-up position one arm at a time while maintaining a rigid core.

mountain climbers

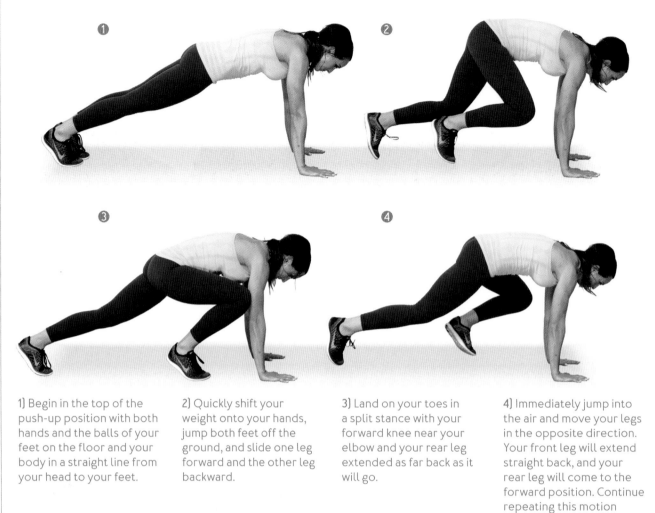

1) Begin in the top of the push-up position with both hands and the balls of your feet on the floor and your body in a straight line from your head to your feet.

2) Quickly shift your weight onto your hands, jump both feet off the ground, and slide one leg forward and the other leg backward.

3) Land on your toes in a split stance with your forward knee near your elbow and your rear leg extended as far back as it will go.

4) Immediately jump into the air and move your legs in the opposite direction. Your front leg will extend straight back, and your rear leg will come to the forward position. Continue repeating this motion rapidly for a set amount of time or number of reps.

plank hold

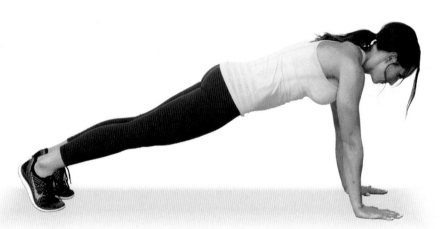

Start in the top of the push-up position. Keep your shoulder blades pulled back and your abs tight. Hold this position for the desired amount of time.

superman

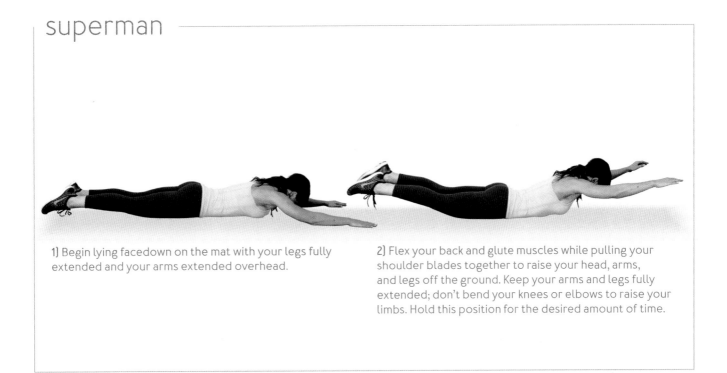

1] Begin lying facedown on the mat with your legs fully extended and your arms extended overhead.

2] Flex your back and glute muscles while pulling your shoulder blades together to raise your head, arms, and legs off the ground. Keep your arms and legs fully extended; don't bend your knees or elbows to raise your limbs. Hold this position for the desired amount of time.

hand-release push-ups

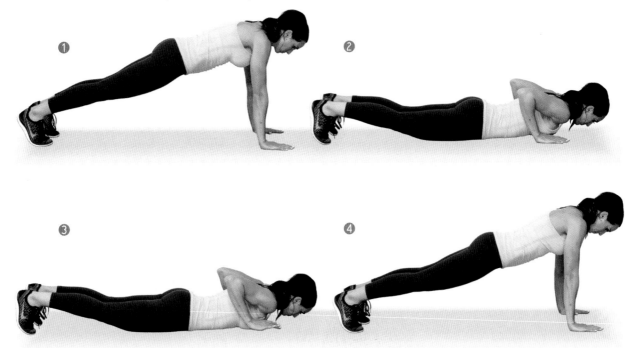

1] Begin in the top of the push-up position. Make sure that your back is in a straight line from your head to your heels and keep your abs tight.

2] Relax your arms and lower your torso to the ground until your chest is flat on the floor.

3] Shift your weight onto your chest and raise your hands completely off the floor. This halts your momentum and forces you to generate more power from the bottom of the push-up, making the exercise more challenging.

4] Place your hands back on the ground, squeeze your back tight, extend your arms, and raise your torso to the top of the push-up position. Repeat the desired number of times.

pike push-ups

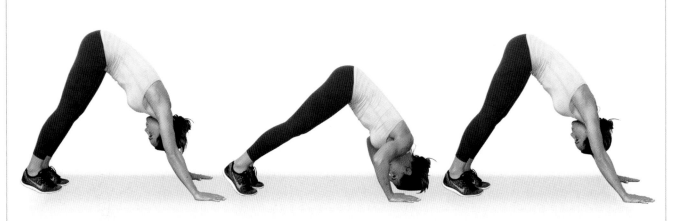

1) Begin in a modified push-up position with your hands and feet flat on the ground. Bend at the waist so that your hips are higher than your shoulders. The higher you raise your hips, the less weight will be loaded onto your hands during the movement.

2) To descend, relax your arms and allow your head to drop all the way to the ground, keeping your back straight. As you move downward, your legs will straighten slightly, transferring more weight onto your hands, making the push-up more challenging as you drop.

3) Flex your triceps and extend your arms, raising your head off the floor and moving back to the start position. Repeat the desired number of times.

push-ups

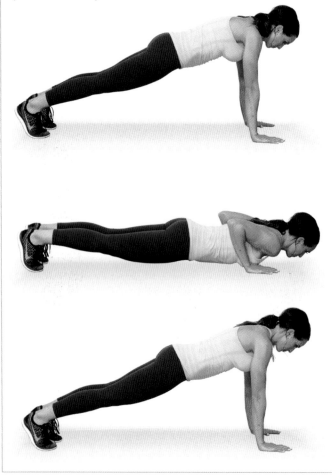

1) Begin in the top of the push-up position with your hands and toes planted on the floor, your abs tight, and your body in a straight line from your head to your feet.

2) To descend, relax your arms and allow your torso to drop until your chest touches the floor. Keep your abs and back tight while descending, and keep your body in a straight line.

3) Flex your triceps and rise to the starting position. Keep your abs tight and your shoulder blades pulled together to keep your back in line and protect your spine.

single-leg deadlifts

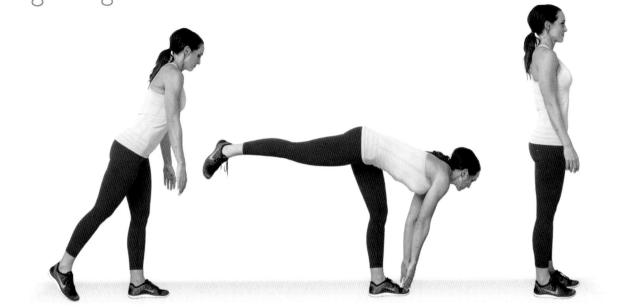

1) Begin standing. Slowly transfer all of your weight to one leg and gradually lean forward while extending the other leg behind your body. Try to maintain a straight line from your head to your heel.

2) Continue bending forward at the waist, being careful to keep your back straight, until you can touch your foot with both fingertips. Your rear leg should rise as your torso drops to counterbalance the movement.

3) Rise back to standing, switch legs, and repeat the movement on the other side. Add weight to make the exercise more challenging.

legs-up-a-wall toe touches

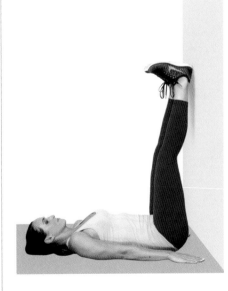
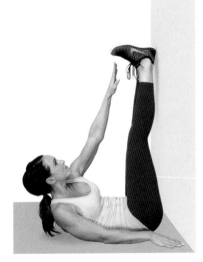
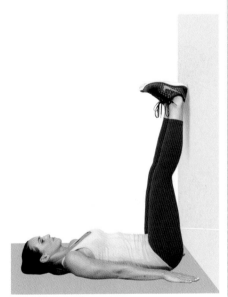

1) Lie flat on your back with your legs straight up a wall. Place both hands on the mat by your hips, palms down.

2) Contract your abs, crunching your shoulders and head up off the mat. At the same time, extend one arm toward your toes. Continue crunching until your fingertips touch your toes.

3) Relax your abs and bring your shoulders back to the mat, keeping your feet in the air. Repeat the movement on the other side.

air squats

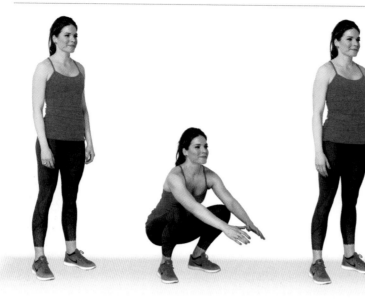

1) Begin standing with your feet about shoulder width apart. Keep your butt clenched and your abs tight.

2) Relax your glutes, push your butt back, and drop into the squat position. Make sure that your weight stays on the balls of your feet and your back stays tight. You can extend your arms forward to counterbalance your weight moving backward.

3) From the bottom of the squat, drive your legs into the ground and force your torso upward. Keep your abs tight throughout the movement and prevent your back from rounding. Repeat this series of movements for the desired number of repetitions.

pistols

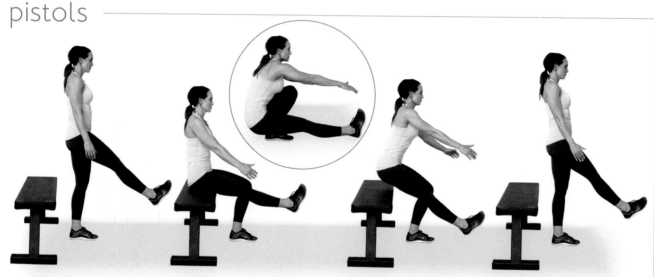

1) Begin standing in front of a bench. Shift your weight onto one leg and extend the other leg in front of your body.

2) Drive your hips back as you extend your arms forward to counterbalance the movement. Continue sitting back until your butt comes to rest on the bench. (You can also do this without a bench and drop until the back of your leg stops your butt.)

3) Lean forward, flex your quad, and extend your hips to rise up off the bench.

4) Come back to standing with your leg still extended in front of you. Either continue with another repetition or switch legs and repeat on the other side.

bulgarian split squats

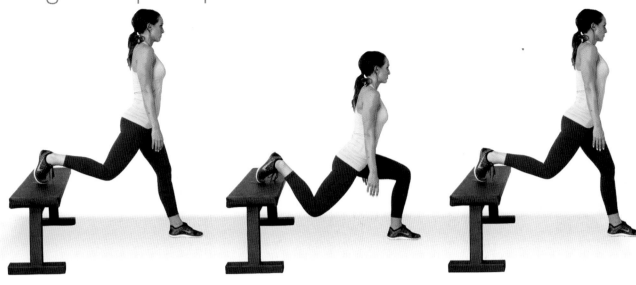

1) Begin standing with a bench 3 to 4 feet behind you. Shift your weight onto one leg, extend your opposite leg behind you, and place the ball of that foot on the bench. This will put you in a split stance, with one foot on the bench and the other on the floor.

2) Squat down until your front knee has a 90-degree bend.

3) Extend your front leg and force yourself back to standing. Your rear leg will be used mainly for balance, while the majority of the work will be transferred onto your front leg. Continue this sequence for the desired number of reps or switch legs and repeat on the other side.

jumping squats

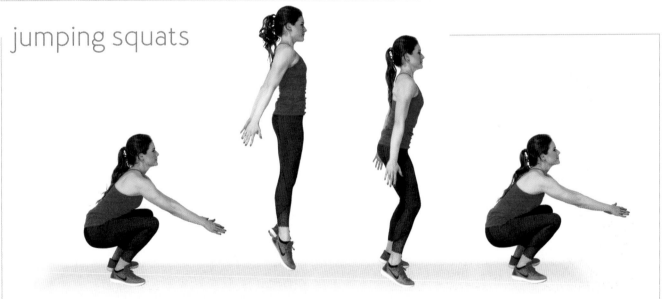

1) Begin standing, then lower down into the squat position. Your abs should be tight and your arms extended in front of your body for balance.

2) Flex your quads, rapidly driving yourself upward. Unlike a standard squat, continue flexing your legs as hard as you can until the very top of the squat. Your momentum will carry your feet off the ground. At that point, flex your toes and drive your hands back for balance as you fly into the air.

3) Land on your toes to absorb your body weight, with your hands at your sides for balance.

4) Immediately relax your legs and drop back into the squat position. Keep your abs tight throughout the movement or you risk losing control of your spine and rounding your back as you drop into the squat. Continue this sequence for the desired number of reps.

knees to squats

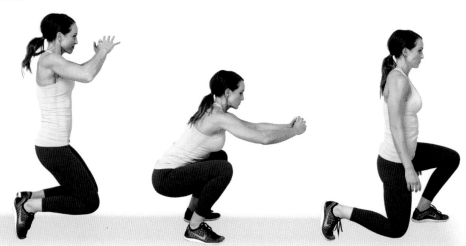

1) Begin on your knees with the balls of your feet on the floor and your hands extended behind your body.

2) Rock your weight back onto your toes and rapidly extend your legs while quickly driving your arms upward. This will cause your torso to rise, bringing your knees off the floor.

3) With your weight completely off your knees, quickly hop your feet forward into the position previously occupied by your knees. This will bring you into the full squat position with your arms extended in front of your body.

4) Step down one leg at a time until both knees are resting on the mat. From the start position, repeat the movement the desired number of times.

one-legged squats

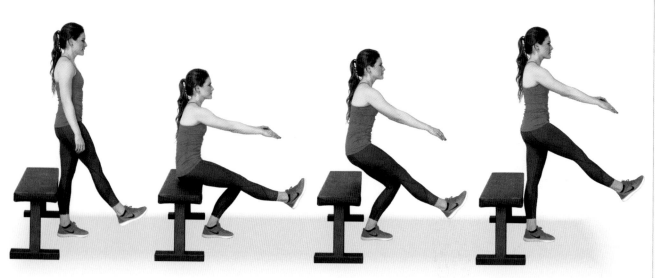

1) Begin standing just in front of a knee-high bench. Shift all your weight onto one leg, then extend the other leg slightly in front of your body.

2) Bend your grounded knee and shift your weight back while extending your arms in front of you for balance. Control your descent until your butt contacts the bench.

3) To come back up, drive your foot into the ground, flex your quad, and elevate your torso. Keep your arms and opposite leg extended for balance.

4) Rise to the standing position. Switch legs and repeat on the other side.

wall ball squats

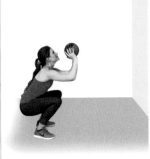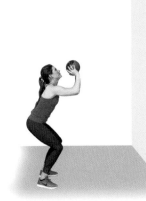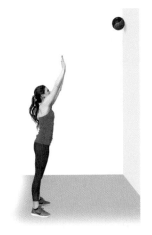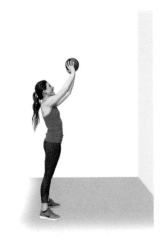

1) Begin in a full squat with a medicine ball in your hands, standing roughly 5 feet away from a sturdy wall.

2) Extend your legs, rapidly driving your hips upward.

3) Extend your arms, timing the extension with the peak of your hip drive, and release the ball at the top of the movement.

4) As the ball bounces off the wall and falls back toward the floor, catch it with both hands and immediately bend your knees, lowering back into the bottom of the squat. Immediately reverse the movement to begin another repetition.

wall sit

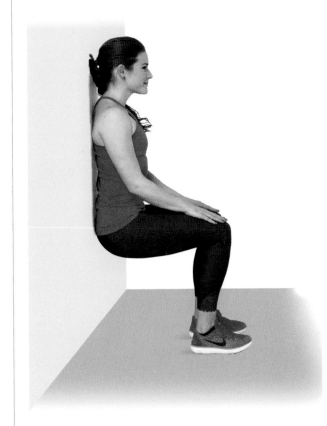

Press your back against a wall and slide your butt downward until your hips are level with your knees. Adjust your feet so that your knees are bent 90 degrees. Squeeze your hips and abs to hold yourself in place. Continue holding for a set amount of time.

recommended equipment

Although many of these exercises can be done with no equipment at all, you may want to pick up one or more of the following (or seek them out at your local gym) to take your workouts to the next level and maximize their benefit.

- AbMat or rolled towel
- Bench or sturdy chair
- Dumbbell (9 pounds for beginner ladies, 15 pounds for ladies or beginner men, 20 pounds for men)
- Kettlebell (23 pounds for beginner ladies, 35 pounds for ladies or beginner men, 45 or 53 pounds for men)
- Medicine ball (9 pounds for beginner ladies, 12 pounds for ladies or beginner men, 15 pounds for men) or sandbag
- Plyometric box for jumps (12-inch for beginner ladies, 20-inch for ladies or beginner men, 24-inch for men)
- PVC pipe
- Speed rope or regular jump rope
- Timer
- Yoga mat

warm-ups

Warming up the body not only helps enhance your performance in a workout, but also helps prevent injury. Here are some sample warm-ups for you to try, as specified in the 28-Day Food & Fitness Plan on pages 90 to 97.

WARM-UP A

- Light jog: 400 meters (or 3 minutes)
- 3 rounds:
  10 push-ups
  10 sit-ups
  10 air squats

WARM-UP B

- 100 jumping jacks
- 7-6-5-4-3-2-1: dips, push-ups, walking lunges (each leg)

WARM-UP C

- 25 burpees
- 3 rounds:
  30-second handstand hold
  30-second plank hold
  30-second air squat hold

WARM-UP D

- 200-meter jog, 100-meter high knees, 100-meter butt kicks, 200-meter jog
- 20 side skater jumps, 20 air squats, 20 pike push-ups, 20 tuck jumps

metabolism-boosting modifications

With some simple swaps and a few pieces of extra equipment, you can really take your workouts to the next level and maximize their benefit. Here are some examples:

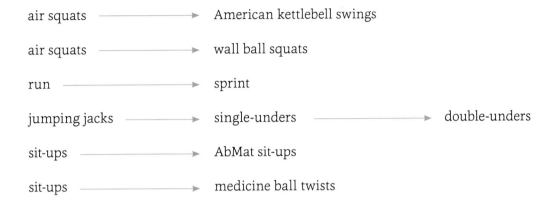

air squats   ⟶   American kettlebell swings

air squats   ⟶   wall ball squats

run   ⟶   sprint

jumping jacks   ⟶   single-unders   ⟶   double-unders

sit-ups   ⟶   AbMat sit-ups

sit-ups   ⟶   medicine ball twists

6-minute mobility

Mobility is crucial to a long, healthy athletic lifestyle. Remember that it's crucial to spend time on mobility—these activities help ensure a speedier recovery and reduce the probability of injury.

For daily mobility, you have several options. You can foam roll, drop into a yoga class, or follow one (or more) of the routines outlined below. Focus on one or all of these groups.

MOBILITY A (LEGS AND HIPS 1)

- 2-minute squat hold: sit in the bottom of a squat, keep your shoulders back and chest up, and push your knees out
- 2-minute (each leg) pigeon holds
- 2-minute (each leg) calf stretches

MOBILITY B (LEGS AND HIPS 2)

- 2-minute (each leg) kneeling quad stretches
- 2-minute (each leg) runner's stretches
- 1-minute (each leg) standing forward folds

MOBILITY C (SHOULDERS)

- 2-minute (each arm) standing shoulder stretches
- 2-minute (each arm) floor shoulder stretches
- 2-minute downward dog

MOBILITY D (CORE)

- 2-minute upward dog
- 2-minute (each side) sitting twists
- 2-minute (each side) L-sit forward folds

workout descriptions

We recognize that not everybody speaks workout-ese, so if the shorthand workouts listed in the 28-Day Food & Fitness Plan on pages 90 to 97 are a little confusing to you, here's a breakdown of what to do in each workout. On the days that have been set aside for rest, either take a break from training and let your body heal, or, if you have the energy and the desire, do some restorative yoga.

DAY 1
After completing warm-up A (page 382), go for a jog. Run at a moderate pace for 2 miles, or for 20 minutes. Then, after a brief rest, move on to part B. This part of the workout consists of 10 jumping squats (page 379), 10 sit-ups (page 354), and 10 hand-release push-ups (page 375). After you complete 10 reps of each exercise, repeat the sequence 3 more times, for a total of 4 rounds. Finish with mobility A (page 383).

DAY 2
After completing warm-up C, do 5 reps of each of the following exercises: burpees (page 358), pike push-ups (page 376), and tuck jumps (page 363). Then repeat the sequence, this time doing 10 reps of each exercise. Continue in this fashion, adding 5 reps of each exercise to each new round, and complete as many rounds as you can in 15 minutes. Finish with mobility C.

DAY 3
After completing warm-up B, go for a 1-mile run. Take a brief rest, then move on to part B, which consists of a 1-minute wall sit (page 381), 1 minute of burpees (page 358), 1 minute of mountain climbers (page 374), and 1 minute of jumping lunges (page 365). Rest for 1 minute, then repeat this sequence 4 more times, for a total of 5 rounds. Finish with mobility A.

DAY 5
After completing warm-up D, begin part A of the workout: 30 push-ups (page 376), 30 box jumps (page 356) or step-ups (page 357) (depending on your personal fitness level), and 30 bench dips (page 355), repeated for 3 rounds. Rest for 2 minutes, then move on to part B: 30 ab leg lifts (page 352), 30 skater jumps (page 363), and 30 dead bugs (page 373), repeated for 3 rounds. Finish with mobility D.

DAY 6
After completing warm-up C, do 10 in-and-out jumps (page 362), 10 walking lunges (page 364) on each leg, and 10 mountain climbers (page 374). Immediately after completing the last rep of mountain climbers, repeat the sequence, but this time do 9 reps of each movement. Continue in this fashion, removing 1 rep of each exercise from each new round, with no break between sets. After you complete the last round consisting of 1 rep of each exercise, immediately restart the circuit, doing 10, then 9, then 8, 7, 6, 5, 4, 3, 2, and 1 rep of each movement, for a total of 3 rounds. Finish with mobility B.

DAY 8
After completing warm-up A, sprint 800 meters. Then immediately do 20 Bulgarian split squats (page 379) on each leg, 20 pike push-ups (page 376), and 20 V-ups (page 355). After your last V-up, begin the sequence again, but this time run 600 meters and do 15 Bulgarian split squats, 15 pike push-ups, and 15 V-ups. Follow that with a 400-meter run and 10 reps of each exercise, and finally do a 200-meter run and 5 reps of each exercise. Finish with mobility B.

DAY 9

After completing warm-up D, do 10 Russian twists (page 353) and 10 legs-up-a-wall toe touches (page 377) on each leg. After your last toe touch, immediately do 20 reps of each exercise, followed by a set of 30 twists and 30 toe touches. After a short break, move on to part B. You'll need a timer. Start the timer and do 14 jumping squats (page 379) followed by 7 burpees (page 358). Rest until the 1-minute mark, at which point you will do 14 more jumping squats followed by 7 more burpees. Do 14 jumping squats followed by 7 burpees every minute on the minute for 18 minutes. At the 18-minute mark, do your final set. Finish with mobility A.

DAY 10

After completing warm-up C, begin part A of the workout. Begin with a lateral box jump (page 357) or jump-over (page 362): As you land on the other side of the box, immediately drop to the ground and do 1 knees to squat (page 380) follow by 1 pike push-up (page 376). Repeat this sequence for 15 minutes, moving back and forth over the box. Take a short break, then move on to part B. This part consists of 10 hand plank to forearm planks (page 373), 10 Supermans (page 375), and 10 V-ups (page 355). Repeat this sequence for 5 minutes, completing as many rounds as you can in that time. Finish with mobility D.

DAY 12

After completing warm-up C, do 5 burpees (page 358), 20 jumping lunges (page 365), 30 Russian twists (page 353), and 20 tuck jumps (page 363). Repeat this sequence, without a break, for 30 minutes straight. Every 2 minutes, do 5 burpees (page 358), then pick up where you left off. Do as many rounds as you can in the 30-minute time frame. Finish with mobility A.

DAY 13

After completing warm-up B, begin part A. Sprint for 400 meters, then rest for 1 minute. Repeat 2 more times, for a total of 3 sprints. After a brief rest, move on to part B. Do 50 legs-up-a-wall toe touches (page 377), 50 high knees (page 360), and 50 sit-ups (page 354) as fast as you can. Rest for 1 minute, then do 40 reps of each exercise, followed by another 1-minute break. Repeat the sequence, doing 30, then 20, and then 10 reps, with a 1-minute break after every round. Finish with mobility D.

DAY 15

After completing warm-up B, begin part A: 20 tuck jumps (page 363) and 10 hand release push-ups (page 375), repeated for a total of 5 rounds. After a short break, move on to part B: 12 slow single-leg deadlifts (page 377) on each leg, 24 bicycle crunches (page 354), and 36 mountain climbers (page 374). Repeat this sequence as many times as you can in a 15-minute time frame. Finish with mobility C.

DAY 16

After completing warm-up A, begin part A: 50 burpees (page 358) as fast as you can do them. After your last burpee, take a break, then move on to part B: 50 flutter kicks (page 352), 40 alternating walking lunges (page 364), and 30 bench dips (page 355). Repeat this sequence of exercises 2 more times, for a total of 3 rounds. Finish with mobility A.

DAY 17

After completing warm-up A, begin the workout: an 800-meter run, 21 burpees (page 358), 21 ab leg lifts (page 352), and 21 jumping squats (page 379). Immediately after your last jumping squat, run 600 meters, then do 18 burpees, 18 leg lifts, and 18 jumping squats. Follow this with a 400-meter run and 15 reps of each exercise, then a 300-meter run and 12 reps of each exercise, a 200-meter run and 9 reps of each exercise, and finally a 100-meter run and 6 reps of each exercise. Finish with mobility B.

DAY 19 After completing warm-up D, begin part A: a 200-meter sprint and 20 push-ups (page 376), repeated for a total of 6 rounds. After a short break, move on to part B, which consists of 30 burpees (page 358) and 30 V-ups (page 355) followed by 30 more burpees done as quickly as possible. Finish with mobility C.

DAY 20 After completing warm-up C, begin the workout: do 21 in-and-out jumps (page 362), 21 V-ups (page 355), and 21 burpees (page 358). For the second round, do 15 in-and-out jumps, 15 V-ups, and 15 burpees. Then do 9 reps of each exercise, then another round of 9 reps of each exercise, then 15 reps of each exercise, and finally 21 reps of each exercise. Finish with mobility D.

DAY 22 After completing warm-up B, begin part A: a 200-meter sprint, with the walk back to the starting line as your rest period. When you reach the starting line, sprint another 200 meters. Continue until you have completed 6 sprints. After a short break, move on to part B: 20 seconds of air squats (page 378) followed by a 10-second break, repeated for 4 minutes. Move immediately into 20 seconds of push-ups (page 376) followed by a 10-second break, repeated for 4 minutes. Finally, do 20 seconds of sit-ups (page 354) followed by a 10-second break, repeated for 4 minutes, until a total of 12 minutes have elapsed. Finish with mobility A.

DAY 23 After completing warm-up D, begin the workout: 20 skater jumps (page 363), 10 hand-release push-ups (page 375), 20 jumping squats (page 379), and 10 V-ups (page 355). With no breaks between rounds, repeat this sequence 8 times. Finish with mobility C.

DAY 24 After completing warm-up A, begin part A: 20 jumping lunges (page 365) and 10 pike push-ups (page 376). Repeat this sequence for a total of 5 minutes, aiming to do as many rounds as you can in that time frame. After a short rest, move on to part B: a 100-meter sprint followed by a 1-minute plank hold (page 374). Repeat this sequence for a total of 7 rounds. Finish with mobility B.

DAY 26 After completing warm-up A, begin the workout: do 12 pistols (page 378) on each leg, 20 sit-ups (page 354), and a 400-meter run. Repeat this sequence 3 times. With no break, move into 20 jumping squats (page 379), 10 V-ups (page 355), and a 400-meter run, repeated for 3 rounds. Finish with 12 Bulgarian split squats (page 379) on each leg, 20 dead bugs (page 373), and a 400-meter run, repeated for 3 rounds, making 9 total rounds of work. Finish with mobility A.

DAY 27 After completing warm-up D, begin part A: 2 minutes of push-ups (page 376), 2 minutes of air squats (page 378), and 2 minutes of sit-ups (page 354), with no breaks between exercises. After these 6 minutes, take a short break, then move on to part B. For this part of the workout, you'll need a timer. Start the timer and run 300 meters. At the end of your run, immediately begin doing burpees (page 358). Do as many burpees as possible until the 3-minute mark, at which point you run another 300 meters, then do as many burpees as possible until the 6-minute mark. Repeat this sequence for a total of 5 rounds or 15 minutes. Finish with mobility A.

glossary

The 28-Day Food & Fitness Plan – A customized plan for which recipes to make and which workouts to do for the 28 days of the Project; see pages 86 to 97. If you prefer to do things your own way, I've also provided a generic daily template for you to follow; see page 103.

AIP – The Autoimmune Protocol; a specific dietary approach to Paleo well suited for individuals who have an autoimmune disease (such as Graves' disease, type 1 diabetes, rheumatoid arthritis, celiac disease, or Hashimoto's thyroiditis), as it excludes possibly irritating foods such as eggs, nuts, seeds, and nightshades. Recipes that are AIP compliant or that include an AIP modification are clearly labeled in this book.

DSN – Daily Sleep Number; the custom amount of sleep (in hours) that an individual needs. You can calculate your DSN by completing the sleep analysis exercise on page 32.

DWN – Daily Water Need; the custom amount of water (in ounces) that an individual needs. You can calculate your DWN by performing the easy calculation on page 37.

FODMAP – Fermentable oligosaccharides, disaccharides, monosaccharaides and polyols; a group of small carbohydrates that in some people are poorly absorbed by the small intestine and are then fermented by the bacteria in the large intestine, causing abdominal bloating, pain, diarrhea, constipation, and/or excess flatulence. Low-FODMAP is a specific dietary approach well suited for individuals who have irritable bowel syndrome, as it excludes FODMAP-containing foods such as garlic, onions, cauliflower, dates, and sausage. Recipes that are low-FODMAP compliant or that include a low-FODMAP modification are clearly labeled in this book.

Foods That Heal – A list of Paleo-friendly foods that promote healing, combat inflammation, and can aid in the loss of excess body fat; see pages 48 to 54.

Foods That Sabotage – A list of foods that harm more than they heal; see pages 44 to 47.

GAPS – Gut and Psychology Syndrome; the GAPS diet is a specific dietary approach similar to Paleo that is well suited for individuals who have chronic digestive inflammation due to a damaged gut, as it excludes possibly irritating foods such as chocolate, cocoa, coffee, okra, and canned vegetables. Recipes that are GAPS compliant or that include a GAPS modification are clearly labeled in this book.

GMO – Genetically Modified Organism; an organism with genetic material that has been modified in a way that is not possible in nature. Many people who are seeking to feed their bodies healing foods prefer to avoid foods made with GMO ingredients.

IFF – Ideal Fitness Fit; a well-rounded fitness routine custom-built by and for you. See page 69 for more information.

Mobility – A proactive anti-injury set of movements that encompasses soft tissue work, stretching, and joint mobilization. Soft tissue includes muscles, tendons, ligaments, and fascia.

Ms. Frizzle – Valerie Felicity Frizzle, the star of the cartoon *The Magic School Bus;* a fictional third-grade teacher who uses fantastic magical devices to teach her students scientific models.

Nightshades – A family of flowering plants that includes tomatoes, eggplant, and bell peppers. Some people feel better when they avoid these foods; they are excluded from the Autoimmune Protocol (AIP).

Portion Compass – A basic portion size recommendation for men and women with approximate nutrition facts for most in-scope foods; see pages 79 to 85.

The Project – The 28-Day Fed & Fit Project and any efforts directed toward designing and fine-tuning a Perfect You Plan.

Projecter – Any rock star who is working through the 28-Day Fed & Fit Project in an effort to develop, live out, and continue to fine-tune his or her Perfect You Plan!

PYP – Perfect You Plan; the custom healthy lifestyle template (which includes your DSN, DWN, personal food scope, and an IFF) designed by and for you using the lessons learned during the 28-Day Fed & Fit Project.

Savvy Seven – The seven exercise pursuits that make up a well-rounded fitness routine: strength, speed, endurance, mobility, rest, fun, and movement. See page 64 for more information.

Scope – "In-scope" speaks to the range of foods that are encouraged within the 28-Day Fed & Fit Project, while "out of scope" speaks to the range of foods that are discouraged.

recipe index

Breakfast Like You Mean It

 140
Bubble & Squeak

 142
Chorizo & Egg
Breakfast Scramble

 143
Cinnamon Sage
Sausage Patties

 144
Jicama
Breakfast Cakes

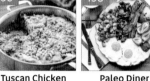 145
Pan-Fried Plantains

 146
Plantain
Protein Pancakes

 148
Sausage & Tomato
Frittata

 150
Smoothies

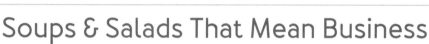 152
Spaghetti Squash
& Dill Egg Cups

154
Sweet Potato
Breakfast Hash
Casserole

156
Tuscan Chicken
Frittata

158
Paleo Diner
Breakfast Plate

Soups & Salads That Mean Business

 162
Chicken
No-Tortilla Soup

 163
Lemony Kale &
Sausage Soup

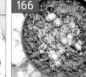 164
A Really Good
Chicken & Sausage
Gumbo

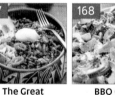 166
Weeknight Leafy
Green & Beef Chili

167
The Great
Beef Taco Salad

168
BBQ Cobb
Chicken Salad

 170
Chicken Caesar
Salad with Potato
Croutons

 172
My Big Fat
Greek Salad

 174
Spring Has
Sprung Salad

 176
Summer Beach
Babe Salmon Salad

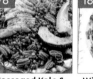 178
Massaged Kale &
Turkey Harvest
Salad

 180
Winter Beef Salad
with Roasted Beet
Vinaigrette

 182
Thai Beef Salad with
Zesty Lime Dressing

Things That Are Stuffed

 186
Olive-Stuffed
Pork Tenderloin

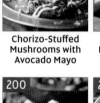 188
Chorizo-Stuffed
Mushrooms with
Avocado Mayo

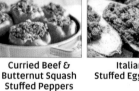 190
Curried Beef &
Butternut Squash
Stuffed Peppers

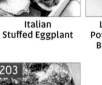 192
Italian
Stuffed Eggplant

 194
Loaded White
Potatoes: Teriyaki
Beef & Broccoli

 196
Loaded White
Potatoes:
Supreme Pizza

198
Loaded Sweet
Potatoes:
Carnitas Street Taco

 199
Loaded Sweet
Potatoes:
Sausage & Kale

 200
Sausage &
Cranberry Stuffed
Acorn Squash

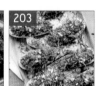 202
Sun-Dried Tomato
Stuffed Chicken
with Pecan Coating

 203
Taco Squash Boats

Set It & Forget It

206
A Very Good Vegetable Beef Soup

208
Garam Masala Beef & Butternut Stew

209
Fork-Tender Balsamic Mustard Pork Chops

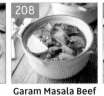
210
Chicken Tikka Masala

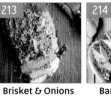
212
Lemon Thyme Chicken & Vegetables

213
Brisket & Onions

214
Barbacoa with Jicama Tortillas

216
Chipotle Carnitas

Casserole Is My Favorite Food

220
BBQ Chicken Potato Casserole

222
Buffalo Chicken Casserole

224
Chile Relleno Enchilada Casserole

226
Creamy Chicken Piccata Casserole

227
Sauerkraut & Brat Bake

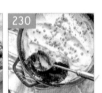
228
Eggplant Lasagna

230
Roasted Garlic Cottage Pie

232
Turkey & Sweet Potato Casserole

234
Zucchini Pizza Casserole

Family Favorite Proteins & Meals

238
Asian-Style Cabbage Rolls

240
Beef Stroganoff with Turnip Noodles

242
Burgers: Buffalo Ranch Bison

243
Burgers: Salmon Cranberry

244
Burgers: Caramelized Onion Balsamic Beef

245
Burgers: Tomatillo Turkey

246
Caramelized Onion Bacon Bison Meatloaf

248
Creole Jambalaya

250
Oven Baby Back Ribs

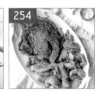
252
The Panang Curry My Husband Loves

254
Rustic Pot Roast

256
Shrimp Fried Rice

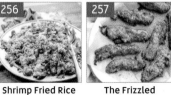
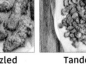
257
The Frizzled Chicken Bake

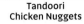
258
Tandoori Chicken Nuggets

Vibrant Veggies

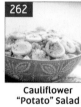
262
Cauliflower "Potato" Salad

264
Cauliflower Rice

266
Crispy Garlic Green Beans

267
Lemon Garlic Spaghetti Squash

268
Sautéed Lemon Garlic Spinach

269
Lemony Bacon Super Greens

270
Loaded Cauliflower Mac & Cheese

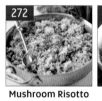
272
Mushroom Risotto

274
N'Orzo Salad

276
Roasted Buffalo Cauliflower

277
Roasted Garlic Cauliflower Mash

278
Scout Cabbage

280
Summer Squash Casserole

281
Tangy New-Fashioned Coleslaw

282
Whole Brussels Bake

283
Zesty Okra Fries

Satisfying Starches

286
Browned Butter Butternut Mash

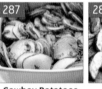
287
Cowboy Potatoes

288
Crispy Garlic Steak Fries

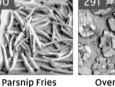

289
Old-Fashioned Mashed Potatoes

290
Parsnip Fries

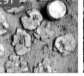
291
Oven-Baked Tostones

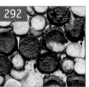
292
Roasted Citrus Beets

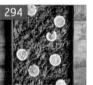
294
Root Veggie Hash

Take It with You

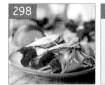
298 Cold Cut Roll-Ups

299 Pesto Chicken Salad Wraps

300 Sonoma Chicken Salad

301 Curried Sardine & Tuna Salad

302 Flax Crackers

304 Cheddar Kale Chips

305 Perfect Hard-Boiled Eggs

306 Protein Bars

308 Teriyaki Beef Jerky

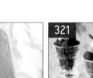
310 Trail Mix

Naturally Sweet

314 Puddings

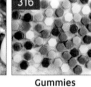
316 Gummies

318 Roasted Fruit Pops

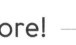

320 Fudgesicles

321 Berries & Cream

I'm Thirsty for More!

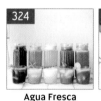
324 Agua Fresca

326 Coffee Creamer

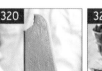
328 Cold-Brew Coffee Concentrate

329 Hibiscus Mint Sparkler

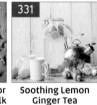
330 Almond, Cashew, or Sunflower Seed Milk

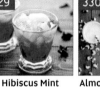
331 Soothing Lemon Ginger Tea

332 Bone Broth— Chicken & Roasted Beef

More Flavor, Please!

336 BBQ Sauce 2.0

337 Buffalo Sauce

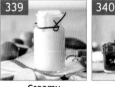
338 3-Ingredient Paleo Ranch

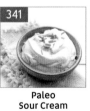
339 Creamy Jalapeño Ranch

340 Ketchup: Classic & Spicy

341 Paleo Sour Cream

342 Pico de Gallo

343 Guacamole

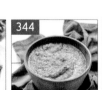
344 Salsa Verde

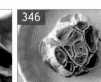
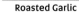
345 Salsa Rojo

346 Roasted Garlic

348 Roasted Garlic Pesto 2.0

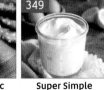
349 Super Simple Paleo Mayo

general index